AF687768

Nutrition Science: Concepts and Applications

Nutrition Science: Concepts and Applications

Isabella Ross

MURPHY & MOORE
www.murphy-moorepublishing.com

Nutrition Science: Concepts and Applications
Isabella Ross
ISBN: 978-1-63987-406-4 (Hardback)

© 2022 Murphy & Moore Publishing

MURPHY & MOORE
Published by Murphy & Moore Publishing,
1 Rockefeller Plaza,
New York City, NY 10020, USA

Cataloging-in-Publication Data

Nutrition science : concepts and applications / Isabella Ross.
p. cm
Includes bibliographical references and index.
ISBN 978-1-63987-406-4
1. Nutrition. 2. Physiology. 3. Health. 4. Food. I. Ross, Isabella.
QP141 .N88 2022
613.2--dc23

This book contains information obtained from authentic and highly regarded sources. All chapters are published with permission under the Creative Commons Attribution Share Alike License or equivalent. A wide variety of references are listed. Permissions and sources are indicated; for detailed attributions, please refer to the permissions page. Reasonable efforts have been made to publish reliable data and information, but the authors, editors and publisher cannot assume any responsibility for the validity of all materials or the consequences of their use.

Trademark Notice: All trademarks used herein are the property of their respective owners. The use of any trademark in this text does not vest in the author or publisher any trademark ownership rights in such trademarks, nor does the use of such trademarks imply any affiliation with or endorsement of this book by such owners.

For more information regarding Murphy & Moore Publishing and its products, please visit the publisher's website www.murphy-moorepublishing.com

Table of Contents

Preface

The branch of science which is concerned with the physiological and biochemical process of nutrition is called nutrition science. It focuses on the impact of nutrients on growth, reproduction and immunity of a living organism. The sub fields of nutrition science include community nutrition, nutrition education and exercise science. Nutrients are classified into macronutrients and micronutrients. Macronutrients which provide organisms with energy can be ingested in large quantities. These include carbohydrates, proteins, fatty acids and fats. Nutrient which don't act as an energy source but are still essential for effective functioning of the body are referred to as micronutrients. Vitamins and minerals are its common examples. Diseases such as anemia, cretinism, and blindness can result from the deficiency of essential nutrients. The topics included in this book on nutrition science are of utmost significance and bound to provide incredible insights to readers. Some of the diverse topics covered herein address the varied branches that fall under this category. Those in search of information to further their knowledge will be greatly assisted by this book.

To facilitate a deeper understanding of the contents of this book a short introduction of every chapter is written below:

Chapter 1- The physiological and biochemical process by which an organism takes food and utilizes it to support its life is known as nutrition. Four types of nutrition explained in this chapter are autotrophic nutrition, heterotrophic nutrition, saprophytic nutrition and holozoic nutrition. This is an introductory chapter which will introduce briefly all the significant aspects of nutrition.

Chapter 2- Proteins are the macromolecules which are made up of one or more long chains of amino acid residues. They are important for growth and repair of body cells. Various animal and plant sources of proteins are explained in this chapter. It has been carefully written to provide an easy understanding of the varied facets of proteins.

Chapter 3- Carbohydrate is a large group of organic compounds that mainly include sugars and starch which are broken down into glucose. There are many foods that contain healthy carbohydrates like vegetables, whole fruits, legumes and nuts. This chapter discusses in detail the carbohydrates, their sources and functions in the body.

Chapter 4- A vitamin is an organic molecule that is required in the diet for the normal growth of the body since our body cannot synthesize it. Vitamins are classified as water-soluble and fat-soluble. The topics elaborated in this chapter will help in gaining a better perspective about the types, digestion and absorption of vitamins.

Chapter 5- Minerals are chemical elements required in small amounts as essential nutrients by organisms to perform normal metabolism. Minerals are of two types; macrominerals and trace elements. Minerals and other related topics are discussed at lenght in this chapter.

Chapter 6- The sum of usual food consumed by a person or other organism is known as diet. This chapter explains diet, dietary supplements, nootropics and raw foodism in an easy-to-understand manner. It closely examines the key concepts of nutrition and diet to provide an extensive understanding of the subject.

I owe the completion of this book to the never-ending support of my family, who supported me throughout the project.

Isabella Ross

1

An Introduction to Nutrition

The physiological and biochemical process by which an organism takes food and utilizes it to support its life is known as nutrition. Four types of nutrition explained in this chapter are autotrophic nutrition, heterotrophic nutrition, saprophytic nutrition and holozoic nutrition. This is an introductory chapter which will introduce briefly all the significant aspects of nutrition.

Nutrition

Nutrition is the sum of all processes involved in the intake, assimilation, and utilization of the proper amounts of nutrients to maintain health, well-being, and productivity. Good nutrition relies on a diverse, adequate diet and is essential for the development and maintenance of the body from infancy to old age. Nutritional status can be both the "cause" and the "outcome" of good or poor health.

The terms "nutrition" and "food" are closely related but not interchangeable. Nutrition is a process of events, while food is a product that is eaten or taken into the body. Food is essential because it contains nutrients that the body needs for the following:

- Developing, growing, maintaining, replacing, and repairing cells and tissues.
- Resisting and fighting infection and recovering from illness.
- Producing energy, warmth, movement, and work.
- Carrying out chemical processes such as digestion.

Nutrition Basics

Nutrients are the substances in food that the body uses to function properly. Nutrients are divided into macronutrients and micronutrients. Macronutrients are nutrients needed by the body in relatively large quantities (many grams per day and include carbohydrates, fats, and proteins.

Micronutrients are nutrients needed by the body in very small quantities (usually less than 1 gram per day) and include vitamins and minerals. The body ingests, assimilates, and utilizes the nutrients in food to meet its needs for macronutrients and micronutrients. The body's physical and chemical process of breaking down food and converting it into a useful form of energy is called metabolism. The energy produced by metabolism is essential to maintain the body's functions and daily activities. The ability to metabolize food may vary from person to person and may be affected by illness or disease. Balancing the body's ability to metabolize food with an appropriate quantity of nutrients and food types will help ensure good health.

Each person processes and uses nutrients differently. The body responds either positively or negatively when it absorbs a nutrient or group of nutrients. The response affects the body's condition and health status. The body's response to nutrients and the subsequent outcome is called nutritional status. The amount and type of food and drink a person eats is called the diet. A nutritious or balanced diet includes a variety of foods and the proper nutrients in the correct amounts and combinations to meet the body's functional needs. A healthy and balanced diet should contain food free of harmful substances and in the optimal amounts and mixtures.

Eating a variety of foods is key to good health, especially for people with special needs, such as infants and young children, pregnant and lactating women, and the elderly. Eating a wide assortment of foods increases the likelihood of getting the necessary nutrients. Except for breast milk, no single food provides all the nutrients the body needs to function properly. Good nutrition involves eating a variety of safe and appropriate foods in the correct quantities to meet the body's needs for health and well-being.

The Essential Nutrient Groups

To function properly, the body must maintain a proper balance of the following key nutrients:

- Carbohydrates
- Proteins
- Fats
- Vitamins
- Minerals
- Water

Sports Nutrition

Sports nutrition is a broad interdisciplinary field that focuses on the science behind and application of proper nutrition during exercise.

- The areas of interest are: body's use of nutrients during athletic competition; the need, if any, for nutritional supplements among athletes; and the role of proper nutrition and dietary supplements in enhancing an athlete's performance.

- The psychological dimension of sports nutrition is concerned with eating disorders and other psychiatric conditions related to nutrition among athletes.

Macronutrients

Macronutrients are nutrients that provide calories or energy to the body. The purpose of macronutrients is to promote healthy cellular growth, metabolism, and to maintain normal bodily functions. The macronutrients, as suggested by the name "macro," are needed in the body in large amounts to provide the full and proper effect. There are three types of macronutrients:

- Carbohydrates
- Proteins
- Fats

Carbohydrates are organic materials composed of hydrogen and oxygen atoms which bond together to form monosaccharides or simple sugar molecules. Carbohydrates are found to form either a simple carbohydrate, composed of one monosaccharide, or a complex (composite) carbohydrate, composed of two or more monosaccharide molecules. When broken down, both simple and complex carbohydrates form glucose, which is the body's main source of energy. In addition, carbohydrates form an important part of waste elimination and intestinal health; Carbohydrates can be found in most fruits, vegetables and grains and provide the body with 4 calories per gram.

Proteins are nitrogenous organic compounds which are involved with many of the body's most crucial functions including:

- Providing the primary workforce in the cells.
- Making hormones and enzymes.
- A high involvement with tissue repair.

Proteins also provide energy when there are not enough carbohydrates available as well as sustain lean body mass. Just as carbohydrates are composed of monosaccharides, proteins are composed of chains of amino acid molecules. Also just like carbohydrates, proteins provide the body with 4 calories per gram. Proteins are most commonly found in animal products, nuts, and beans.

Fats, which are collectively referred to as triglycerides, are molecules comprised of fatty acids and glycerol. Fats provide essential elements of cell membranes and also provide the body with the ability to absorb fat-soluble vitamins A, D, and E. As fats are the most energy-dense macronutrient, they also provide the highest calorie count, providing the body with 9 calories per gram instead of the 4 provided by one gram of either carbohydrate or protein. The three primary types of fat include:

- Saturated fat

- Unsaturated fat
- Trans fat

Saturated fat, such as that found in butter and cream, as well as trans-fat, which is found in snack foods and fried foods, have been shown to increase the risk for heart disease. While in turn, unsaturated fats, which are found in olive oil and canola oil, has been shown to decrease the risk of developing heart disease. In regards to athletes, the knowledge of what carbohydrates, proteins, and fats provide the body with will allow them to make the best dietary decisions regarding their performance goals.

Micronutrients

Micronutrients are chemical elements comprised of thirteen organic essential vitamins and seven inorganic minerals. When consumed in the human body, micronutrients play an important role in energy production, haemoglobin synthesis, healthy growth, bone and immune health, and maintain normal metabolism. Despite the importance of maintaining the correct level of these vitamins and minerals in the body, as the name "micro" suggests, these chemical elements are only required to exist in the body in small amounts to provide ample effect.

The thirteen essential vitamins fall into one of two categories, water-soluble and fat-soluble. The water-soluble vitamins, the eight vitamins which compose the vitamin B complex and vitamin C, must be consumed daily as the body is unable to store what it does not immediately use. In contrast, the fat-soluble vitamins, vitamin K, A, D and E, can be stored in the body's adipose tissue and therefore does not have to be consumed on daily basis to maintain the correct levels in the body.

Minerals are inorganic nutrients that also play a key role in ensuring an athlete's health. The seven minerals needed to maintain accurate energy and hydration levels include:

- Calcium
- Iron
- Zinc
- Magnesium
- Sodium
- Chloride
- Potassium

These are important because proper hydration prior, during, and after an activity is crucial in the effect on an athlete's performance.

According to multiple sources, the most important vitamins and minerals for athletes include:

- Calcium.
- Iron.
- Zinc.
- Magnesium.
- The vitamin B complex.
- Vitamins C, D and E due to their role in the efficiency of muscle contraction; both smooth and cardiac muscle.

These vitamins and minerals can be obtained in a wide variety of food or through added supplementation.

Nutritional Recommendations for Athletes

Nutrition is very important to every athlete, and at high levels, where talent and training are relatively equal; it can be the difference between winning and losing. We are advised to take a careful look at their daily intake of food to make sure their body is getting the nutrients it needs to repair, maintain, and build muscle. There are many recommendations for what athletes should be eating.

Overall, the most important recommendation is that an athlete needs to track the amount of energy they are expending each day and make sure they are replacing this energy with a balanced diet of carbohydrates, protein, and fat. The recommended replenishment for maintaining carbohydrate levels in the body is eating 0.68 grams per pound of bodyweight within the first 30 minutes after training and again every two hours for four hours. For example, if a 180 lb. athlete completes their training for the day they need to have a meal/snack with about 122 g of carbohydrates, which could be a multi-grain bagel with peanut butter and an oatmeal bar Importantly, studies have shown it is not necessary for athletes who rest one or two days in between training bouts to follow this post-training carbohydrate recommendation as long as they are meeting their daily requirements.

An athlete should never train on an empty stomach. An athlete eats between 200 and 300 g of carbohydrate three to four hours prior to exercising. The USADA says to add in small amounts of protein to help slow the breakdown of carbohydrates and aid in regulating energy levels by sending carbohydrates to muscles at a steadier rate throughout the training. However, they also say this is up to the athlete and the size of the meal they can tolerate before training. Athletes should experiment with different pre-training meals to find what they feel comfortable with and eat that meal at a time consistent to when they eat the pre-training meal before a game.

Research has shown a strong benefit to endurance performance for an athlete performing in events lasting longer than one hour if they eat about 30-60 grams of carbohydrates every hour during the event. This equates to eating a banana, a food bar, or something with equal carbohydrates every hour. It is much more beneficial to the body's energy storage to eat small snacks or bites of carbohydrates every 15-20 minutes (about 10-20 grams each time) rather than waiting and eating 60-120 grams every two hours. The USADA says an athlete can intake 6-12 ounces of a sports drink that has 6-8% carbohydrates to water ratio. Anything greater than a 10% ratio increases the likelihood of cramps and can upset the stomach. High-quality protein consumed pre and post-training at just 0.2 grams per pound of bodyweight, which is about 4 ounces of chicken breast, is enough for a "maximal acute anabolic effect."

An athlete's daily calorie should encompass about, 50-70% carbohydrates, 10-35% protein, and 20-30% fat. Therefore, an athlete needs to plan their day of meals according to these percentages so that they know their total caloric intake for a day encompasses enough of each type.

Carbohydrates

- 1 hour of training per day:
  - 2.5 grams per pound of body wt per hour of training.
- More than 4 hours of training per day:
  - No more than 6 grams per pound of body wt.

Proteins

- Endurance training:
  - 0.54-0.64 grams per pound of body wt.
- Strength training (to gain muscle mass):
  - 0.72-0.81 grams per pound of body wt.
- Strength training (to maintain wt):
  - 0.54-0.64 grams per pound of body wt.

Fats

- 20% of daily calories.

They do not recommend a specific value of grams per pound of fats because of the wide variety a person can consume. Almost all athletes do not need to make an attempt to consume more because foods an athlete is eating has fat in it, so the athlete just needs to be careful that he or she is choosing foods that have an adequate amount of fat.

For the athlete looking for nutritional recommendations, the primary point of agreement between all researchers is that while there is some flexibility in the optimal timing of nutrients, the most important factor for maximizing the benefits of training is to consistently meet your daily carbohydrate, protein, and fat needs.

Nutrient Timing and Sport

Nutrient timing became popular about 15-20 years ago and is defined as intentionally eating specific foods before, during, and after training. Before this time athletes were not as concerned with their nutrition, let alone when they should eat certain foods. Ivy and Portman state that nutrient timing "will allow you to build more strength and lean muscle mass in less time than ever before." They set out to debunk the fact that, if protein is good for the body then more protein must be that much better to build muscle.

Muscles have a very specific 24-hour growth cycle that involves the muscle producing energy, recovering, and building and athletes need to provide specific nutrients at each of these phases. They break these phases down into the energy phase (occurs during training), the anabolic phase (occurs within 45 minutes after training), and the growth phase (occurs after the 45 minutes and until the next training session). During the energy phase, the muscles use its glycogen stores so the athlete needs to already have eaten carbohydrates and protein to aid the protein synthesis after training. During the anabolic phase, the athlete needs to follow the recommendations and eat enough carbohydrates because the "muscle cell membranes are more permeable to glucose...this results in faster rates of glycogen storage". Finally, during the growth phase, the athlete needs to consume carbohydrate meals with increased glycemic indexes because that helps the glycogen stores for the next workout. This new, at the time, physiological research gave athletes something scientific they could look at and convinced a lot of them that nutrition was an important aspect of training that they have been missing.

Fluids and Hydration

Dehydration not only negatively alters performance but also causes serious complications. Dehydration of 1% to 2% body weight negatively influences performance and dehydration of greater than 3% further decreases physiological function and increases an athlete's risk of developing exertional heat illness or worse. When intense exercise is combined with elevated temperatures or restricted heat loss, core temperature may rise by 2-3 °C and also result in exertional heat illness. Total water intake should be approximately in the 3.0 L (liter) range. Researchers found when dehydration increased, work capacity decreased by as much as 35% to 48%, and work capacity decreased even when maximal aerobic power did not change.

Water is the most important nutrient for athletic performance and the biggest component of the human body, accounting for approximately 73% of lean body mass. Trained athletes have higher total body water percentage values by virtue of high muscle mass and low body fat, because fat-free mass is roughly 75% water, while adipose tissue is only 10% water. Individual characteristics like body weight, genetics, metabolic proficiency, and heat acclimatization tendency will influence sweat rates.

Each pound of weight lost during exercise represents 1 pint (0.5 L) of fluid loss. Electrolytes regulate water distribution in various components of the body, with sodium being imperative to fluid regulation. The major electrolytes lost during exercise are mainly sodium chloride and some potassium. Sweat evaporation provides is the primary means of heat loss during vigorous exercise in hot weather. The goal of fluid replacement should be to prevent dehydration in excess of 2% body mass from occurring.

Before Exercise

The goal of hydrating before exercise is to start the physical activity hydrated with normal electrolyte level. Studies recommended 500-600 mL (17-20 fluid ounces (fl oz)) of water two to three hours prior to exercise and 200-300 mL (7-10 fl oz) 20 minutes before activity.

During Exercise

The goal of hydrating during exercise is to prevent excessive dehydration and electrolyte imbalances that could hinder athletic performance. Studies recommended about 200-300 mL (7-10 fl oz) ever 10-20 minutes during physical activity. Athletes should make sure carbohydrate-loaded drinks have a 4-6% concentration.

After Exercise

The goal of hydrating after exercise is to fully replenish any fluid or electrolyte deficits. The athlete should ideally complete rehydration within 2 hours for hydration restoration, ingest carbohydrates (CHO) to replenish glycogen stores, and include electrolytes to prompt rehydration. Sodium in post-exercise beverages conserves fluid volume and stimulates thirst, while CHOs replenish glycogen stores.

Performance Implications:

- Dehydration has little to no effect on muscle strength or ballistic power but impairs the ability to perform aerobic exercise.
- 12-15 year-old basketball players with a water deficit of ~2% body mass made fewer shots and were significantly slower at sprinting and lateral movement tests.
- The players attempted fewer shots and were less able to make shots linked with movement when dehydration had increased to 3%. Stationary shooting was consistent up to 4% loss.
- Soccer players with modest dehydration during games perceived exercise as more difficult compared to when fluids were consumed with a higher internal temperature. Performance times were worse on running tests that mimicked play, as well.

- 66% of 139 college athletes surveyed recognized that body mass change is an effective method to evaluate hydration practices, but only 15% actually check their body mass.

Hyperhydration

Excessive hydration that surpasses sweating rate increases the potential of exercise-associated hyponatremia (EAH), a potentially lethal condition.

Ergogenic Aids and Performance

An ergogenic aid is defined as any means that supports in enhancing energy and utilization. Athletes use ergogenic aids to maximize performance separate themselves from the competition. Studies classified ergogenic aids as mechanical, psychological, physiologic, and more studied pharmacological and nutritional. The general public seems mostly concerned with anabolic steroids, but a vast array of other ergogenic aids have come under scrutiny in athletics. In 2013, 0.7% of male athletes and 0.1% of female athletes reported using anabolic steroids in the last 12 months. Human growth hormone (HGH) is a commonly used aid in athletics, despite no evidence that says it improves strength, power, or performance. Amphetamines, creatine, erythropoietin (EPO), and androstenedione are several other ergogenic aids that are widely used that will be covered below. Numerous studies reported the use of performance-enhancing substances (PES) in athletes as variable and range from 5% to 31%. 15.1 % of athletes noted the usage of cognitive doping to increase focus, determination, and memorization.

Anabolic Steroids

The main benefits of steroids are increased muscle size, strength, and lean body mass. Studies randomly assigned 21 male weight-training subjects to either a testosterone or a placebo group over a 12-week period and found those in the testosterone group had significantly greater increases in muscle strength and circumference and decreases in abdominal skinfold measurements than the placebo group. Common side effects include acne, testicular atrophy, gynecomastia, cardiovascular disease, arrhythmias, stroke, blood clots, liver dysfunction, and cancer. Anabolic steroids are banned in all major sporting associations and events.

HGH

HGH is released in the anterior pituitary gland and stimulates growth through the actions of insulin-like growth factor-1 which promotes lipolysis and protein anabolism to decrease fat and increase lean muscle. Although HGH leads to an increase in muscular size, it does not lead to an increase in strength or athletic performance. Common side effects from prolonged fluid accumulation can lead to arthralgias and carpal tunnel syndrome among others.

Amphetamines/Stimulants

Commonly used stimulants include amphetamines, ephedrine, caffeine, phenylephrine, and methamphetamines. Stimulants release norepinephrine, which results in vasoconstriction, increased blood pressure, mood elevation, resistance to fatigue, and even an increase in anaerobic capacity. A lower level of caffeine is the only accepted stimulant with drug testing.

Beta-Hydroxy-Beta-Methylbutyrate (HMB)

HMB is becoming increasingly more popular in supplementing training regimens. It is a precursor to cholesterol and is believed to diminish protein breakdown. Researchers found upper body strength and peak torque generation showed decent improvements after HMB supplementation in untrained individuals, but bench press gains and leg press one-repetition maximums in trained athletes were not affected. HMB is not tested for and completely safe.

Creatine

Creatine monohydrate is a naturally occurring compound that serves as an energy substrate for muscle contraction and is consumed in most diets. It increases in strength, power, sprint times, total work to fatigue, peak force, and peak power. Of 21,000 students, the NCAA reported 14% usage among all athletes , with other studies reporting a 41% to 48% usage among college males. Caution should be observed in extreme, long-term usage, due to liver and kidney disease.

Vitamins

Athletes primarily use vitamin E, C, and A. These vitamins were antioxidants and therefore able to act as free-radical scavengers.

L-carnitine

L-carnitine slowed muscle glycogen breakdown and led to a decrease in lactic acid production during exercise, which was proved inconclusive. Large doses of L-carnitine can cause excessive diarrhea.

Androstenedione

As a natural precursor to testosterone, androstenedione is thought to allow for conversion to testosterone, but the majority of studies showed no significant increases in composition, strength, and testosterone concentrations. Most researchers found androstenedione lowered HDL levels, which increases the risk of cardiovascular issues, as well as the potential for the down-regulation of endogenous testosterone synthesis. Androstenedione is banned in all major sporting associations and events.

Erythropoietin (EPO)/Blood Doping

Endurance athletes benefit from improved delivery of oxygen to their tissues. One method which athletes attempt this is by living or training at high altitudes and another is through blood doping. Blood doping transfusions artificially increase the hematocrit, which increases the oxygen-carrying capacity of blood. An alternative to doping, the drug EPO, which is produced mostly in the kidneys, increases hematocrit levels when administered in recombinant form. In response to hypoxic exposure, the body produces a greater amount of EPO.

After an autologous transfusion of 750 mL of red blood cells, the VO2 max increased by 12.8 %, and times on a treadmill test to exhaustion improved significantly . With blood doping, researchers found a 34% increase in time to exhaustion at 95% VO2 max, and a 44-second improvement in a five-mile treadmill run time performance.

Eating Disorders and Body Image in Athletes

Athletes may have a more positive body image than non-athletes. A meta-analytic review found a small effect size which indicated athletes had a more positive body image than non-athletes. The review found no difference between females or males, the type of athlete, age or body mass index. Those who exercise regularly like athletes have been found to have a more positive body image than those who do not.

Despite athletes overall having a more positive body image than non-athletes, they may be more likely to develop an eating disorder. Common eating disorders include anorexia nervosa, bulimia nervosa, and anorexia athletica. Studies compared the prevalence of eating disorders between 1620 male and female elite athletes with 1696 male and female controls. They found 13.5% of athletes had eating disorders compared with 4.6% of the controls. Female athletes were also more likely to have eating disorders than males. Those in aesthetic sports such as gymnastics, dancing, figure skating, aerobics and diving or sports with weight classes were more likely to have an eating disorder than those in endurance, technical or ball game sports. Another medical condition female athletes who compete in sports which emphasize leanness are at risk of developing is the female athlete triad.

The treatment of athletes with eating disorders requires a multidisciplinary approach. Coordination and support ideally should be provided from sports medicine professionals, athletic trainers, and dieticians, psychiatrists, coaching staff, teammates and those close to the athlete. Cognitive behavioural therapy, psychodynamic psychotherapy and medications such as selective serotonin reuptake inhibitors and atypical antipsychotics may also be used. Eating disorders should be treated like sports injuries and require prevention, screening programs, correct treatment and timely support.

Child Nutrition

Child nutrition involves making sure that children eat healthy foods to help them grow and develop normally, as well as to prevent obesity and future disease. The traditional or mainstream approach to good childhood nutrition is to follow suggestions based on dietary guidelines that are appropriate for a child's age and development level and that have been developed and recommended by government, research, and medical professionals. The guidelines include selections from different food groups to provide the vitamins and minerals young bodies need for natural growth and activity. The U.S. Department of Agriculture's (USDA's) Food Guide Pyramid recommends how many servings a day a child should eat of each food group, such as milk, vegetables, fruits, fats, and meats, and asserts that by sticking closely to the guidelines, parents can ensure their children get a well-balanced diet that supplies the vitamins, minerals and calories they need to support growing bodies and active lifestyles. However, in this age of what has been called "advanced medicine," there are those who seek to understand why so many among us, especially children, suffer from so much serious illness.

In spite of recommendations, the diet quality of most children is not what it should be. The USDA surveyed American children age two to nine in 1998 and found that up to 8% of them had a poor diet; while as many as 80% of those ages seven to nine had a diet that needed improvement. The Centers for Disease Control (CDC) defines childhood obesity at a level above the 95th percentile of body mass index for his or her age group. Body mass index (BMI) is a measurement system used to assess if a child (or adult) is underweight, overweight, or at risk for becoming overweight. Pediatricians use height and weight measurements taken at a child's regular checkups to determine his or her BMI. To help guide parents and others in making good nutritional choices to keep BMI in line with normal growth and just to keep children healthy, the American Medical Association (AMA) suggests the following food choices for children, based on the USDA guidelines.

Children: Two to Five Years of Age

The AMA and USDA recommend food guidelines for young children similar to those for older children and adults, but with smaller portions. When looking at a range of portion sizes, parents and those who care for young children should choose the smaller portion sizes for children age two or three, and go with a slightly larger portion for children who are age four or five. Daily recommendations include:

- Four to five servings of breads, cereals, rice, pasta.
- Two or more servings of vegetables.
- Two or more servings of fruit.
- Three to four servings of dairy products.
- Two or three servings of meat, fish, poultry, legumes (beans, lentils, peas).

After age two, a child needs less fat than an infant—about 30% of daily calories. After age three, fiber becomes more important in a child's diet and can impact future heart health.

Calcium requirements steadily increase as children get older, from 500 mg a day at age three to 800 mg a day at age four to eight. There is more calcium in the body than any other mineral. Calcium works together with phosphorus (two parts calcium to one part phosphorus) for healthy bones and teeth and works together with magnesium (two parts calcium to slightly over one part magnesium) to prevent cardiovascular (blood vessels of the heart) and other degenerative diseases. In order for calcium to be absorbed by the body, it must also have sufficient amounts of vitamins C, D and A. In addition to food sources, an hour of sunshine each day can also provide a child with his/her daily vitamin D requirement.

Children: Six to Twelve Years of Age

By the time children reach age five or six, they begin to tell parents what foods they like. Parents and those who care for the children can help select foods from each recommended group that a child will enjoy. Calorie requirements and portion sizes increase as children get older: between ages six and ten, boys and girls need between 1,600 and 2,400 calories each day. Because of puberty and adolescent growth, between ages 10 and 12, girls need about 200 more calories a day. Boys will begin needing about 500 more calories a day after age 12. The following servings per day are recommended for children ages six to twelve:

- Six to 11 servings of breads, cereals, rice, pasta.
- Three to five servings of vegetables.
- Two to four servings of fruit.
- Three or four servings of dairy products.
- Two or three servings of meat, fish, poultry, legumes.

By age six, children still need only about 30% of calories from fat. Nutritionists say that by adding five to the child's age, parents can estimate the number of fiber grams a child needs each day. Calcium requirements continue to rise, from 800 mg a day at age four to eight to 1,300 mg each day for children beginning at age nine.

Preparations

Getting children to eat the right foods is easy if they begin good eating habits at a young age and if they are offered a variety of healthy foods. Many books, magazines, and web sites offer tips on making healthy foods interesting. Some suggestions for each food group follow:

- Breads, cereals, and pastas including whole grain breads, unsweetened cereals, unrefined rice, whole grain crackers, cornbread, rice cakes.

- Vegetable servings from cooked or raw vegetables such as asparagus, beets, broccoli, carrots, corn, green and red peppers, green beans, kale, peas, pumpkin, squash, sweet potato, tomato, zucchini, or vegetable juice.
- Good fruit choices such as apples, applesauce, bananas, cantaloupe, apricots, peaches, unsweetened fruit cocktail, plums, grapefruit, kiwi, nectarines, strawberries, watermelon, and fresh fruit juices.
- Milk, low-fat yogurts and cheeses are good dairy sources, as are low-fat cottage cheese, custard, ice milk, and occasional ice cream servings.
- Meat, fish, poultry, and legume choices include lean meats, dried beans, peanut butter, shellfish, dried peas, lentils, tofu, and reduced-fat cold cuts.

To reduce fat in a child's diet, parents can switch to low-fat or non-fat milk; remove skin from poultry or trim fat from red meat; reduce use of margarine and butter; use low-fat cooking methods such as baking, broiling, and steaming; and serve foods rich in fiber. Fresh salads can improve fiber in diet, as can adding oat or wheat bran to baked foods. Good, easy-to-assimilate sources of calcium for children, besides milk and cheeses, are tofu made with calcium sulfate; soup made with fish, fowl or beef bones and one tablespoon of wine vinegar to draw out the calcium into the broth; canned salmon and sardines with bones; sesame seeds and tahini (ground sesame seed butter); beans and nuts; calcium-fortified fresh orange juice; greens, especially broccoli, collards, kale, mustard, turnip tops, parsley, watercress and dandelion; and cooked sea vegetables if children like them.

White sugar, like white rice and white flour, goes through an industrial refining process: its juice is extracted from sugar cane, then filtered and boiled until it has been separated from all of its water, minerals, vitamins, protein and fiber, all of which the body needs to digest and metabolize the sugar. Because it lacks those nutrients, refined sugar becomes what Colbin calls a "naked carbohydrate," and so the body will draw them from other foods in the same meal or the body's tissues. Thus when refined white sugar is consumed, there is loss of stored B vitamins, calcium, phosphorus, iron, and other nutrients from the body. The loss of calcium stored in teeth weakens them and makes them more susceptible to bacterial attack/cavities. Also, this nutrient loss from refined sugar consumption can produce hunger for the missing nutrients and provoke great sugar-eating binges. On food labels, sugar is often identified as lactose, maltose, fructose, sucrose, and others. Glucose is the name of sugar found in the blood.

Colbin points out that if you eat meat, you need to digestively balance it with white sugar and vice versa, and that serious problems arise when the amount of sugar eaten is more than the amount needed to balance the meat. Sugar is as addictive as a drug because eating a small amount creates a desire for more sugar and because quitting sugar "cold turkey" brings on withdrawal symptoms that can last for an extended period of time. Typical withdrawal symptoms include strong cravings, fatigue, depression, mood swings, and sometimes headaches. Excessive sugar consumption is believed to be involved in such very common problems as hypoglycemia or hyperinsulinism, diabetes, heart disease, dental caries, high cholesterol, obesity, indigestion, myopia (nearsightedness), seborrheic dermatitis, gout, genetic narrowing of pelvic and jaw structures, crowding and malformation of teeth, hyperactivity, lack of concentration, depression, and anxiety. These problems result when the sugar intake provides more "naked carbohydrates" than are needed to balance the animal protein intake. Since white flour also provides additional "naked carbohydrates," only a small amount of sugar can create an excess amount in the body.

It is important that children eat three meals a day and not skip breakfast. Studies have shown that children and teens that skip breakfast have more trouble concentrating, do not perform as well in school, and often have later problems with heart disease. Obesity is common in children who skip breakfast.

While the obesity problem in today's youth can be blamed on a number of factors, including larger food portions for adults and children, convenient salty and sugary snack foods, and cheap and convenient fast food, much attention has been focused on the role of the nation's schools. There are fewer physical education classes because of more emphasis on academic classes and those gym classes that remain have too much standing around and not enough activities that interest the children, say some experts. School lunches generally have not provided healthy or balanced nutrition but instead have consisted of highly refined, processed foods that are full of additives and simple carbohydrates, which do not provide good nutrition or energy. In addition, many schools also offer "snack bars" or vending machines with sodas and sugary, fatty, or salty snacks. Many children have been choosing these snacks over the prepared school lunches.

To counter this problem in schools, the Healthy Schools Summit was held in October 2002. It consisted of representatives from more than 30 national education, fitness, nutrition, and health organizations, as well as 450 school administrators, government leaders, food service directors, counselors, dietitians, nurses, and health and fitness teachers. Since that time, many school districts around the country have been working to improve their physical education programs and to remove or change the selections in vending machines and snack bars on school campuses. Parents can check with their children's schools or pack healthy lunches from home with foods their children like to ensure they eat well while at school.

Children who are very active and participate in organized sports need a particularly healthy diet. For extended energy, they should eat many complex carbohydrates, such as unrefined rice, whole grain pasta and bread, and whole grain cereal. While all children need to drink plenty of water, those who participate in sports need to drink even more. Some experts say an easy formula to remember is one cup of fluid for every one-half hour of physical activity.

At home, some parents choose convenient snack and fast foods because often, both parents work long hours. Along with bigger portions and increased time spent in front of the television instead of out being physically active, today's youth are becoming obese from receiving and growing accustomed to less nutritional foods. Many experts say that getting children up off the couch and watching their snack choices helps. Also, many sources can help parents find healthier alternatives to fast food meals for their families. Suggestions include cooking healthy meals on weekends and freezing them for busy weekdays and looking for cookbooks or online sources of quick and healthy recipes. Simply cooking with less fat and using baking, roasting or poaching methods instead of frying helps children and adults. Also, offering children healthy snacks to last them until mealtime will keep them from reaching for poor snack choices and make them less likely to overeat at the evening meal.

For a variety of reasons, some children follow vegetarian diets. Some people are concerned that a vegetarian diet is harmful for children, but generally, if a child aged two or older still follows the recommended Food Guide Pyramid and makes good food choices, a vegetarian diet can be healthy. In fact, 2% of children ages six to 17 never eat meat, fish, or poultry. If a vegetarian child needs a vitamin or mineral supplement, a physician or professional nutritionist can help determine the proper level of supplement needed.

Precautions

Parents are sometimes cautioned by nutritional experts not to turn mealtimes and eating into a battle of wills. Offering a variety of healthy choices allows children to select favorite foods from among those that are good for them and to balance foods containing a number of vitamins and minerals. Research in 2004 showed that taste for certain foods probably develops while people are still infants. In fact, infants in the study who had been exposed to the flavor of carrots through their mothers' breast milk later ate more of a carrot-flavored cereal that those who had not been exposed to carrots as infants. The researchers said that encouraging children to eat more fruits and vegetables as early as possible was helpful.

Many physicians and medical researchers have cautioned parents not to turn to fad diets for their children's weight problems. Many of the diets and diet products on the market have not been proven by clinical studies to be effective in the long term for adults and therefore they certainly have not been proven safe or effective as a solution to weight problems in children. The best solution for childhood obesity is a combination of activity, a balanced diet that follows the AMA/USDA guidelines for food groups and portions, and involvement of a physician, dietician, or other trained professional as needed. A further caution concerning dieting is the concern that as young children enter adolescence, too much worry about weight and appearance can cause social anxieties and lead to eating disorders such as anorexia and bulimia.

When changing a young child's diet, it should be done slowly, particularly when introducing fiber, and with the help of a physician, dietician, or nutritionist Too much fiber can interfere with the body's absorption of vitamins and minerals.

Children who do not eat enough food and do not get enough nutrition suffer from severe undernourishment, or malnutrition. Each year, more than six million children under the age of five years die around the world as a result of hunger. Malnutrition also can make a child more susceptible to a number of diseases. Worldwide, it is estimated that food insecurity affects 815 million households, mostly in developing countries. However, in 2003, a report showed that at least 10% of U.S. households also don't have enough food and about 3% report hunger at home. It is not the sort of hunger a person feels when they eat a late lunch but the kind of painful sensation someone gets from repeated or involuntary lack of food.

There are parents and health professionals, both traditional and alternative, who feel children, should have vitamin/mineral supplements to stay healthy. However, there are also parents and health professionals who believe that when children eat a balanced diet of wholesome foods, they seldom need vitamin supplements; that individual vitamins and minerals should be taken, like medicine, when a deficiency has been created by a diet imbalance; and that when such a deficiency has been corrected, they should be discontinued.

If children are not eating a healthy diet and are being given a vitamin/mineral supplement, it is important to keep chewable vitamins out of reach of young children, as their appealing taste may be irresistible and dosage needs to be controlled according to directions. Children with poor appetites or erratic eating habits also may benefit from vitamins and minerals. It is best to check with a pediatrician, dietician or nutritionist for dosing.

Some parents and health professionals feel that vegetarian children may benefit from vitamin/mineral supplementation because they may lack some iron and zinc normally obtained through meat products and/or fish. Other substantial sources of iron are eggs, whole-grain breads and cereals, leafy and other vegetables, potatoes, fruit and milk. Foods containing vitamin C (broccoli, Brussels sprouts, collards, kale, parsley, sweet peppers, strawberries, grapefruit, melons, tangerines, potatoes, and more) will increase absorption of iron in non-animal foods. Vegetarian sources of zinc are eggs, legumes, and whole grains. Zinc deficiency has been found in populations whose intake is derived solely from cereal sources, but in recent studies, vegetarians had adequate zinc levels. Those children who avoid dairy products, although it is difficult to get enough, may get calcium from broccoli, leafy green vegetables like kale, canned salmon and sardines including the bones, and soy products. If a child's physician or qualified nutritionist feels a supplement is necessary, he/she should recommend the dosage.

Children often don't recognize feelings of thirst and have to be encouraged to drink before becoming thirsty. If a child's urine is clear or the color of pale lemonade, he or she is drinking enough fluids. Dark urine the color of apple juice indicates too little hydration and the child is in danger of dehydration or heatstroke.

Side Effects

Only the fat-soluble (capable of being dissolved in fat or oil) vitamins A, D, K and E has side effects that are potentially, though rarely, toxic (poisonous).

“The facts are that only a few vitamins and minerals have any known toxicities, all of which are reversible, with the exception of vitamin D. Anything can be harmful if you take enough of it—even pure water. But vitamins and minerals are among the safest substances on earth. The amounts needed to become toxic are enormous.” They add that being on medication or having a medical condition can influence vitamin/mineral requirements and indicate that when one’s physician is not well-versed in nutrition, it is ideal to have him work with a qualified nutritionist.

With regard to vitamin D, they indicate, “According to several studies, up to 1,000 IU per day of vitamin D appears to be safe. Both the beneficial and adverse effects of exceeding this amount are controversial. Overdosing of vitamin D is irreversible and *may be fatal*. Symptoms of too much vitamin D are nausea, loss of appetite, headache, diarrhea, fatigue, restlessness, and calcification of the soft tissues (insoluble lime salts in tissue) of the lungs and the kidneys, as well as the bones.” Vitamin D (400 IU) is usually sold with vitamin A (5,000 IU) in a tiny tablet or capsule.

Active vitamin A from fish liver oil or synthetic palmitate is stored in the liver; that 15,000 IU would cause problems in infants; but that 100,000 IU of active vitamin A would have to be taken daily for months before any signs of toxicity (state of being poisonous) appear. Vitamin A in the form of beta-carotene can be taken without any risk of toxicity.

At doses of 800–1,200 IU per day, Lieberman/Bruning found no well-documented toxicity of vitamin E. At doses of over 1,200 IU per day, adverse effects such as flatulence, diarrhea, nausea, headache, heart palpitations, and fainting have been reported, but were completely reversible when dosage was reduced.

Vitamin K is easily obtained by the body from a healthy diet and deficiencies are rare, especially in children. It is given prophylactically to newborn infants to prevent hemorrhage and before surgery to people with blood-clotting problems. Lieberman/Bruning describes the major effect of too much vitamin K as an anemia where red blood cells die more quickly than usual and cannot be replaced by the body.

Some children have severe food allergies. It is important to watch for signs of allergies in very young children in particular, since they are eating many foods for the first time. Signs of food allergies can range from mild to severe. A child may, for instance, eat peanuts or shellfish and immediately show signs of a severe reaction, such as swelling and trouble breathing. Other food allergies may be less obvious but may occur from common foods found in many everyday products such as milk, eggs, wheat, or soy. If a child appears to have a severe reaction and has trouble breathing, the parent or caregiver should seek immediate medical attention, since the allergic reaction may be serious. If a child has ongoing problems such as eczema or other allergic reactions or signs of intolerance to foods, the parent may choose to seek help from a registered dietician and/or an allopathic physician who specializes in allergies. The allopathic physician may test the child first to determine the source of the allergies. The dietician will work with the family to help plan ways to meet nutritional needs while avoiding foods that cause allergic reaction or intolerance.

The parent of an allergic child can also choose to seek help from a homeopathic or naturopathic physician. Andrew Weil, M.D. believes that the body can heal itself and believes allergies are learned responses of the immune system to environmental agents that are not necessarily harmful. Weil says treatment should focus on calming an over-reactive immune system in order to alleviate allergy symptoms. Allergies can and are frequently "healed." However, traditional allergy medications tend to be "more or less" toxic to the body and can increase an allergic response over time.

To increase the likelihood of spontaneous healing, Dr. Weil made the following recommendations. Dietary modification to reduce allergic responses: following a low-protein diet; cutting down on animal protein in general; eliminating cow's milk and products made from it because they are known to irritate the immune system; and eating organically grown foods as much as possible to avoid agricultural chemicals that cause immune system reaction. Regular use of quercetin, a natural product from buckwheat and citrus fruits, that stabilizes cell membranes that release histamine, which is involved in many allergic reactions. Quercetin is a preventative and Dr. Weil recommends it be used regularly. The recommended dose is 400 mg twice a day between meals. For hay fever, the freeze-dried extract of the herb stinging nettle, one to two capsules every two to four hours as needed, he says will control symptoms with none of the toxicity of anti-histamines or steroids. He also recommends a safe nasal spray, Nasalcrom, which works like quercetin. In the home, environmental methods like installing air filters can reduce allergic effects on and relieve the immune system. And finally, some allergic reactions indicate that high brain levels are involved in misdirected immune system response, and mind/body intervention is suggested.

Autotrophic Nutrition

Auto = self, Trophic = nutrition. The exact meaning of this word is self-nutrition. Autotrophic nutrition is a process in which the organism produces their food from the simple inorganic materials such as water, carbon dioxide and mineral salts in the presence of sunlight. All the green plants have an autotrophic mode of nutrition.

The autotrophic organisms have a green colored pigment named "chlorophyll" which helps in catching energy from the sun. They make their own food with the help of the water, solar energy, and carbon dioxide by the method of photosynthesis. This results in the making of glucose. Plants such as blue-green algae and cyanobacteria could be considered as some examples of autotrophic nutrition.

Nutrition in Plants

Every living organism wants some kind of energy and nutrient substances to ensure that the life processes run smoothly. Besides, this energy needed is acquired from the food.

Plants and their Nutrition Requirements

Plants are also a part of living things that require some form of energy. They have cells and tissues. They also grow in girth and size. And they are the creators of the ecosystem. So, in order to create food, they do have nutrient necessities. Of course, the kind of nutrient requirements differs.

This type of nutrition in plants is so-called the "autotrophic mode of nutrition". What does this actually stand for? It means that plants have the special ability to make their own food, with the help of simple inorganic substances to harvest organic substances. They get energy sources from non-living things like sun and carbon dioxide CO_2.

Plants also contain chlorophyll in them, the green color pigment. With the help of all these above elements, plants can yield simple carbohydrates. The carbohydrates thus made are utilized by the plants and gives it energy. When there is a surplus of carbohydrates in the plants, then it is used as a backup for later use.

Types of Autotrophic Nutrition

According to the kind of energy source used, autotrophic nutrition in plants can be of two kinds. They are Photo-autotrophic nutrition (where sunlight is the energy is the only source) and Chemoautotrophic nutrition (where chemicals are the energy is the only source).

Photosynthesis

Plants that can produce their food are called autotrophs. But, there are some plants that cannot and are known as heterotrophs. The method by which plants produce their own food is known as photosynthesis. The photosynthesis process happens mostly in the leaves of the plant which are also known as the 'kitchen of the plant'. In certain cases, even the stems have the potential to carry out photosynthesis.

Photosynthesis is a method to transform solar energy into chemical energy to produce starch. Different parts of a plant play different roles to complete the photosynthesis, such as:

- Leaves – They are the food factories of the plant.
- Stomata– It is present in the lower epidermis of the leaf which uses carbon di-oxide CO_2 from the air.
- Roots – They absorb minerals and water from the soil and carry it to different parts of the plant.

Leaves of the vascular plants have a superior structure called chloroplasts which possess chlorophyll. Plants manufacture glucose with the help of carbon dioxide and water in the existence of sunlight. The stomata existing in the leaf releases oxygen and water as a by-product through the daytime. The manufactured food is conveyed to different parts of the plant for storage and utilization. These green plants make proteins using nitrogen which could be acquired from the soil.

All the minerals which are dissolved in water are used to transform sugar into proteins, fats, and carbohydrates. These food constituents act as the source of energy for other heterotrophic animals and plants. Glucose is manufactured by this process and transformed into different compounds like cellulose and starch which is stored in different parts of the plant.

The Leaf

The procedure of photosynthesis happens in the leaf of a plant. The leaf is anatomically separated into many layers. Photosynthesis happens in the mesophyll layer of the leaf, the middle layer also called palisade parenchyma. These mesophyll cells are rich in special cell organelles known as chloroplasts which are responsible for the photosynthesis process.

Leaves also have small openings on their undersurface called 'stomata' which are responsible for gaseous exchange and are the source of CO_2 that enters the leaf.

The Chloroplast

These are unique organelles inside which the photosynthesis process occurs. Chloroplasts are double-membrane organelles. The Chloroplast contains disc-shaped thylakoids that are arranged together. Stacked thylakoids are known as 'grana'. It is in the membrane of the thylakoid that pigment chlorophyll is also present.

Photosynthesis Process

Photosynthesis process can be separated into two stages:

- Light reaction
- Dark reaction

Light Reaction

This reaction is a light-dependent reaction and it is required to generate energy molecules like ATP and NADPH. This reaction happens in the thylakoid membrane of the chloroplast where the sunlight activates of the reaction of chlorophyll pigment.

The stimulated chlorophyll releases an electron which is taken by the H2 of water after its splitting. The reactions that occur are redox reactions and eventually lead to the manufacture of energy molecules- ATP and NADPH which are then required for the subsequent synthesizing reactions that happen in the dark reaction.

Dark Reaction

This reaction does not literally happen in the dark but is named so because it is independent of light (no light is needed). This reaction can happen both in the presence and absence of sun rays. Due to the scientists who worked to find out this cycle, this reaction is also known as the Calvin-Benson-Bassham cycle.

This reaction happens in the stroma which is present in the chloroplast. This reaction uses the energy molecules produced in the light phase of photosynthesis and transforms CO_2 into glucose. The photosynthesis method can be summarized by the following equation:

$$6CO + 6HO \rightarrow CHO + 6O \; (in\ the\ presence\ of\ sunlight)$$

Factors Affecting Photosynthesis Process

There are some factors that encourage or inhibit photosynthesis depending on their concentration:

- Light
- Temperature
- Oxygen
- CO_2

Purpose of Photosynthesis

For the plants, photosynthesis helps produce glucose to be able to produce energy to perform other functions such as transport of water and minerals throughout the plant and respiration. Plants require energy also to make other biological and biochemical methods to enable it to multiply. For other organisms, plants serve as food.

Chemoautotrophic Nutrition

The organism that can make their own food with the help of chemical energy and they do not need sunlight. This nutrition can only be possible at night time. Example: Nitrosomonas, hydrogen bacteria, etc.

Sources for Chemoautotrophic Nutrition:

- Energy Source: Chemicals (Chemo).
- Carbon Source: Environmental Carbon Dioxide.
- Example: Extremophiles.
- Halophiles (salt-loving bacteria). Halophiles are organisms that thrive in very high salt concentrations. They are a kind of extremophile organism. (The name derives from the Greek word means "salt-loving").
- Methanogens.
- The bacteria and archaea that live in the deep sea ocean.

Heterotrophic Nutrition

"Heterotroph is an organism that is unable to synthesize its own food, and therefore, has to rely on other sources, specifically plant and animal matter." All animals and non-photosynthetic plants are classified as heterotrophs since they are unable to prepare food. So these organisms resort to other various forms of nutrition. Hence, from an ecological perspective, heterotrophs are always secondary or tertiary consumers in a food chain.

Humans and other vertebrates rely on converting organic, solid or liquid food into energy. Other organisms such as fungi rely on converting dead organic matter into nutrients. In essence, heterotrophs break down complex food into its readily usable constituents.

Types of Heterotrophic Nutrition

In nature, organisms exhibit various types of heterotrophic nutrition. They are as follows:

- Holozoic Nutrition
- Saprophytic Nutrition
- Parasitic Nutrition

Holozoic Nutrition

Holozoic nutrition involves the ingestion and internal processing of solid and liquid food in an organism. This involves the steps of ingestion, digestion, absorption, assimilation and excretion. Ingestion is the intake of food, which is broken down into simpler organic matters by a process called digestion. After extraction of useful components, the unwanted and undigested particles are excreted out. Examples of animals that exhibit holozoic nutrition include all vertebrates. Even some unicellular organisms such as amoeba also exhibit holozoic nutrition.

Holozoic Nutrition in Amoeba

Amoeba exhibits holozoic nutrition. The process takes place in the following steps:

- The amoeba projects its pseudopodia and encircles the food. It then engulfs the food by the process of phagocytosis.
- The food vacuoles of amoeba are rich in digestive enzymes, which help break the food into simpler substances. This process is known as digestion.
- The digested food is absorbed into the cytoplasm leaving behind the undigested materials. This absorbed food is utilized to produce energy for the growth and development of the cell.
- The undigested food material is ejected out by the rupturing of the cell membrane.

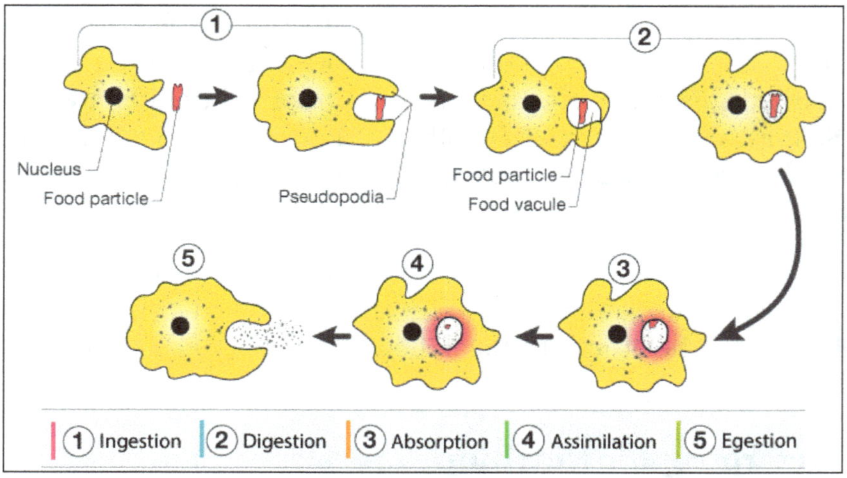

Figure: An amoeba exhibiting heterotrophic nutrition.

Types of Holozoic Organisms

Holozoic organisms can be divided into three types:

- Herbivores: These organisms depend upon plants for their food. Cows, buffaloes, deer, elephants are herbivores.

- Carnivores: These animals feed on other animals for their food. Lions, tigers and leopards are carnivores.
- Omnivores: These animals can survive on either plants or animals for their food. Cockroach, pig, chimpanzees, raccoons and ant are some examples of omnivores.

Saprophytes (animals which follow saprophytic nutrition) feed on dead and decayed organisms for energy. They are an important part of the ecosystem as they help to keep our environment clean and recycle nutrient back into the ecosystem. Some examples of saprophytes are fungi and certain types of bacteria. These are also responsible for the staling of bread and other similar food products. Saprophytes release certain enzymes to act on the complex organic matter. It works by breaking it down into its constituents, which can be easily consumed by them.

Parasitic Nutrition

Organisms that live in or on other organisms and acquire food at the expense of its host are called parasites. Most parasites are harmful to the hosts' health; sometimes, they even kill the host. Both animals and plants may serve as a host. Unlike commensalism, the parasite causes some harm to its host. A few examples of parasites are louse on a human head, Cuscuta plant and tapeworms.

Cymothoa exigua is an unusual parasite. It is also known as the tongue-eating louse and is aptly named so as it is found in the mouth of the marine fish Lithognathus. It essentially severs the fish's tongue, cutting off the blood supply and causing the tongue to fall off. The louse then attaches itself to the remains of the tongue and essentially acts as the fish's new tongue.

Saprophytic Nutrition

Saprophytes are the living organisms that live and feed on dead and decaying organisms. They are considered extremely important in soil biology. They break down the complex organic matter into simpler substances that are taken up by the plants for various metabolic activities. Thus, saprophytes play a significant role in the ecosystem. Fungi and a few bacteria are saprophytes. Saprophytes have certain characteristic features:

- They produce filaments.
- They are devoid of leaves, roots and stem.
- They cannot perform photosynthesis and are heterotrophs.
- They can produce spores.

The saprophytes secrete digestive juices and breakdown the organic matter around them. The fungi grow tubular structures known as hyphae that branch into the dead matter and produce digestive enzymes.

Saprophytes undergo extracellular digestion to digest the dead and decaying matter. They secrete digestive substances into the surrounding environment and break down the organic matter into simpler substances. The nutrients thus produced are absorbed directly through the cell membranes of the organisms.

In saprophytic nutrition, the proteins are digested into amino acids, starch is broken down into simple sugars, and fats are broken down into glycerol and fatty acids. These end products are transported through the cell membranes. Following are a few examples of saprophytes:

- Mucor: Mucor, also known as mould, is a saprophytic fungus that grows on decayed organic matter, especially those that are rich in carbohydrates. Mucor is majorly found on stale bread, vegetables and dung. It reproduces by sexual and asexual means.
- Yeast: Yeast is commonly found on sugary substances. It is present in grape juice, flower nectar, and vineyards, in large amounts. It reproduces by budding under favourable conditions.
- Penicillium: Penicillium grows on the decayed matter such as bread, jam, jellies, fruits, vegetables and also on damp leather and shoes.

Saprophytes are decomposers since they feed on the dead and decaying matter. Suitable conditions are required for the optimum growth of saprophytes. If they have access to sufficient water, they grow well. Saprophytes do not thrive under alkaline conditions. They grow well in neutral or slightly acidic soil. There must usually be oxygen present as the majority of saprophytes cannot grow under anaerobic conditions.

Holozoic Nutrition

Holozoic nutrition takes place in those organisms which take solid or liquid food through the mouth inside their body Examples of organisms having holozoic mode of nutrition are human beings, dog, cat, lion, deer, crow, frog and fish etc. This process takes place in following steps:

- Ingestion: The process of taking food inside the body is called ingestion.
- Digestion: In digestion the ingested food is converted into simple form with the help of digestive enzymes.
- Absorption: In this stage the food digested in second step is absorbed into the cells of body.

- Assimilation: Assimilation is the process of utilizing the food absorbed in third step by various cells of the body.
- Egestion: Egestion is the final step of holozoic nutrition in which the undigested food is removed from the body.

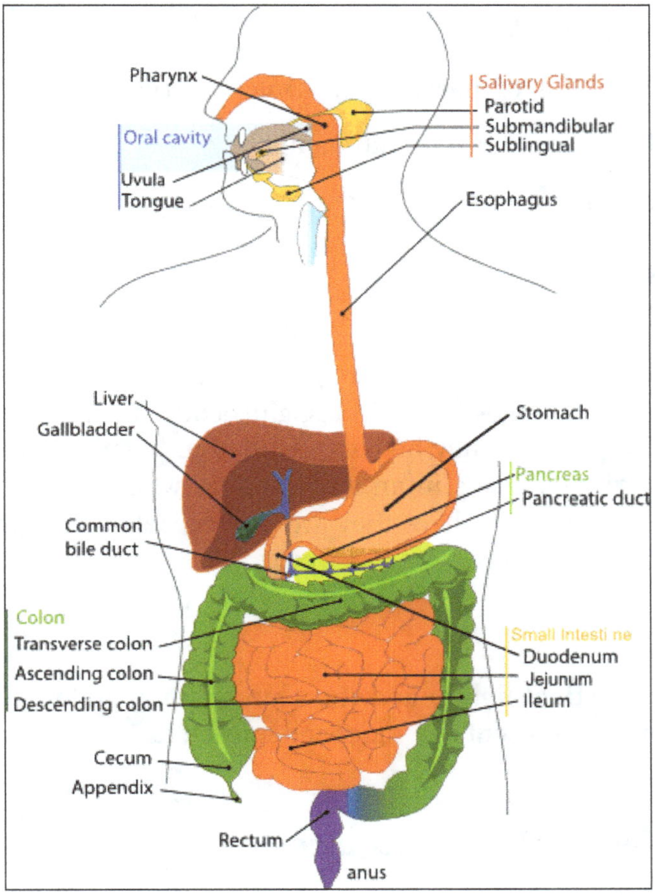

Malnutrition

Malnutrition is a common, under-recognised and undertreated problem facing patients and clinicians. It is both a cause and consequence of disease and exists in institutional care and the community. Approximately 5% of the UK population are underweight with a body mass index (BMI) below 20 kg/m, although obese individuals who unintentionally lose weight and subsequently have a BMI within the normal range are also at risk of malnutrition. Other patients become at risk as a result of an acute event (e.g. small bowel infarction), leaving them unable to meet their metabolic requirements both in the short and longer term. The prevalence of malnutrition increases by at least twofold in the elderly and those with chronic disease, and threefold in individuals living in institutional care.

Causes of Malnutrition

Malnutrition in developed countries is unfortunately still more common in situations of poverty, social isolation and substance misuse. However, most adult malnutrition is associated with disease and may arise due to:

- Reduced dietary intake.
- Reduced absorption of macro- and/or micronutrients.
- Increased losses or altered requirements.
- Increased energy expenditure (in specific disease processes).

Dietary Intake

Probably the single most important aetiological factor in disease-related malnutrition is reduced dietary intake. This is thought to occur due to reductions in appetite sensation as a result of changes in cytokines, glucocorticoids, insulin and insulin-like growth factors. The problem may be compounded in hospital patients by failure to provide regular nutritious meals in an environment where they are protected from routine clinical activities, and where they are offered help and support with feeding when required.

Mal-Absorption

For patients with intestinal failure and those undergoing abdominal surgical procedures, mal-absorption represents an independent risk factor for weight loss and malnutrition

Increased Losses or Altered Requirements

In some circumstances, such as enter cutaneous fistulae or burns, patients may have excessive and/or specific nutrient losses; their nutritional requirements are usually very different from normal metabolism.

Energy Expenditure

It was thought for many years that increased energy expenditure was predominantly responsible for disease-related malnutrition. There is now clear evidence that in many disease states total energy expenditure is actually less than in normal health. The basal hyper metabolism of disease is offset by a reduction in physical activity, with studies in intensive care patients demonstrating that energy expenditure is usually below 2,000 kcal/day. The exception is patients with major trauma, head injury or burns where energy expenditure may be considerably higher, although only for a short period of time.

Consequences of Malnutrition

Malnutrition affects the function and recovery of every organ system.

Muscle Function

Weight loss due to depletion of fat and muscle mass, including organ mass, is often the most obvious sign of malnutrition. Muscle function declines before changes in muscle mass occur, suggesting that altered nutrient intake has an important impact independent of the effects on muscle mass. Similarly, improvements in muscle function with nutrition support occur more rapidly than can be accounted for by replacement of muscle mass alone.

Down-regulation of energy dependent cellular membrane pumping, or reductive adaptation, is one explanation for these findings. This may occur following only a short period of starvation. If, however, dietary intake is insufficient to meet requirements over a more prolonged period of time the body draws on functional reserves in tissues such as muscle, adipose tissue and bone leading to changes in body composition. With time, there are direct consequences for tissue function, leading to loss of functional capacity and a brittle, but stable, metabolic state. Rapid de-compensation occurs with insults such as infection and trauma. Importantly, unbalanced or sudden excessive increases in energy intake also put malnourished patients at risk of de-compensation and re-feeding syndrome.

Cardio-Respiratory Function

Reduction in cardiac muscle mass is recognised in malnourished individuals. The resulting decrease in cardiac output has a corresponding impact on renal function by reducing renal perfusion and glomerular filtration rate. Micronutrient and electrolyte deficiencies (eg thiamine) may also affect cardiac function, particularly during re-feeding. Poor diaphragmatic and respiratory muscle function reduces cough pressure and expectoration of secretions, delaying recovery from respiratory tract infections.

Gastrointestinal Function

Adequate nutrition is important for preserving GI function: chronic malnutrition results in changes in pancreatic exocrine function, intestinal blood flow, villous architecture and intestinal permeability. The colon loses its ability to reabsorb water and electrolytes, and secretion of ions and fluid occurs in the small and large bowel. This may result in diarrhoea, which is associated with a high mortality rate in severely malnourished patients.

Immunity and Wound Healing

Immune function is also affected, increasing the risk of infection due to impaired cell-mediated immunity and cytokine, complement and phagocyte function. Delayed wound healing is also well described in malnourished surgical patients.

Psychosocial Effects

In addition to these physical consequences, malnutrition also results in psychosocial effects such as apathy, depression, anxiety and self-neglect.

Assessment of Nutritional Status

Identification of patients at risk of malnutrition at an early stage of hospital admission (or attendance to the outpatient clinic) allows for early intervention with nutritional therapy.

The Malnutrition Universal Screening Tool (MUST)

MUST is a simple, rapid and easy method to screen patients and has been proven to be reliable and valid. It aims to identify those at risk by incorporating:

- Current weight (BMI).
- History of recent unintentional weight loss.
- Likelihood of future weight loss.

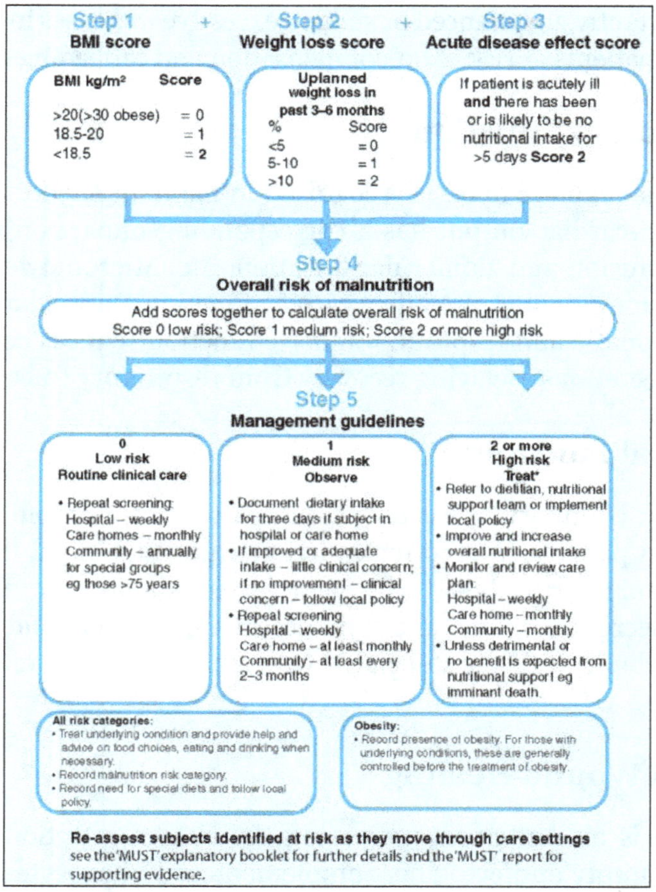

Figure: The Malnutrition Universal Screening Tool (MUST) BMI = body mass index.

Screening

The screening process identifies patients who require a more detailed assessment and formulation of an individualized stepwise management plan by a nutrition specialist. In vulnerable patient groups the simple provision of regular meals or food with better nutritional content may be enough to address nutritional risk. Additional measures may include broader menu choices or providing assistance with feeding. Patients in whom these 'social' interventions are insufficient to ensure that nutritional requirements are met need the addition of oral nutritional supplements or enteral tube feeding under dietetic supervision. Patients rarely require parenteral nutrition (PN). Need for PN usually occurs in the context of an inaccessible or non-functioning GI tract. Re-screening of inpatients at seven-day intervals throughout a hospital admission alerts clinicians to those who have lost weight and require greater intervention.

References

- Holozoic-nutrition: funscience.in, Retrieved 12, July 2020
- Heterotrophic-nutrition, biology: byjus.com, Retrieved 08, April 2020
- Saprophytes, biology: byjus.com, Retrieved 11, August 2020
- Autotrophic-nutrition, biology: vedantu.com, Retrieved 24, May 2020
- Sports-Nutrition: physio-pedia.com, Retrieved 10, March 2020

2

Proteins

Proteins are the macromolecules which are made up of one or more long chains of amino acid residues. They are important for growth and repair of body cells. Various animal and plant sources of proteins are explained in this chapter. It has been carefully written to provide an easy understanding of the varied facets of proteins.

Proteins are highly complex substance that is present in all living organisms. Proteins are of great nutritional value and are directly involved in the chemical processes essential for life. The importance of proteins was recognized by chemists in the early 19th century. Proteins are species-specific; that is, the proteins of one species differ from those of another species. They are also organ-specific; for instance, within a single organism, muscle proteins differ from those of the brain and liver.

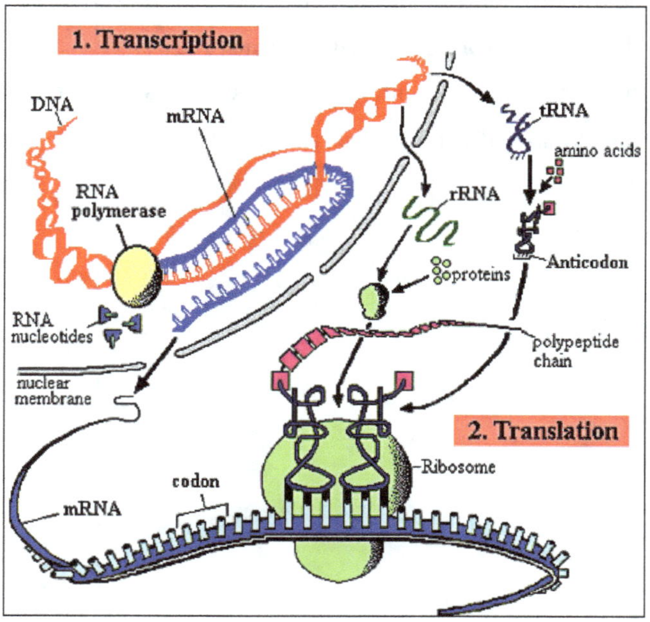

Figure: Protein synthesis.

A protein molecule is very large compared with molecules of sugar or salt and consists of many amino acids joined together to form long chains, much as beads are arranged on a string. There are about 20 different amino acids that occur naturally in proteins. Proteins of similar function have similar amino acid composition and sequence. Although it is not yet possible to explain all of the functions of a protein from its amino acid sequence, established correlations between structure and function can be attributed to the properties of the amino acids that compose proteins.

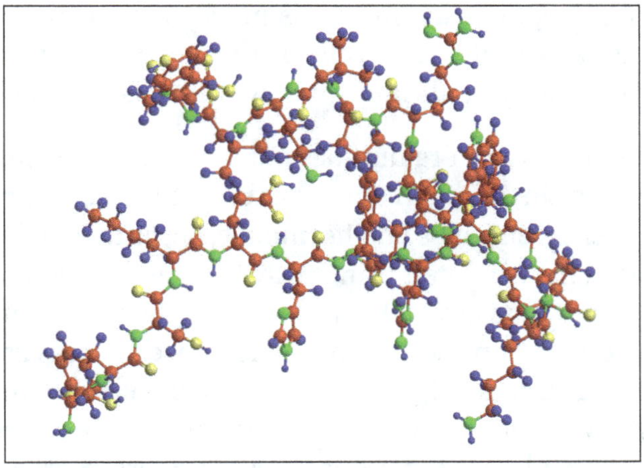

Figure: The molecular structure of a peptide (a small protein) consists of a sequence of amino acids.

Plants can synthesize all of the amino acids; animals cannot, even though all of them are essential for life. Plants can grow in a medium containing inorganic nutrients that provide nitrogen, potassium, and other substances essential for growth. They utilize the carbon dioxide in the air during the process of photosynthesis to form organic compounds such as carbohydrates. Animals, however, must obtain organic nutrients from outside sources. Because the protein content of most plants is low, very large amounts of plant material are required by animals, such as ruminants (e.g., cows), that eat only plant material to meet their amino acid requirements. Nonruminant animals, including humans, obtain proteins principally from animals and their products—e.g., meat, milk, and eggs. The seeds of legumes are increasingly being used to prepare inexpensive protein-rich food.

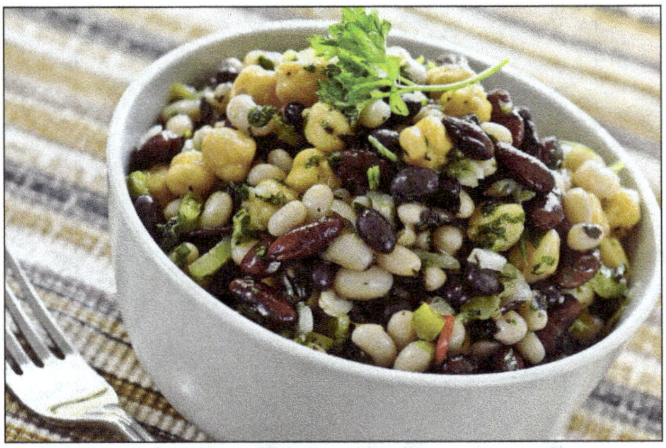

Figure: Legume; amino acid.

Legumes—such as beans, lentils, and peas—are high in protein and contain many essential amino acids. The protein content of animal organs is usually much higher than that of the blood plasma. Muscles, for example, contain about 30 percent protein, the liver 20 to 30 percent, and red blood cells 30 percent. Higher percentages of protein are found in hair, bones, and other organs and tissues with low water content. The quantity of free amino acids and peptides in animals is much smaller than the amount of protein; protein molecules are produced in cells by the stepwise alignment of amino acids and are released into the body fluids only after synthesis is complete.

The high protein content of some organs does not mean that the importance of proteins is related to their amount in an organism or tissue; on the contrary, some of the most important proteins, such as enzymes and hormones, occur in extremely small amounts. The importance of proteins is related principally to their function. All enzymes identified thus far are proteins. Enzymes, which are the catalysts of all metabolic reactions, enable an organism to build up the chemical substances necessary for life—proteins, nucleic acids, carbohydrates, and lipids—to convert them into other substances, and to degrade them. Life without enzymes is not possible. There are several protein hormones with important regulatory functions. In all vertebrates, the respiratory protein hemoglobin acts as oxygen carrier in the blood, transporting oxygen from the lung to body organs and tissues. A large group of structural proteins maintains and protects the structure of the animal body.

Hemoglobin

Hemoglobin is a protein made up of four polypeptide chains (α1, α2, β1, and β2). Each chain is attached to a heme group composed of porphyrin (an organic ring like compound) attached to an iron atom. These iron-porphyrin complexes coordinate oxygen molecules reversibly, ability directly related to the role of hemoglobin in oxygen transport in the blood.

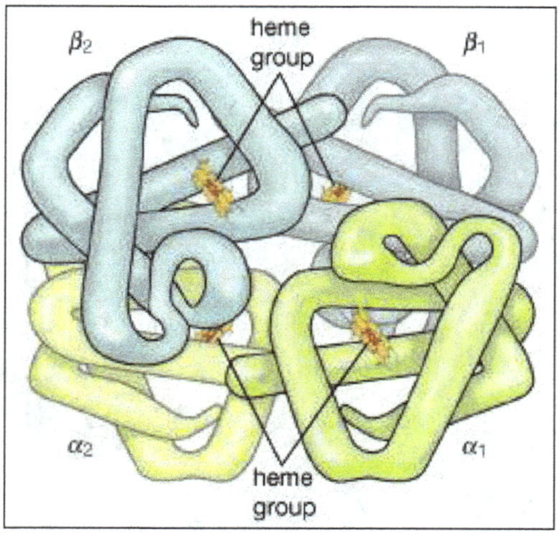

Levels of Structural Organization in Proteins

Primary Structure

Analytical and synthetic procedures reveal only the primary structure of the proteins—that is, the amino acid sequence of the peptide chains. They do not reveal information about the conformation (arrangement in space) of the peptide chain—that is, whether the peptide chain is present as a long straight thread or is irregularly coiled and folded into a globule. The configuration, or conformation, of a protein is determined by mutual attraction or repulsion of polar or nonpolar groups in the side chains (R groups) of the amino acids. The former have positive or negative charges in their side chains; the latter repel water but attract each other. Some parts of a peptide chain containing 100 to 200 amino acids may form a loop, or helix; others may be straight or form irregular coils.

The terms secondary, tertiary, and quaternary structure are frequently applied to the configuration of the peptide chain of a protein. A nomenclature committee of the International Union of Biochemistry (IUB) has defined these terms as follows: The primary structure of a protein is determined by its amino acid sequence without any regard for the arrangement of the peptide chain in space. The secondary structure is determined by the spatial arrangement of the main peptide chain without any regard for the conformation of side chains or other segments of the main chain. The tertiary structure is determined by both the side chains and other adjacent segments of the main chain, without regard for neighboring peptide chains. Finally, the term quaternary structure is used for the arrangement of identical or different subunits of a large protein in which each subunit is a separate peptide chain.

Secondary Structure

The nitrogen and carbon atoms of a peptide chain cannot lie on a straight line, because of the magnitude of the bond angles between adjacent atoms of the chain; the bond angle is about 110°. Each of the nitrogen and carbon atoms can rotate to a certain extent, however, so that the chain has a limited flexibility. Because all of the amino acids, except glycine, are asymmetric L-amino acids, the peptide chain tends to assume an asymmetric helical shape; some of the fibrous proteins consist of elongated helices around a straight screw axis. Such structural features result from properties common to all peptide chains. The product of their effects is the secondary structure of the protein. Matrix proteins are large molecules tightly bound to form extensive networks of insoluble fibers. These fibers may even exceed the size.

Tertiary Structure

The tertiary structure is the product of the interaction between the side chains (R) of the amino acids composing the protein. Some of them contain positively or negatively charged groups, others are polar, and still others are nonpolar. The number of carbon atoms in the side chain varies from zero in glycine to nine in tryptophan. Positively and negatively charged side chains have the tendency to attract each other; side chains with identical charges repel each other. The bonds formed by the forces between the negatively charged side chains of aspartic or glutamic acid on the one hand, and the positively charged side chains of lysine or arginine on the other hand, are called salt bridges. Mutual attraction of adjacent peptide chains also results from the formation of numerous hydrogen bonds.

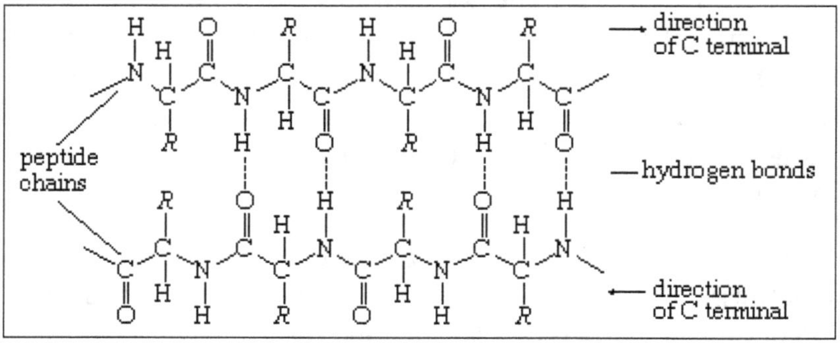

Hydrogen bonds form as a result of the attraction between the nitrogen-bound hydrogen atom (the imide hydrogen) and the unshared pair of electrons of the oxygen atom in the double bonded carbon–oxygen group (the carbonyl group). The result is a slight displacement of the imide hydrogen toward the oxygen atom of the carbonyl group. Although the hydrogen bond is much weaker than a covalent bond (i.e., the type of bond between two carbon atoms, which equally share the pair of bonding electrons between them), the large number of imide and carbonyl groups in peptide chains results in the formation of numerous hydrogen bonds. Another type of attraction is that between nonpolar side chains of valine, leucine, isoleucine, and phenylalanine; the attraction results in the displacement of water molecules and is called hydrophobic interaction.

In proteins rich in cystine, the conformation of the peptide chain is determined to a considerable extent by the disulfide bonds (–S–S–) of cystine. The halves of cystine may be located in different parts of the peptide chain and thus may form a loop closed by the disulfide bond.

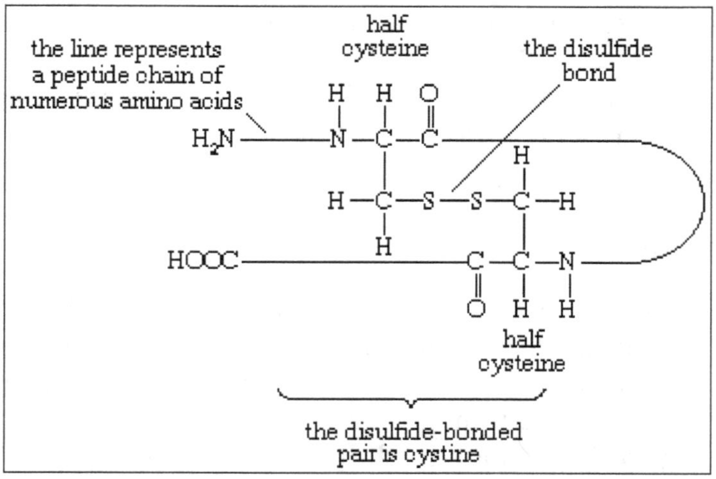

Figure: The disulfide bridge between two cystine halves in an amino acid chain showing how loops in the chain are formed by this amino acid.

If the disulfide bond is reduced (i.e., hydrogen is added) to two sulfhydryl (−SH) groups, the tertiary structure of the protein undergoes a drastic change—closed loops are broken and adjacent disulfide-bonded peptide chains separate.

Quaternary Structure

The nature of the quaternary structure is demonstrated by the structure of hemoglobin. Each molecule of human hemoglobin consists of four peptide chains, two α-chains and two β-chains; i.e., it is a tetramer. The four subunits are linked to each other by hydrogen bonds and hydrophobic interaction. Because the four subunits are so closely linked, the hemoglobin tetramer is called a molecule, even though no covalent bonds occur between the peptide chains of the four subunits. In other proteins, the subunits are bound to each other by covalent bonds (disulfide bridges).

The amino acid sequence of porcine proinsulin is shown below. The arrows indicate the direction from the N terminus of the β-chain (B) to the C terminus of the α-chain (A).

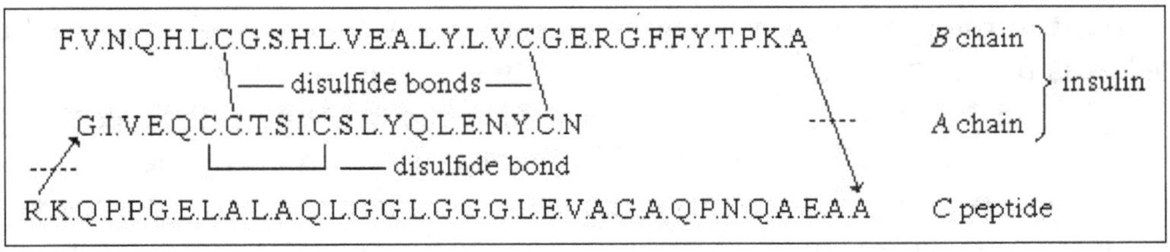

Special Structure and Function of Proteins

Despite its weaknesses, a functional classification is used here in order to demonstrate, whenever possible, the correlation between the structure and function of a protein. The structural, fibrous proteins are presented first, because their structure is simpler than that of the globular proteins and more clearly related to their function, which is the maintenance of either a rigid or a flexible structure.

Structural Proteins in Scleroproteins

Collagen

Collagen is the structural protein of bones, tendons, ligaments, and skin. For many years collagen was considered to be insoluble in water. Part of the collagen of calf skin, however, can be extracted with citrate buffer at pH 3.7. A precursor of collagen called procollagen is converted in the body into collagen. Procollagen has a molecular weight of 120,000. Cleavage of one or a few peptide bonds of procollagen yields collagen, which has three subunits, each with a molecular weight of 95,000; therefore, the molecular weight of collagen is 285,000 (3 × 95,000). The three subunits are wound as spirals around an elongated straight axis. The length of each subunit is 2,900 angstroms, and its diameter is approximately 15 angstroms. The three chains are staggered, so that the trimer has no definite terminal limits.

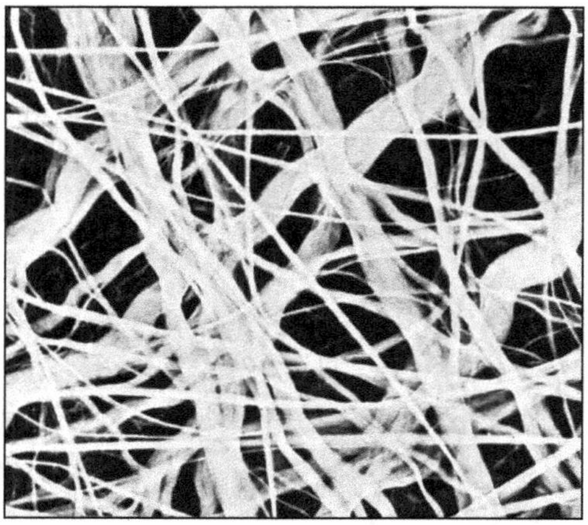

Figure: Collagenous fibers, randomly oriented collagenous fibers of varying size in a thin spread of loose areolar connective tissue (magnified about 370 ×).

Collagen differs from all other proteins in its high content of proline and hydroxyproline. Hydroxyproline does not occur in significant amounts in any other protein except elastin. Most of the proline in collagen is present in the sequence glycine–proline-X, in which X is frequently alanine or hydroxyproline. Collagen does not contain cystine or tryptophan and therefore cannot substitute for other proteins in the diet. The presence of proline causes kinks in the peptide chain and thus reduces the length of the amino acid unit from 3.7 angstroms in the extended chain of the β-structure to 2.86 angstroms in the collagen chain. In the intertwined triple helix, the glycines are inside, close to the axis; the prolines are outside.

Native collagen resists the action of trypsin but is hydrolyzed by the bacterial enzyme collagenase. When collagen is boiled with water, the triple helix is destroyed, and the subunits are partially hydrolyzed; the product is gelatin. The unfolded peptide chains of gelatin trap large amounts of water, resulting in a hydrated molecule.

When collagen is treated with tannic acid or with chromium salts, cross links form between the collagen fibres, and it becomes insoluble; the conversion of hide into leather is based on this tanning process. The tanned material is insoluble in hot water and cannot be converted to gelatin. On exposure to water at 62° to 63° C (144° to 145° F), however, the cross links formed by the tanning agents collapse, and the leather contracts irreversibly to about one-third its original volume.

Collagen seems to undergo an aging process in living organisms that may be caused by the formation of cross links between collagen fibres. They are formed by the conversion of some lysine side chains to aldehydes (compounds with the general structure RCHO), and the combination of the aldehydes with the ε-amino groups of intact lysine side chains. The protein elastin, which occurs in the elastic fibres of connective tissue, contains similar cross links and may result from the combination of collagen fibres with other proteins. When cross-linked collagen or elastin is degraded, products of the cross-linked lysine fragments, called desmosins and isodesmosins, are formed.

Keratin

Keratin, the structural protein of epithelial cells in the outermost layers of the skin, has been isolated from hair, nails, hoofs, and feathers. Keratin is completely insoluble in cold or hot water; it is not attacked by proteolytic enzymes (i.e., enzymes that break apart, or lyse, protein molecules), and therefore cannot replace proteins in the diet. The great stability of keratin results from the numerous disulfide bonds of cystine. The amino acid composition of keratin differs from that of collagen. Cystine may account for 24 percent of the total amino acids. The peptide chains of keratin are arranged in approximately equal amounts of antiparallel and parallel pleated sheets, in which the peptide chains are linked to each other by hydrogen bonds between the carbonyl and imino groups.

Reduction of the disulfide bonds to sulfhydryl groups results in dissociation of the peptide chains, the molecular weight of which is 25,000 to 28,000 each. The formation of permanent waves in the beauty treatment of hair is based on partial reduction of the disulfide bonds of hair keratin by thioglycol, or some other mild reducing agent, and subsequent oxidation of the sulfhydryl groups (−SH) in the reoriented hair to disulfide bonds (−S−S−) by exposure to the oxygen of the air.

The length of keratin fibres depends on their water content. They can bind approximately 16 percent of water; this hydration is accompanied by an increase in the length of the fibres of 10 to 12 percent.

The most thoroughly investigated keratin is hair keratin, particularly that of wool. It consists of a mixture of peptides with high and low cystine content. When wool is heated in water to about 90° C (190° F), it shrinks irreversibly. This is attributed to the breakage of hydrogen bonds and other noncovalent bonds; disulfide bonds do not seem to be affected.

Others

The most thoroughly investigated scleroprotein has been fibroin, the insoluble material of silk. The raw silk comprising the cocoon of the silkworm consists of two proteins. One, sericin, is soluble in hot water; the other, fibroin, is not. The amino acid composition of the latter differs from that of all other proteins. It contains large amounts of glycine, alanine, tyrosine, and serine; small amounts of the other amino acids; and no sulfur-containing ones. The peptide chains are arranged in antiparallel β-structures. Fibroin is partly soluble in concentrated solutions of lithium thiocyanate or in mixtures of cupric salts and ethylene diamine. Such solutions contain a protein of molecular weight 170,000, which is a dimer of two subunits.

Little is known about either the scleroproteins of the marine sponges or the insoluble proteins of the cellular membranes of animal cells. Some of the membranes are soluble in detergents; others, however, are detergent-insoluble.

Role of Proteins in Food

In addition to having many vital functions within the body, proteins perform different roles in our foods by adding certain functional qualities to them. Protein provides food with structure and texture and enables water retention. For example, proteins foam when agitated. (Picture whisking egg whites to make angel food cake. The foam bubbles are what give the angel food cake its airy texture.) Yogurt is another good example of proteins providing texture. Milk proteins called caseins coagulate, increasing yogurt's thickness. In cooked proteins add some color and flavor to foods as the amino group binds with carbohydrates and produces a brown pigment and aroma. Eggs are between 10 and 15 percent protein by weight. Most cake recipes use eggs because the egg proteins help bind all the other ingredients together into a uniform cake batter. The proteins aggregate into a network during mixing and baking that gives cake structure.

Protein Denaturation: Unraveling the Fold

When a cake is baked, the proteins are denatured. Denaturation refers to the physical changes that take place in a protein exposed to abnormal conditions in the environment. Heat, acid, high salt concentrations, alcohol, and mechanical agitation can cause proteins to denature. When a protein denatures, its complicated folded structure unravels, and it becomes just a long strand of amino acids again. Weak chemical forces that hold tertiary and secondary protein structures together are broken when a protein is exposed to unnatural conditions. Because proteins' function is dependent on their shape, denatured proteins are no longer functional. During cooking the applied heat causes proteins to vibrate. This destroys the weak bonds holding proteins in their complex shape (though this does not happen to the stronger peptide bonds). The unraveled protein strands then stick together, forming an aggregate (or network).

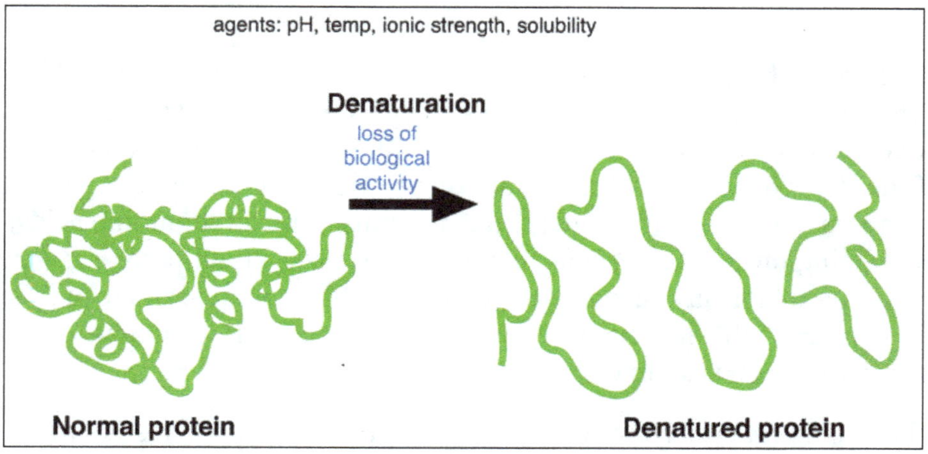

Figure: When a protein is exposed to a different environment, such as increased temperature, it unfolds into a single strand of amino acids.

Animal Protein

Adults require about 0.8 or 0.9 grams of protein per healthy kilogram of bodyweight per day. Does it matter if that protein is from animals or plants? Apparently yes. The adverse effects associated with long-term, high protein-high meat diets may include disorders of bone and calcium balance, increased cancer risk, disorders of the liver, and worsening of coronary artery disease.

Researchers followed thousands of healthy women for more than a decade to look for the presence of excess protein in their urine, a sign that kidneys may be starting to fail. The researchers found three dietary components associated with this sign of declining kidney function: animal protein, animal fat, and cholesterol. Each is found in only one place: animal products. No association was found between kidney function decline and intake of plant protein or fat.

High animal protein intake may induce hyper filtration, a dramatic increase in the kidney's workload. Within hours of consuming meat, whether beef, chicken, or fish, our kidneys may rev up into hyper filtration mode, whereas an equivalent amount of plant protein causes virtually no such stress on the kidneys.

Animal protein consumption also appears to trigger the release of insulin-like growth factor 1 (IGF-1), a cancer-promoting growth hormone. IGF-1 levels rise during childhood to power our development and diminish when we reach adulthood. Should the levels remain too high, however, our cells will constantly receive a message to grow, divide, and keep going and growing. Not surprisingly then, the more IGF-1 in our bloodstream, the higher our risk for developing some cancers. Animal protein appears to stimulate IGF-1 production whether it's the muscle proteins in meat, the egg-white protein in eggs, or the milk proteins in dairy. After just 11 days of cutting back on animal protein, however, our IGF-1 levels may drop by 20 percent.

Milk Protein

Milk is an important component of a balanced diet and contains numerous valuable constituents. Considerable acclaimed health benefits of milk are related to its proteins, not only for their nutritive value but also for their biological properties. Scientific evidence suggests that ant carcinogenic activities, antihypertensive properties, immune system modulation, and other metabolic features of milk, are affiliated with its proteins (intact proteins or its derivatives).

Bovine milk is a liquid food (87% water) which contains an average of 13% total solids and about 9% solids-not-fat. Milk is a nutrient-dense food with important nutritional value due to its calcium, vitamin D (especially in fortified form), protein, vitamin B_{12}, vitamin A, riboflavin, potassium, and phosphorus. Sufficient content of the amino acid tryptophan, a niacin precursor, highlights milk as an important source of niacin equivalents. Additionally, it contains different bioactive compounds with medicinal (nutraceutical) effects. Epidemiologic studies have manifested the association of milk and its products consumption in lower risk of metabolic disorders, cardiovascular diseases, hypertension, cancer, and some other diseases with.

Total protein content of bovine milk is approximately 3.5% by weight (36 g/L), providing almost 38% of the total solids-not-fat content of milk, and about 21% of whole milk energy. Milk is known as a major source of high-quality proteins that possesses a wide range of nutritional, functional, and physiological activities. Milk is also a unique source of peptides with biological activity. Peptides derived from casein fractions and whey proteins, including opioid peptides, antihypertensive peptides, casein phosphopeptides (CPPs), Glycomacropeptide (GMP), and lactorphins, possess various physiological roles, such as opioid-like features, immunostimulating activities, anti-hypertensive activities, antibacterial and antiviral impacts and also enhancement of calcium absorption.

Casein and whey protein are the major proteins of milk. Casein constitutes approximately 80%(29.5 g/L) of the total protein in bovine milk, and whey protein accounts for about 20% (6.3 g/L). Casein is chiefly phosphate-conjugated and mainly consists of calcium phosphate- micelle complexes. It is a heterogeneous family of 4 major components including alpha- (α_{s1}- and α_{s2}-casein), beta-, gamma-, and kappa-casein.

Whey protein is a collection of globular proteins with a high level of α-helix structure and the acidic-basic and hydrophobic-hydrophilic amino acids are distributed in a fairly balanced form. Alpha-Lactalbumin (α-LA) and beta-Lactoglobulin (β-LG) are the predominant whey proteins and comprise about 70–80% of the total whey proteins. Among the other types of whey proteins, immunoglobulins (Igs), serum albumin, lactoferrin (LF), lacto peroxidase (LP), and protease-peptones. Whey proteins have substantial levels of secondary, tertiary, and quaternary structures. They are heat-labile stabilizing their protein structure through intermolecular disulfide linkages.

Nutritional Benefits

Bovine milk protein is considered a high-quality, or complete protein, because it contains all 9 of the essential amino acids in proportions resembling amino acid requirements. Due to the high quality of bovine milk protein, it is regarded as a standard reference protein to evaluate the nutritive value of other food proteins. Furthermore, branched-chain amino acid (isoleucine, leucine, and valine) contents in milk proteins are at higher levels than in many other food sources. These amino acids, especially leucine, help to minimize muscle wasting under conditions of increased protein breakdown and can stimulate muscle protein synthesis. Moreover, whey protein has a high content of sulfur-containing amino acids (cysteine and methionine) which are precursors of glutathione, a tripeptide with antioxidant, anticarcinogenic, and immunostimulatory properties.

Therapeutic Benefits

Caseins and whey proteins differ in their physiological and biological properties.

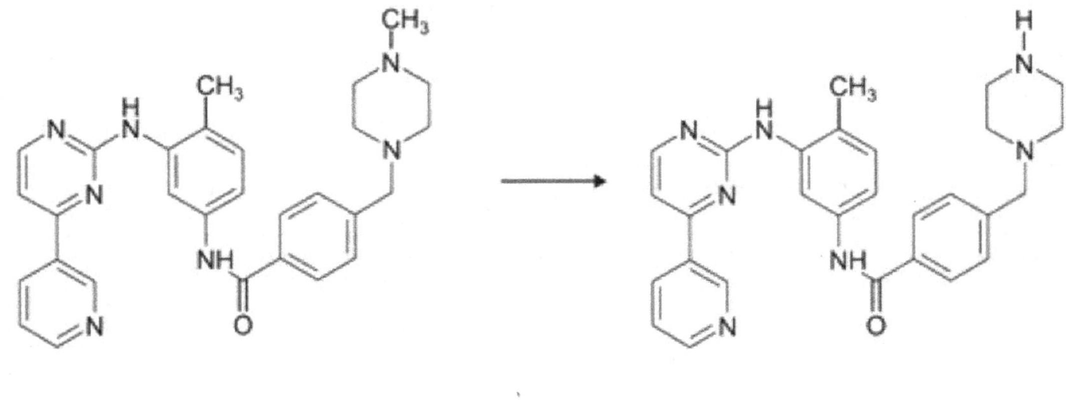

Figure: Molecular structure of imatinib and CGP74588

Table: Selected publications on health benefits of milk proteins.

Type of protein	Biological function	Note
Whey proteins Whey protein concentrate	Anti-carcinogenic activity	Inhibition of incidence and growth of chemically induced tumors.
	Immunomodulation	Higher mucosal antibody responses to antigens.
		Impact on T-cell populations, increase in the T-helper cells concentration and T-helper cells/T-suppressor cells ratio.
β-Lactoglobulin	Anti-carcinogenic activity	Stimulation of the glutathione synthesis.
	Antiviral activity	Inhibition of HIV-1 protease and integrase activities.
α-Lactalbumin	Anti-carcinogenic activity	Antiproliferative action on colon adenocarcinoma cell lines.
	Antibacterial and antiviral activity	Reduction in cell numbers of the infant fecal E. coli.
		Inhibition of HIV-1 protease and integrase activities.
Lactoferrin	Anti-carcinogenic activity	Antiproliferative, anti-inflammatory and antioxidant activities.
	Immunomodulatin	Improving delayed-type hypersensitivity responses to a range of antigens.
		Antimetastatic activity and increase in the numbers of CD4+, CD8+, and NK cells in mice.
	Antibacterial activity and antiviral activity	Inhibitory effect against H. pylori.
		Antibacterial activity against Gram-negative organisms.

		Inhibition of HIV-1 reverse transcriptase, protease and integrase activities.
	Anti-cariogenic activity	Inhibition of the interaction between S. mutans and salivary agglutinin.
		Inhibition of S. mutans adherence to S-HA.
Immunoglobulin	Antibacterial activity	Prevention of shigellosis.
		Protection against oral challenge with enterotoxigenic E.coli.
	Anti-cariogenic activity	Slight inhibitory activity against S. mutans adherence to S-HA.
Casein Whole casein	Anti-carcinogenic activity	Protect against colon cancer.
		Decreasing the incidence of chemically induced intestinal tumors.
		Anti-mutagenic effect in the small intestine.
	Anti-cariogenic activity	Reduction in the hydroxyapatite dissolution rate.
	Hypocholesterolemic effects	Reduction in the total cholesterol, LDL-C, HDL-C and lipoprotein (a) concentrations.
k-Casein	Anti-cariogenic activity	Reduction in the activity of the plaque-promoting enzyme.
		Inhibiting the adherence of S. mutans to the S-HA surfaces of teeth.
β-Casein	Hypocholesterolemic effects	Reduction in blood cholesterol levels.
Bioactive peptides Lactoferricin	Anti-carcinogenic Activity	Cytotoxic, antitumor, and apoptotic activity against cancer cell lines.
		Inhibition of tumor angiogenesis mediated by growth factors in mice.
	Immunomodulation	Increase in Igs (IgM, IgG, and IgA) production. Decrease in the IL-6 response in a monocytic cell line. Increasing the phagocytic activity of human neutrophils.
	Antibacterial activity	Growth inhibition of diverse range of Gram-positive and Gram-negative bacteria.
	Antihypertensive activity	Inhibition of ACE activity and ACE-dependent vasoconstriction.
Lactorphin	Antihypertensive activity	Decrease in blood pressure in hypertensive rats.
Casein-phosphopeptides	Anti-cariogenic activity	Stabilization of calcium phosphate, decreasing the mineral loss during cariogenic episode.
Kappacin	Antibacterial activity	Inhibition of S. mutans, Porphyromonas gingivalis and E. coli.
Caseicidin	Antibacterial activity	Antibacterial activity against staphylococci, sarcina, B. subtilis, Diplococcus pneumoniae and Streptococcus pyogenes.
Caseicins	Antibacterial activity	Inhibitory activity against Enterobacter sakazakii.

Glycomacropeptide	Antiviral activity	Inhibition of against human influenza virus and Epstein Barr virus.
	Immunomodulation	Indirect anti-inflammatory effect of intestinal by Promotion host defense against microorganisms. Enhancing of proliferation and phagocytic activities of human macrophage-like cells.
Casomorphin peptides	Anticarcinogenic activity	Decrease in proliferation of prostatic cancer cell lines Promotion of apoptosis in human leukemia cells (HL-60).

Therapeutic Benefits of Whey Proteins

Anticarcinogenic Effects

Several studies suggest that milk proteins, especially whey proteins, may protect the human body against some cancers (colon, breast, and prostate gland) probably through their ability to enhance cellular levels of glutathione as well as promoting hormonal and cell-mediated immune responses. It has been indicated that whey proteins such as LA, LG, LF, LP, and Igs possess anticarcinogenic activity.

LF, an iron-binding glycoprotein from the transferrin family, has antiproliferative, anti-inflammatory, and antioxidant features. Based on in vivo studies, oral administration of LF to rodents significantly decreased the chemically induced carcinogenesis in various organs such as breast, esophagus, tongue, lung, liver, colon, bladder, and hindered angiogenesis. However, the mechanisms of LF action is yet to be understood besides there are some evidences to support its capability to interact with some receptors and to modulate the genetic expression of several molecules which are vital to the cell cycle and apoptosis mechanisms.

The majority of findings suggesting the anticancer traits of whey proteins, have been acquired from in vitro studies using carcinoma cell lines or in vivo studies using animal models. In vitro studies examining chemically induced tumor formation have reported the inhibitory effect of whey protein supplementation on the incidence and growth of the tumors, as induced by 1, 2-dimethylhydrazine (DMH) and azoxymethane (AOM), and might reduce the risk of developing colorectal cancer. Hakkak *et al.* found that the incidence of mammary tumors induced by dimethylbenz-[α]-anthracene, a chemical substance used to produce mammary adenocarcinoma, was approximately 50% lower in female rats fed with 14% (w/w) whey protein compare to casein-fed rats, and approximately 30% less than soy-fed rats after 4 months. In another study by McIntosh et al., rats on whey protein diet (20 g protein/100 g body weight) showed improved protection against dimethylhydrazine-induced intestinal tumors compared to animals fed an equal amount of soy protein or red meat.

β-LG, as a rich source of cysteine, stimulates glutathione synthesis, an anticarcinogenic tripeptide produced by liver to protect against intestinal tumors. Moreover, in vitro growth inhibition of MCF-7 human breast cancer cell by bovine serum albumin (BSA) has been reported. Also, bovine α-LA, in a concentration of 5 to 35 microg /mL, exerted an antiproliferative and apoptotic activity against some types of human colon cancer cell lines such as Caco2 and Ht-29.

Immunomodulatory Effects

Various in vitro and in vivo studies have proven that milk whey proteins are able to positively influence immune responses. Mice fed with whey protein concentrate (for 12 weeks) showed significantly higher mucosal antibody responses to ovalbumin and cholera toxin compared to those fed a normal diet.

Ingestion of bovine whey proteins (for 5 to 8 weeks) was recognized to improve footpad delayed-type hypersensitivity responses and in-vitro concanavalin A-induced spleen cell proliferation in mice. The influence of whey protein concentrate on T-cell populations has also been reported. Mice fed with 25 g undenatured whey protein concentrate (for 4 weeks) exhibited higher numbers of L3T4+ cells (helper cells) and a higher ratio of L3T4+/Lyt-2+ cells (helper/suppressor) compared to those fed an isocaloric casein diet. A significant increase in total white blood cells, CD4+ and CD8+ lymphocyte counts, and concanavalin A-stimulated interferon-gamma (IFN-γ) production by spleen cells has also been observed in alpha whey fraction-fed mice compared to mice fed with casein and soy protein isolate.

One study announced a dose-dependent improvement of delayed-type hypersensitivity responses to a range of antigens, including ovalbumin, sheep red blood cells, and Calmette- Guerin bacillus in mice, after oral or parenteral administration of bovine LF.

An in-vitro study reported that modified whey protein concentrate (mWPC) suppressed T and B lymphocyte proliferative responses to mitogens in a dose-dependent manner, while it also suppressed alloantigen-induced lymphocyte proliferation during a mixed leukocyte reaction. Additionally, cytokine secretions, IFN-γ and interleukin-4 (IL-4), and the percentage of activated CD25+ T cell blasts following mitogen stimulation, were suppressed by the mWPC. It has been observed that oral administration of bovine LF promoted antimetastatic activity and strongly increased the numbers of CD4+, CD8 +, and natural killer (NK) cells in the lymphoid tissues, small intestine, and peripheral blood of tumor-bearing mice. Moreover, it enhanced the cytotoxic activities of these cells against Yac-1 lymphoma cell and colon 26 carcinoma. In addition, it significantly augments production of IL-18, IFN-γ, and caspase-1 in the small intestine.

In cancer patients, prescription of whey protein (30 g daily for 6 months) has been demonstrated to normalize the number of blood leukocytes. Also, supplementation with whey protein has been reported to increase plasma glutathione levels and natural killer (NK) cell activity in patients with chronic hepatitis B.

Antimicrobial and Antiviral Effects

Intact whey contains a number of unique components with broad antimicrobial activity. Several studies have demonstrated the inhibitory activity of whey proteins against Helicobacter pylori (H. *pylori*) in infected subjects. In a study in fifty-nine healthy subjects, Okuda et al. revealed that twice daily oral administration of LF tablets (200 mg) for 12 weeks decreased the ability of H. pylori to form colonies, but complete eradication was not achieved. In a large multicentered trial, the eradication rate of H. pylori in the infected patients receiving LF (200 mg) twice a day for 7 days was 73%.

LF has been shown to render direct bactericidal activity against Gram-negative organisms due to its ability to bind to the lipid A part of bacterial lipopolysaccharides and to increase membrane permeability. It was found that LF (1 mg/mL) significantly protected cultured epithelial cells (isolated from patients suffering from pharyngitis) against in vitro invasion by group A Streptococcus (GAS) and intensely prevented invasiveness of GAS pretreated by erythromycin or ampicillin. The efficacy of bovine milk Ig concentrate against Shigella flexneri and protection against shigellosis among healthy adult subjects has been reported by Tacket et al. Furthermore, bovine milk-derived Igs could protect against oral challenge with enterotoxigenic Escherichia coli (E. coil) in healthy adult volunteer. A significant reduction in growth and cell numbers of an infant fecal microorganism, E. coil 2348/69, in infants fed with a formula supplemented with α-LA was reported by Brücket al.

Moreover, some studies showed antiviral activity of whey proteins. Some research has examined the inhibitory activity of whey proteins against human immunodeficiency virus (HIV). LF, α-LA, and β-LG have shown inhibitory activities against HIV-1. LF exhibited strong inhibitory activity against HIV-1 reverse transcriptase activity, but weak inhibitory activity against HIV-1 protease and integrase, while α-LA and β-LG exerted inhibitory activity against HIV-1 protease and integrase but did not inhibit HIV-1 reverse transcriptase. LF was more effective during the early stage of HIV infection.

Anticariogenic Effects

There is much scientific evidence that supports protective impacts of whey proteins against dental caries. It has been indicated that whey might have a topical anticariogenic impact by its buffering capacity. Mitoma et al. Demonstrated that bovine LF can be firmly bound to salivary agglutinin and therefore inhibit the interaction between protein antigen of *Streptococcus mutans* (*S. mutans*) and salivary agglutinin. In another study, inhibition of *S. mutans* adherence to saliva-coated hydroxyapatite (S-HA) by milk components was demonstrated. Bovine LF showed the strongest inhibitory activity. Other components, such as LP and IgG revealed moderate inhibitory activities. Also, LP and lysozyme synergistically provided anticariogenic effects through restricting glucose metabolism by *S. mutans* and therefore reduced acid production in the dental plaque environment.

The Impact of Whey Proteins on Satiety, Food Intake, and Weight Loss

The effects of milk and milk products on the regulation of food intake and satiety have been attributed to several components. Among milk components, proteins possess the greatest potential to provide satiety signals and milk proteins are more satiating than other protein sources. Whey proteins contribute to the short-term and long-term food intake regulation by inducing satiety signals. One study showed that consumption of 45 g whey protein, in the form of sweetened beverages, suppressed food intake more than egg albumin and soy protein at a pizza meal 60 min later. In another study, drinks containing 400 Kcal and 48 g of whey stimulated subjective satiety, and reduced food intake at a buffet meal 90 min later, more than the drinks containing the same amount of casein. A high-protein breakfast (58.1% of energy from protein and 14.1% of energy from carbohydrate) consisting of dairy products enriched with whey protein isolate raised glucagon-like peptide-1 levels over 3 h more than a high-carbohydrate breakfast (19.3% of energy from protein and 47.3% of energy from carbohydrate) consisting of plain yogurt.

After 23 weeks of consumption of supplemental whey protein, soy protein, and an iso-energetic amount of carbohydrate, body weight and body fat among the whey protein group were lower than the group consuming carbohydrate. Waist circumference was also smaller in the subjects receiving whey protein than in the other groups. Moreover, fasting ghrelin was lower in subjects receiving whey protein in comparison with soy protein or carbohydrate.

Feeding insulin-resistant obese rats with whey protein has been shown to reduce calorie intake, to decrease body fat, and therefore to result in a significant improvement in insulin sensitivity in comparison with a red meat diet. Furthermore, in rats receiving high-protein diets ad libitum over a 25-day period, milk protein fractions (whole milk protein, whey protein, or β-LG-enriched fraction) reduced calorie intake, body weight, and body fat. β-LG was the most efficient fraction.

Therapeutic Benefits of Casein Proteins

Anticarcinogenic Effects

Evidence indicates that casein might protect the body against some cancers. Casein inhibits fecal beta-glucuronidase; an enzyme produced by intestinal bacteria and deconjugates procarcinogenic glucuronides to carcinogens. Casein might also protect against colon cancer through its influence on the immune system, specifically by stimulating phagocytic activities and increasing lymphocytes.

Lower incidence of DMH-induced colorectal cancer was found in rats fed a casein diet compared to rats fed other sources of protein such as soybean and red meat. The intracellular concentration of glutathione in the liver was also greater in the casein-fed rats. A reduced incidence of colon tumors was also observed in rats fed a mixture of casein and wheat protein compared to those fed with the equivalent amount of wheat and chickpea protein. In an investigation, rats treated with 10 weekly injections of 7.4 mg/Kg body weight of AOM, received synthetic isoenergetic diets with different amount of protein content including 25% casein (normal-protein diet), 10% casein (low-protein diet), or 5% casein (very-low-protein diet). Administration of a diet containing 25% casein resulted in a fewer incidence of colon tumors in rats than isoenergetic diets containing 10 and 5% casein after 30 weeks.

In-vitro and in-vivo studies have demonstrated the impact of caseinate and soy protein on the mutagenic potential of N-methyl-N′-nitro-N-nitrosoguanidine (MNNG). Of these 2 dietary proteins, only casein presented antimutagenic activity against MNNG in the small intestine of mice treated with this mutagen. In addition, the antimutagenic potential of casein was assessed against different mutagens, including some food-related mutagens. Casein showed the most antimutagenic activity against benzo[a]pyrene, N-methylnitrosourea, and nitrosated 4-chloroindole, and the least antimutagenic activity against sodium azide and N-nitroquinoline-1-oxide.

Anticariogenic Effects

Some studies indicate that casein might contribute to the beneficial effects of milk on oral health. Kappa-casein (k-casein) may protect against dental caries by decreasing the activity of glucosyltransferase, a plaque-promoting enzyme produced by *S. mutans*, and the ability of this enzyme to adhere to dental surfaces or S-HA. -Casein has also been revealed to reduce the adherence of *S. mutans* to the S-HA surfaces of teeth.

A study in rats infected by mixed bacterial suspensions of Streptococcus sobrinus *OMZ 176* and Actinomyces viscosus Ny1indicated that consumption of powdered milk micellar casein could reduce the formation of advanced dental fissure and smooth surface lesions, and inhibit colonization of Streptococcus sobrinus (S. sobrinus). In another study whole casein was combined with a citric acid solution in order to assaying the impact of soft drinks on the hydroxyapatite dissolution rate. Adding 0.02% (w/v) casein to citric acid solutions significantly decreased the hydroxyapatite dissolution rate by approximately 50–60%.

Hypocholesterolemic Effects

Some investigators have studied the effect of casein on blood cholesterol. In a crossover study, 11 normal participants received diets providing 20% of calories from casein or soy protein. The mean of cholesterol intake was 500 mg/d. An initial reduction in plasma cholesterol and low-density lipoprotein cholesterol (LDL-C) was observed in both diets. In another crossover study, normolipidemic non-obese healthy men consumed 2 liquid-formula diets containing casein or soy protein. After 30 days on each diet, the lipoprotein (a) concentration was reduced by approximately 50% with the casein diet compared to the soy-protein diet. Total cholesterol, LDL- C, and high-density lipoprotein cholesterol

(HDL-C) concentrations also were lowered with both diets. In hypercholesterolemic subjects who consumed 2 doses of casein (30 or 50 g) in the form of beverage, total cholesterol concentrations were reduced during 16 weeks. One study in Australian individuals at high risk of developing heart disease showed daily supplementation with 25 g of beta-casein (β-casein) A1 or A2 could significantly reduce blood cholesterol concentrations.

Therapeutic Benefits of Bioactive Peptides Derived from Milk Proteins

Milk contains different bioactive components, including bioactive peptides with physiological functionality. Peptides generated from milk include a variety of substances which are potent modulators of various regulatory processes in the body and exhibit multifunctional bioactivities. Biologically active peptides hidden within the intact milk proteins are released and activated by gastrointestinal digestion of milk, fermentation of milk by proteolysis starter cultures, or hydrolysis by proteolytic enzymes. Bioactive peptides derived from casein and whey proteins, including opioid peptides, antihypertensive peptides, CPP, lactorphins, and albutensin have been demonstrated to play physiological roles such as opioid-like features, immunostimulation, angiotensin I-converting enzyme (ACE) inhibition, anti-hypertensive property, and antimicrobial activity.

Therapeutic Benefits of Bioactive Peptides Derived from Whey

Hydrolysis of whey proteins generates bioactive peptides .Experimental findings have revealed that bioactive peptides can be purified from α-LA, β-LG, bovine LF, and BSA. Some of these peptides have been given particular names such as α- and β-lactorphin, β-lactotensin, serophin, albutensin A, lactoferricin (Lfcin), and lactoferrampin. Most of these peptides have not been characterized to the extent of casein-derived peptides. Recently, whey-derived peptides have received special attention, because of their preventive and therapeutic characteristics.

Anticarcinogenic Effects

Peptides derived from the N-terminal region of LF have been investigated in order to identify sequences with potential antitumor activity. Roy et al. isolated 4 peptides from pepsin hydrolysates of lactoferrin with Antiproliferative and apoptotic property. The sequence corresponding to residues 17–38 of bovine LF showed the highest apoptotic activity in human leukemia cells (HL-60). Eliassen et al. reported that bovine Lfcin, exhibited cytotoxic activity against Meth Afibrosarcoma, melanoma, and colon carcinoma cell lines, and significantly lowered the size of solid Meth A tumors. Also, Lfcin displayed antitumor activity against MDA-MB-435 breast cancer cells by inducing apoptosis and cytotoxic activity in-vitro and in-vivo against neuroblastoma cells by destabilization of the cytoplasmic and the mitochondria membranes.

Lfcin B could also inhibit angiogenesis mediated by vascular endothelial growth factor and fibroblast growth factor in mouse models, as well as to mediate Antiproliferative andantimigratory activities against proangiogenic factor-induced human umbilical vein endothelial cells.

In-vitro studies suggest treatment with Lfcin B induced apoptotic death in several different human leukemia and carcinoma cell lines by stimulating the mitochondrial pathway of apoptosis via the production of reactive oxygen species and activation of caspase-9 and caspase-3. In addition, it has been observed that bovine Lfcin can trigger mitochondrial-dependent apoptosis in Jurkat T-leukemia cells by cell membrane damage through binding to the cell membrane, increasing permeabilization of the cell membrane, and the subsequent disruption of the mitochondrial membrane.

Immunomodulatory Effects

Whey includes several potent immunomodulatory peptides that are hidden within the intact structure of whey proteins. The impact of peptides liberated by tryptic digestion of bovine β-LG on various immune functions in mice was studied by Pecquet et al. The tolerance to β-LG was enhanced in mice fed β-LG hydrolysates or fractions of the hydrolysate. A reduction in serum and intestinal IgE levels was also observed. Furthermore, β-LG-specific delayed-type hypersensitivity and proliferative responses of splenic cells were suppressed.

Prioult et al. announced that hydrolaysate of β-LG with Lactobacillus paracasei peptidases generated a number of small immunomodulatory peptides. These peptide sequences reduced lymphocyte proliferation and enhanced immunosuppressant interleukin-10 production.

Several studies have revealed the immunomodulary properties of Lfcin. Hydrolysis of bovine LF with pepsin produced some immunostimulatory and immunoinhibitory peptides. The hydrolysate significantly enhanced proliferation and Igs (IgM, IgG, and IgA) generation in murine splenocytes and also proliferation and IgA production in Peyer's patch cells in-virto. Bovine LF and Lfcin B were found to reduce the IL-6 response in THP-1 human monocytic cells after stimulating by lipopolysaccharide. In addition, Lfcin B augmented the phagocytic activity of human neutrophils through direct binding to the neutrophils and opsonin-like activity.

Antimicrobial Effects

LF-derived peptides have been identified to present antimicrobial properties. The antibacterial features of enzymatic hydrolysates of bovine LF were investigated by Tomita et al. Hydrolysates prepared with cleavage of LF by porcine pepsin, cod pepsin, or acid protease from Penicillium dupontiexerted intense antibacterial activity against Escherichia coli.

It was shown that Lfcin B inhibited or inactivated various ranges of Gram-positive and Gram-negative bacteria, including E. coli, Salmonella enteritidis, Yersinia enterocolitica, Klebsiella pneumoniae, Proteus vulgaris, Pseudomonas aeruginosa, Campylcbacter jejuni, Staphylococcus aureus, Staphylococcus haemolyticus, Streptococcus thermophilus,S. mutans, Clostridium perfringens, Corynebacterium diphtheriae, Listeria monocytogenes, Bacillus subtilis (B. subtilis), and Bifidobacterium infantis.

Proteolytic cleavage of α-LA generated 3 antibacterial peptide fragments including LDT1, LDT2, and LDC. These sequences were effective against Gram-positive bacteria, while they presented weak activity against Gram-negative bacteria. Furthermore, 4 peptide fragments were isolated by tryptic digestion of bovine β-LG. Released fragments revealed bactericidal activity against Gram-positive bacteria.

Antihypertensive Effects

It has been recognized that *in-vitro* incubation of milk proteins with gastrointestinal protease, including pepsin, trypsin, and chymotrypsin, can yield a large number of fragments with ACE inhibitory activity. The ACE inhibitory peptides are produced during gastrointestinal transport. Bacterial and plant proteinases can be applied to produce such peptides as well.

Nurminen et al. examined the antihypertensive activity of alpha-lactorphin, a tetrapeptide (Tyr-Gly-Leu-Phe) originating from milk α-LA, in conscious spontaneously hypertensive rats (SHR) and in normotensive Wistar Kyoto rats. α-Lactorphin lowered blood pressure in SHR and Wistar Kyoto rats dose-dependently. Enzymatic cleavage of the whey protein by proteinase K released 6 potent ACE inhibitory peptides. These peptides possessed antihypertensive activity in SHR. Of these 6 peptides, the fragment Ile-Pro-Ala, originally derived from β-LG, exhibited the most ACE inhibitory feature.

Mullally et al. investigated the ACE inhibitory activity of a tryptic cleavage of bovine β-LG. The β-LG fraction gave an ACE inhibition index of 84.3%. In another investigation, some ACE-inhibitory peptides were isolated by hydrolysis of bovine whey proteins with an enzyme combination, including pepsin, trypsin, and chymotrypsin, or with trypsin alone. The generated peptides were α-LA fragments, and β-LG fragments. ACE activity was 50% suppressed by the whey hydrolysates at the concentration ranges of 345-1733 μg/mL.

In addition, enzymatic digestions of LF released some antihypertensive peptides with molecular masses lower than 3 kDa. These fractions showed inhibitory activity against ACE and endothelin-converting enzyme (ECE) in-vitro.

Ruiz-Giménez et al. reported that a set of 8 LfcinB-generated peptides could inhibit ACE activity *in-vitro*. Of these peptides, 7 exerted *ex-vivo* inhibitory activity against ACE-dependent vasoconstriction. Only Oral administration of LfcinB and one of its fragments, F1, reduced blood pressure in SHR.

Moreover, in a controlled study with prehypertensive or stage 1 prehypertensive human volunteers, blood pressure was significantly lower in the treatment group that consumed 20 g/day hydrolyzed whey protein isolate rich in bioactive peptides than in the control group that consumed the same amount of unhydrolyzed whey protein isolate.

Therapeutic Benefits of Bioactive Peptides Derived from Casein

Casein, in either milk or dairy foods, is a main source of bioactive peptides. Casein-derived peptides reveal different bioactive roles.

Anticarcinogenic Effects

According to various cytochemical studies, there is some evidence for the possible anticarcinogenic activity of casein-derived peptides. *In-vitro* examinations have indicated that casein-based peptides isolated after microbial fermentation of milk could protect against colon cancer through changing cell kinetics. Kampa *et al.* described that several casomorphin peptides, a group of opioid peptides derived from α- and β-casein, suppressed the proliferation of some prostatic cancer cell lines, including LNCaP, PC3, and DU145, via involving opioid receptors. Also, apoptosis of HL-60 cells was promoted by the opioid peptide β-casomorphin-7 and the phosphopeptide β-CN 4P. Moreover, purified peptides, corresponding to bioactive fractions of casein, showed modulatory effects on cell viability, proliferation, and apoptosis in various human cell culture models, including human peripheral blood lymphocytes, HL-60, polymorphonuclear leukocytes, and Caco-2 cells.

Immunomodulatory Effects

Some experiments have been conducted to consider the effect of casein-derived bioactive peptides on immune function. It was found that in-vitro digests of casein produced by peptidases of Lactobacillus rhamnosus inhibited protein kinase C translocation and downregulated IL-2 mRNA expression. These findings demonstrated in-vitro suppression of T cell activation by casein digests. Sütaset al. reported that bovine caseins hydrolyzed with enzymes produced by Lactobacillus GG inhibited IL-4 production of peripheral blood mononuclear cells in atopic children. In another study, Sütas et al. showed that digestion of caseins with proteasesgenerated from Lactobacillus casei (L. casei) GG, produced some fractions with suppressive effects on lymphocyte proliferation in-vitro. Hata et al. demonstrated that caseinophosphopeptides β-CN(f1–25)4P and α_{s1}-CN(f59–79)5P possessed immunostimulatory effects via increasing IgG production in mouse spleen cell cultures. Moreover, CPPs derived from bovine αs2- and β-casein exerted immuno-enhancing activity by enhancing the level of serum and intestinal antigen-specific IgA in mice fed with a CPPs preparation.

Bovine GMP can stimulate human monocytes and secretion of tumor necrosis factor, IL-1β and IL-8 from human monocytes, through effects on mitogen-activated protein kinase and nuclear factor-kappaB signaling pathways. GMP might have an indirect intestinal anti-inflammatory impact through enhancing host defenses against invading microorganisms. GMP and its derivatives generated by peptic hydrolysis can stimulate proliferation and phagocytic activities of the human U937 macrophage-like cells.

Antimicrobial and Antiviral Effects

There is some evidence regarding antimicrobial properties of casein-derived peptides. McCann et al. discovered a novel fragment from bovine α_{S1}-casein, purified by enzymatic digestion of bovine sodium caseinate with pepsin. This fragment exhibited inhibitory activity against Gram-positive and Gram-negative bacteria.

Kappacin, the monophosphorylated fragment Ser(P)149 k -casein -A produced by endoproteinase Glu-C digestion of CPP, displayed inhibitory activity against S. mutans, Porphyromonas gingivalis, and E. coli. Caseicidin, a defense peptide purified by chymosin hydrolysis of casein at neutral pH, showed inhibitory activity against staphylococci, Sarcina spp, B. subtilis, Diplococcus pneumoniae, and Streptoco ccus pyogenes. The immunomodulatory peptide isolated from bovine β-casein, β-CN peptide, promotes the antimicrobial activity of mouse macrophages via up-regulation of MHC class II antigen expression and enhancement of phagocytic activity. The antimicrobial property of caseicins has been well demonstrated. Caseicins A and B, corresponding of bovine α_{s1}-casein, showed an intense activity against Enterobacter sakazakii.

In-vitro studies have revealed that casocidin-I, a C-terminal fragment of bovine α_{S2}-casein, inhibited the growth of E. coli and Staphylococcus strains. Antibacterial and antiviral features of GMP have also been demonstrated. The ability of GMP to inhibit binding of cholera toxin to normal Chinese hamster ovary cells was reported by Kawasaki et al. Furthermore, it showed similar inhibitory activity against E. coli heat-labile enterotoxins LT-I and LT-II, associated with colonization factor antigen CFA/I and CFA/II, respectively, in the Chinese hamster ovary model. GMP could also inhibit hemagglutination by 4 strains of human influenza virus at concentration ranges from 10^{-2} to 10^{-3}. Dosako et al. demonstrated the ability of GMP to inhibit the morphological transformations in peripheral blood lymphocytes induced by Epstein Barr virus.

Anti-Cariogenic Effects

Some researchers have assayed the ability of casein's bioactive peptides to inhibit demineralization and to enhance remineralization of tooth enamel. Milk-derived bioactive peptides such as CPP and GMP may be responsible for the cariostatic properties of cheese via suppressing the growth of cariogenic bacteria, concentrating calcium and phosphate in plaque, reducing enamel demineralization, and enhancing remineralization.

The anti-cariogenic impacts of CPPs have been demonstrated in animal and human experiments. It was suggested that CPPs stabilized calcium phosphate by forming casein phosphopeptide-calcium phosphate complexes (CPP-CP) and increasing the uptake of calcium and phosphate by dental plaque. In addition, CPP and amorphous calcium phosphate (ACP) bind to plaque, providing a potential source of calcium within the plaque and decreasing the diffusion of free calcium. Therefore, CPP-ACP can protect against dental caries by reducing mineral loss during a cariogenic episode and supplying a rich source of calcium for subsequent remineralization. Additionally, CPPs might exert an anti-cariogenic impact by competing with plaque-forming bacteria for binding to calcium.

Neeser et al. investigated the ability of milk casein components to restrict the adhesion ability of some odontopathogenic bacteria to tooth surface. Sodium caseinate, CPP, and GMP inhibited adherence of potential dental pathogens, including Streptococcus sobrinus OMZ 176 as well as Streptococcus sanguis (S. sanguis) OMZ to S-HA beads. In a similar study, Schüpbach et al. considered GMP and CPP as adhesion inhibitors of oral bacteria. Adhesion ability of S. sobrinus to salivary pellicle was decreased 49%, 75%, and 81% by GMP, CPP, and the combination of GMP and CPP, respectively.

Antihypertensive Effects

Considerable research has been performed to investigate the impact of biologically active peptides obtained from casein on blood pressure. In a single-blind, placebo-controlled study with Japanese adults having high-normal blood pressure or mild hypertension, receiving a casein hydrolysate containing bioactive peptides (for 6 weeks), led to significant reduction in systolic blood pressure from 1.7 to 10.1 mm Hg, in a dose-dependent fashion. A study in normotensive and mildly hypertensive patients showed consumption of 10 gr of a tryptic digest of casein (twice daily for a 4-week period) had an antihypertensive influence. In another investigation, daily ingestion of 800 mg/Kg body weight of a casein hydrolysate product for 6 weeks decreased the development of hypertension and increased the eNOS expressionin SHRs.

In a placebo-controlled study, daily consumption of 95 mL sour milk containing two ACE-inhibitory peptides from β-casein, and significantly attenuated the blood pressure of hypertensive participants after 4–8 weeks. It has been reported that casein-derived peptides by *L. helveticus* proteases indicated ACE inhibitory activities. ACE inhibitory activity of the casein-based tripeptides Ile-Pro-Pro and Val-Pro-Pro has also been revealed by Nakamura *et al.*

In a placebo-controlled double-blind crossover study, consumption of a product containing casein-derived tripeptides (Ile-Pro-Pro and Val-Pro-Pro) and plant sterols acutely reduced blood pressure in individuals with mild hypertension.

In conclusion, milk is the oldest and one of the most widely consumed nutritious foods worldwide. It is highlighted as a source of high-quality proteins and one of the most important sources of bioactive peptides. Milk proteins have high nutritive value and remarkable medicinal properties. They are known as potential ingredients of health-promoting functional foods, and the dairy industry has already commercialized many milk proteins and peptide-based products which can be consumed as part of a regular daily diet. They are consumed by infants, the elderly and immune-compromised people. They are also consumed to maintain good health status and prevent diet-related chronic diseases such as obesity, cardiovascular disease, and cancer. Milk-derived peptides are commonly ingested both in functional foods and drugs. They exhibit various well-defined pharmacological effects, for example, in the treatment of diarrhea (casomorphins), hypertension (casokinins), thrombosis (casoplatelins), dental diseases, mineral malabsorption (CPPs), and immunodeficiency (immunopeptides). These findings introduce new perspectives in the nutritional and technological evaluation of milk products and encourage utilization of these substances for production of food and new health promoting products. More studies related to the mechanisms by which these proteins exert their effects are required to achieve further substantial evidence.

Egg Protein

The chicken eggs have always been recognized as an excellent source of human nutrition, especially for the dietary protein. The chemical composition of an egg has always fascinated human mind, may be due to the compartmentalized structure of the whole egg. However, only in recent years, with the help of innovative research tools, scientists have revealed the structural and functional diversity of the different components in eggs. These revelations diversify the use of eggs in various processed food products and increase the commercial value of an egg. Egg proteins are well-known for its functional properties and are massively used as an ingredient to enhance the texture or flavor of variety of food products. Additionally, egg proteins are also a potential source of bioactive proteins and peptides. The bioactive egg proteins and peptides can exhibit health beneficial effect above and beyond their known nutritional value. Subsequently, egg proteins, especially proteins from egg white, are known as a major allergen affecting nearly 2.5% young children in the USA. The egg consists of three major portions; a) eggshell, b) egg white, and c) egg yolk. Protein is one of the major components present in all three parts of the egg, and egg white is the prime source of proteins.

Egg Shell Proteins

The eggshell is the outermost layer of an egg and is mainly composed of a foamy layer of cuticle, a calcium carbonate layer, and then two flexible membranes (inner and outer membrane). This whole structure together retains the egg white or albumen and egg yolk inside the egg and also prevents the invasion of any pathogenic bacteria.

The organic matter of chicken eggshell and eggshell membrane comprises of a complex mix of proteins and polysaccharides, out of which proteins constitute almost 70% of the total organic matter. The eggshell membrane has been found to contain many bacteriolytic enzymes, such as N-acetylglucosaminidase and lysozyme, and other components which might have a role in preventing the invasion of Gram-negative and Gram-positive bacteria. Moreover, the eggshell membrane hydrolysates have been found to contain hydroxyproline suggestive of the presence of collagen in the membrane layers the collagen constitutes almost 10% of the total proteinaceous matter in the eggshell.

Eggshell mainly comprises of various ubiquitous proteins which are extensively expressed in different organs. Osteopontin, a phosphorylated glycoprotein, is found in kidney, bones and many body secretions and it was found to be expressed in the uterus epithelial cells during the calcification of the eggshell. This protein is mainly confined to the mammillae, core of the non-mineralized shell membrane fibers, and the outermost segment of the shell palisade layer. Osteopontin inhibits the precipitation of calcium carbonate in the eggshell, and the protein loses its inhibitory activity upon dephosphorylation with alkaline phosphatase. This suggests that osteopontin might have a role as a modulator in the precipitation of calcium carbonate in the uterine fluid or even as an inhibitor during the termination of the calcification process.

Clusterin is another ubiquitous eggshell secretory protein which is a heterodimeric glycoprotein bonded with disulfide linkages. This particular protein is found in many tissues and is also present in all the calcified regions of the eggshell. In the uterus, it is secreted by the tubular gland cells into the uterine fluid, irrespective of the shell calcification stage. Clusterin might have a role in preventing premature aggregation and precipitation of eggshell proteins by acting as an extracellular chaperone in the uterine fluid. There are specific proteins which are unique to the eggshell and are secreted only by the tissues present in the shell. These proteins have been identified in domestic hens only.

Ovocleidin-17 (OC-17) is a 142 amino acid long phosphorylated protein having a C-type lectin domain, and it was the first protein to be purified to homogeneity. This protein is also present as a 23 kDa glycosylated protein in a minor form. The tubular gland cells of the uterus secrete OC-17 throughout the calcified part of the shell during the entire calcification period. OC-17 modifies the shape of calcium carbonate crystals in vitro.

Ovocleidin-116 (OC-116) is an 80 kDa protein with 742 amino acids, and it was the first eggshell protein which was cloned. The protein comprises of two disulfide bonds and two N-glycosylations. OC-116 was named ovoglycan and it forms the protein core of the primary proteoglycan of the shell. The carbohydrates of OC-116 comprises of 17 different oligo-structures. Eight of them were hybrid-type, four were the high-mannose type, and the rest five had a complex-type structure. When present in the uterine fluid, OC-116 exists as a 116 kDa protein due to glycosylation modification and as a 190 kDa protein after glycation. This protein is thought to have a role in the modulation of calcite growth. Ovocalyxin-32 (OCX-32) is released in the uterine fluid by the surface epithelial cells of the uterus during the end of the calcification phase and thus it is mainly confined to the outer regions of the shell, i.e., the vertical crystal layer, cuticle, and the palisade layer. Therefore, it has been suggested that this protein has a role in the termination of the calcification process of the eggshell. Ovocalyxin-36 (OCX-36) is found in abundance in the uterine fluid during the calcification process, and the expression of this protein is highly up regulated. This protein has been cloned as well.

OCX-36 has homologous similarities with proteins involved in innate immune responses such as bactericidal permeability increasing proteins, lipopolysaccharide binding proteins, and Plunc family proteins, which suggests the fact that OCX-36 may also be involved in the defence mechanisms to keep the egg pathogen free.

Ovocalyxin-25 and -21 are also two other eggshell proteins which are exclusively detected in tissues undergoing mineralization. Database analysis reported that Ovocalyxin-21 has remarkable homologies with brichos domain-containing proteins. The Brichos domain consists of nearly 100 amino acids and comparing the similarities, several functions of the ovocalyxin-21 proteins were postulated including chaperon-like functions. Ovocalyxin-25 contains two protease inhibitory domains, one of which is the WAP-type. The matrix protein from the nacreous layer of the pearl and shell of molluscs, known as lustrin A, also has the same inhibitory WAP-type domains.

Egg White Proteins

The egg white is made up of four individual layers: chalaziferous layer, thin layer, thick layer, and the chalazae cord. The thin layer accounts for about 23.3% of egg white, which is further separated into two layers, i.e., inner and outer thin layers. The thin inner layer (16.8% of egg white) is attached to the chalaziferous layer, which accounts for about 2.7% of egg white, whereas, the thin outer layer is connected to the inner eggshell membrane. The outer and inner thin layers are separated by the thick or viscous layer which accounts for the most substantial portion of egg white, i.e., 57.3%. Water is the primary constituent of egg white which accounts for about 84% to 89% of the total egg white or albumen weight. Among albumen solids, proteins are the major constituents (10%–11%), while the minor components include carbohydrates (0.9%), lipids (0.03%), vitamins and minerals. Egg proteins are well known for their high nutritional quality, excellent digestibility and comprise of all the essential amino acids necessary for the human nutrition and development (Friedman, 1996). Egg albumen consists of several different protein components which have been identified and characterized through modern high-resolution analytical techniques. In a study, 78 egg white proteins were detected using 1-dimensional electrophoresis and liquid chromatography tandem mass spectrometry (LC-MS/MS). However, among egg white proteins, ovalbumin, ovotransferrin, ovomucoid, ovomucin, and lysozyme have been studied extensively due to their abundant presence in egg albumen. Physicochemical characteristics of major egg white protein are provided in Table below.

Protein	Dry weight of albumen (g/kg)	Isoelectric point (PI)	Molecular weight (kDa)	T_d °(C)
Major proteins				
Ovalbumin	540	4.5	45	84
Ovotransferrin	120	6.1	76	61
Ovomucoid	110	4.1	28	77
Ovomucin	35	4.5-5.0	5500-8300	-
Lysozyme	34	10.7	14.3	75

Minor proteins				
Ovoglobulin	40	(6.1-5.3)	30-45	92.5
G_2 globulin	40	5.5	-	-
G_3 globulin	15	4.8	49	-
Ovoinhibitor	10	5.1	24.4	-
Ovoglycoprotein	8	3.9	32	-
Ovoflavoprotein	5	4.0	769	-
Ovomacroglobulin	0.5	4.5	12.7	-
Cystatin	0.5	5.1	68.3	-
Avidin		10		

'–' represents not determined.

Ovalbumin

Ovalbumin constitutes about 54% of the total egg albumen and thus it is the primary protein present in egg white. It is a phosphorylated glycoprotein made up of complete three subunits having different phosphate groups along with a carbohydrate group attached to its N-terminal. Ovalbumin is a member of the serpin (serine protease inhibitors) superfamily despite lacking the inhibitory activity unlike the other serpin-like proteins. The molecular weight of ovalbumin is 45 kDa and is composed of 386 amino acids along with two genetic polymorphisms seen at 290 (Glu/Gln) and 312 (Asn/Asp) . Among all other egg albumen proteins, ovalbumin is a unique protein as it contains six cysteine residues, two of which are involved in a disulfide bond between Cys74 and Cys121, while the rest four include free sulfhydryl (eSH) groups. One out of the four eSH group is reactive only when the protein is denatured; however, the other three are masked in the native state. The amino acid composition analysis of egg albumen revealed that 50% of the total amino acids are hydrophobic while 30% are acidic and charged amino acids, the latter contributing to the acidic isoelectric point (pI) of 4.5. Ovalbumin has a unique amino acid distribution as compared to other glycoproteins. It lacks an N-terminal ladder sequence but contains an acetylated glycine and proline in the N- and C-terminal, respectively, along with carbohydrate moiety attached to the amino acids in the N-terminal.

Ovalbumin-Y is a chimeric glycoprotein with an amino acid sequence very similar to the native ovalbumin and a carbohydrate group identical to ovomucoid. Ovalbumin-Y protein was first identified and characterized by Nau et al. by 2-Dimensional PAGE and peptide mass fingerprinting. Ovalbumin Y is not phosphorylated unlike ovalbumin; however, it is glycosylated. Three isoforms of ovalbumin Y protein and five isoforms of ovalbumin-related Y protein have been identified via electrophoresis, each protein differing in their pIs. However, this polymorphism could not be explained by genetic variations or by phosphorylation or glycosylation levels.

Ovalbumin in its native form is resistant to digestion by trypsin but once it is heat denatured or given an acid or pH change treatment, it becomes susceptible to trypsin digestion. With high pH and temperature dependent denaturation, ovalbumin converts into a thermally stable form known as S-ovalbumin. Sugimoto et al. demonstrated that storage temperature influences this conversion more than the storage time, where longer storage time at 20–25 C did not affect the conversion. However, Huang et al. demonstrated that during storage, the conversion of ovalbumin to S-ovalbumin had been attributed to an increase of pH and change of pH has a direct effect on the conversion rather than temperature. Therefore, despite temperatures of 4 C, long time storage of eggs may increase the conversion of native ovalbumin to S-albumin by 81%.

Ovalbumin is also the primary allergen in egg white which is responsible for IgE-mediated allergic reactions. The ovalbumin epitopes which bind IgE consists of mainly polar, charged and hydrophobic amino acids and these sequences are mostly made up of b-sheet and b-turn structures. The only allergenic epitope which comprises of an alpha helix is Asp95-Ala102.

Ovotransferrin

Ovotransferrin is a monomeric glycoprotein which is involved in the transfer of ferric ions to the developing embryo from the hen's oviduct. Ovotransferrin accounts approximately 12% of the entire egg white protein. Ovotransferrin belongs to the transferrin protein family and has been reported to have around 50% homology with mammalian lactoferrin and transferrin. Ovotransferrin can bind 2 mol of different metal ions per mole of protein. For, ovotransferrin, lactoferrin and serum transferrin, each lobe binds one carbonate anion and one Feþ3 atom. Such iron complex formation in ovotransferrin inhibits microbial growth that requires iron.

The N and C lobes of ovotransferrin consist of a single iron-binding site located in a deep cleft along with 15 disulfide bridges which maintain the globular structure of the protein. The N- and C- terminal lobes of ovotransferrin form two sulfide bonds where Ala1-Tyr72 in the N-terminal segment acquires a local-native like confirmation. This interaction between the two lobes is very critical for iron acquisition. The various metal and anion-binding properties of the iron binding sites of ovotransferrin can be attributed to the presence or absence of basic amino acid residues.

The process of in-vitro Fe^{+3} uptake and release by ovotransferrin are reported to be very similar, but not identical, to lactoferrin and serum transferrin. The Feþ3 is bound very tightly by the four protein ligands in a closed interdomain cleft. Ovotransferrin efficiently binds Feþ3 at pH greater than 7 and releases any bound Feþ3 at a pH lesser than 4.5. On uptake of Fe^{+3}, the transferrins undergo a major conformational transition from the apo structure (open-form/iron-free) to the closed/iron-bound holo formation, suggesting that initial binding occurs in the open form. Both these forms have significantly different physiochemical properties, for instance, the holo-form emits a salmon pink color due to the presence of iron whereas the apo-form does not have any color. Moreover, the apo-form is more prone to physical and chemical changes as compared to the holo-form.

Apart from the iron-binding capacity, several recent studies have investigated other structural and functional features of ovotransferrin that might be associated with various biological properties. For instance, the embryos of mammal and bird's egg are susceptible to oxidative stress, and thus maintenance of a constant, reducing environment during the development of the embryo can provide protection and although much knowledge is not present currently, however egg white is suggested as the primary target for this. Ovotransferrin is capable of auto cleavage at specific sites once it gets reduced by thiol reducing agents. This auto cleavage occurs due to a unique chemical reaction between the four tripeptide motifs present on both sides of the two disulfide domains (115–211 and 454–544 residues) of ovotransferrin protein. It has been found that many auto-processing proteins contain these reduction-scissile sequences (His/Cys-X-) which suggest that this sequence is evolutionarily conserved.

Ovomucoid

Ovomucoid is a glycoprotein which belongs to the Kazal family of protein inhibitors. It constitutes 11% of the total egg white proteins and is thermally stable. The protein consists of 186 amino acids with a molecular mass of 28 kDa. It consists of 9 disulfide bonds and has three different domains which are cross linked only by the intra-domain disulfide bonds. Ovomucin has trypsin inhibitory effect, and the active site for the trypsin inhibitory activity lies within the Domain II of the protein. However, considerable variations in the inhibitory activities and specificities of the domains have been reported from different avian species. Chicken ovomucoid is one of the significant egg white allergens, and it plays a crucial role in the pathogenesis of IgE-mediated allergic reactions. This allergenic potential could be attributed to its higher stability towards gastrointestinal digestion and heat treatment. The digestibility of ovomucoid by pepsin is much better over the pH range of 1.5–2.5. However, the digestibility loses at a pH of 3.0 or higher. Moreover, pepsin-digested fractions of ovomucoid retain its trypsin-inhibitory activities. The epitopes on ovomucoid which were responsible for the IgE binding were present only on the protein backbone and not the carbohydrate groups. Nine IgE epitopes (5–16 amino acids) and eight IgG epitopes (5–11 amino acids) were identified within the primary ovomucoid sequence. Through mutational studies of the epitopes, it was found that charged amino acids (lysine, glutamic acid, and aspartic acid), polar amino acids (cysteine, tyrosine, threonine, and serine), and hydrophobic (glycine, leucine, and phenylalanine) are crucial for antibody binding. Numerous studies have been conducted to alter the composition and structure of the ovomucoid epitopes responsible for the allergenicity. Some of the attempts made include heating in the presence of wheat flour, gamma irradiation along with heating, deglycosylation by endo-beta-N-acetylglucosaminidases, and genetic modifications. However, none of these modifications made any significant changes to the allergenic epitopes of ovomucoid, suggesting that the epitopes were extremely resistant to any modifications.

Ovomucin

Ovomucin contributes to about 3.5% of the total egg white proteins. It is a sulfated glycoprotein which is responsible for the jellylike structure of egg white. The protein consists of two parts: soluble part (8,300 Da), which is the main component of the inner and outer egg white, and the insoluble part (220–270 kDa), which is responsible for the insoluble gel-like fraction of thick albumen. Both fractions are made up of two subunits, a-ovomucin and b-ovomucin, but have different carbohydrate contents. The soluble fraction consists of 40 a- and three b-subunits, while the insoluble fraction contains 84 a- and 20 b-subunits. There are two distinct subunits of the a-subunit, i.e., a1 and a2, and both the a-subunits have lesser carbohydrate groups than b-subunits. Acidic amino acids such as glutamic acid and aspartic acids mainly make up the a-subunit whereas; serine and threonine primarily make up the b-subunit. The quality of eggs could be positively correlated with the amount of ovomucin present in the thick albumen. However, a higher concentration of highly glycosylated b-ovomucin containing hexoses, sialic acid, and hexosamines, signifies the inferior quality of eggs. Ovomucin is responsible for many of the functional and biological properties of egg white. It has a significant role in thinning of egg white during prolonged storage. Studies have shown that thinning of egg white can be either due to disruption of the ovomucin-lysozyme complex or the reduction of disulfide bonds leading to the degradation of ovomucin. Moreover, it is known for its exceptional emulsifying and foaming properties.

Lysozyme

Egg white lysozyme consists of 129 amino acids and is a 14.4 kDa protein with a pI of 10.7. Lysozyme present in the egg is unique as it is highly soluble and stable as compared to lysozyme present in other foods. Although the lysozyme present in egg exists as a monomer, it is also frequently found as a dimer which leads to its thermal stability. Four unique disulfide bonds stabilize the tertiary structure of egg lysozyme. Lysozyme tends to bind to negatively charged proteins in the egg albumen such as ovalbumin, ovomucin, and ovotransferrin. The chalaza and the chalaziferous layer mainly consist of the lysozyme–ovomucin complex. The complete structure with a resolution of 2 A° and the amino acid composition of lysozyme had been established in the 1960s. However, still much research is carried out to investigate its structure and function further. Three-dimensional structural analysis, at the resolution of 1.46 A, revealed the hexagonal crystal form of lysozyme. Various studies have also been conducted to investigate the structural changes of lysozyme induced by different conditions, such as aqueous-organic solvent mixtures, pH variations, co-crystallization in presence of different alcohols, sorbitol, in presence of thiol reagents, and supercritical CO_2 treatment followed by heat treatment. The first purification of lysozyme was done using the high concentration of ammonium sulfate, however, it led to the modification of the characteristics and morphology of the protein due to the high salt concentration used during extraction. The purification technique which is commonly used nowadays for lysozyme is cation exchange chromatography which makes use of the high pI value of the protein.

However, due to the small size of the resin granules used in the chromatography, the flow rate is low which makes it a time-consuming process. Crystallographic structures of some of the three major egg white proteins are listed in Figure below.

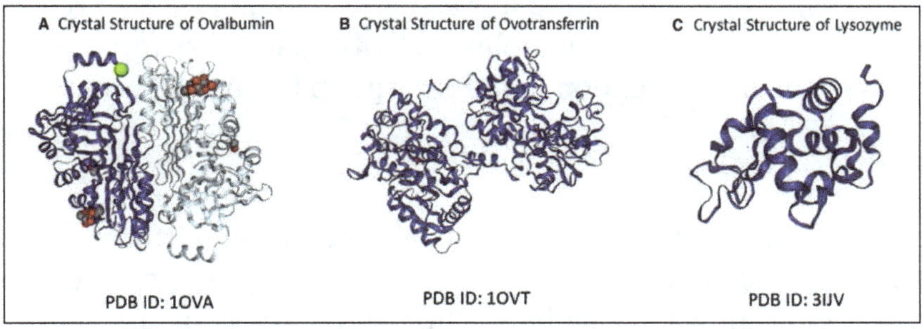

Figure: Crystallographic structure of major egg white proteins. Protein Data Bank.

Minor Proteins in Egg White

Egg white contains more than 50 proteins, among which the five major ones are described above. However, there are some other proteins, which although are present in very small amount, play a crucial role in determining the physicochemical and structural properties of the egg.

Ovoglobulin

Ovoglobulin constitutes 4% of the total egg white proteins and is a minor protein. The protein is made up of two subunits G2 and G3, with molecular weights of 36 kDa and 45 kDa respectively. Ovoglobulin was reported to be completely soluble in high and low ionic strength salt solution and coagulated with heat treatment; these properties were very similar to ovalbumin. Ovoglobulin G2, present in chicken eggs, shows polymorphism. Ovoglobulin has been reported to be crucial for the foaming properties of egg white, even though other biological functions are not well known yet. The competitive adsorption of the five major egg white proteins described above, along with ovoglobulin was studied, at low and high ionic strengths, and it was found that at 0.1 ionic strength, only ovoglobulin and ovalbumin were able to adsorb at the interface, while the other proteins were excluded from the interface.

Cystatin

Cystatin is a cysteine proteinase inhibitor which inhibits the action of thiol proteases, for instance, papain and ficin. Cystatin of the chicken egg contains two disulfide bonds near the carboxy-terminal along with a reactive site which is highly conserved. The pI of phosphorylated cystatin is 5.6, whereas it is 6.5 for the non-phosphorylated form, with a molecular weight of 13kDA. In a study, the effects of storage conditions of eggs, the age of hens, and heat treatment of albumen on the cystatin activity was investigated. The cystatin present in eggs laid by hens, either older than 60 weeks or younger than 30 weeks, had the lowest activity, while eggs laid by hens aged 40–50 weeks had the highest cystatin activity. Furthermore, the eggs stored for 28 days at 15 C showed a 4%–12% decrease in the cystatin activity. Thermal treatments also decreased the activity. Apart from having proteinase inhibitor activity, cystatin has been reported to have bioactive properties, such as, antimicrobial activity against bacterial pathogens, and inhibitor of bone matrix degradation in the resorption lacunae adjacent to osteoclasts.

Avidin

Avidin is well known for its biotin-binding activities and is essentially a tetrameric glycoprotein from egg albumen. All the four monomers of the protein are capable of binding biotin and establishing a strong interaction with a dissociation constant of 10–15 M. The protein constitutes approximately 0.05% of the total proteins in egg white. Each avidin chain comprises of 128 amino acids which are arranged as eight-stranded antiparallel beta-barrel, where the D-biotin binding site is defined by the inner regions. The secondary structure of avidin mainly comprises of beta-sheets and extended beta-turns (66%), while the rest is made up of b-turns and disordered structures. Avidin has been shown to have insecticidal and antimicrobial activity. The insecticidal activity has been used with genetically engineered and host plant resistance against Colorado potato beetle. Bacteriostatic effect of avidin has been reported against Salmonella typhimurium. However, the effect is lost on biotin addition. Terminal mannose and N-acetylglucosamine residues of avidin are capable of binding to lectins. Tumor cells express lectins on their cell surface at various levels, which acts as an important biomarker. Thus binding of avidin and cytotoxic agents can be easily detected via cell surface lectins. This mechanism was considered for tumor treatments, and avidin served as a potential vehicle for transport of toxins, drugs, therapeutic genes, and radioisotopes.

Ovoflavin

Ovoflavin, also known as riboflavin-binding protein or ovo-flavoprotein, is a phosphoglycoprotein which is present in both egg yolk and white in equal amounts. This protein is bind with riboflavin or vitamin B2 and the protein contains the highest selenium (Se) content (1800 ng/g) as compared to other egg proteins. Ovoflavin in egg white constitutes 219 amino acids with the presence of pyroglutamic acid at the amino terminus 96 although the biological function of ovoflavin is not fully understood its ability to bind minerals and vitamins suggests that it may be involved in nourishing the embryo with vitamins and minerals during development.

Egg Yolk Proteins

Egg yolk is composed of plasma and granules, located between the thin and thick albumen, supported by the chalazae. Yolk plasma constitutes 80% of the yolk fraction, and its protein content is of 23% on a dry basis, composed of Low-Density Lipoprotein (LDL) (15%) and globular glycoproteins (15%). Proteins such as livetins present as ϒ- livetins are mainly IgY antibodies, whose functions have been applied as immunological supplements in foods and several other industries. Yolk granules nonetheless have a higher concentration of lipids (33%) and proteins (58%) in comparison with plasma. Their structure formation is mainly composed of non-soluble HDL-phosvitin complexes. Therefore a medium ionic strength has shown to modify its solubility. Protein composition is also dependent on factors such as feed intake and environment during the hen's productive life. Molecules such as pigments or vitamins determine the color of the egg yolk. Studies supplementing herbs, quercetin, and TSAA with lysine, improved the color, oxidative stability, and reduced yolk protein respectively. Also, egg lipid and protein content vary throughout the productive cycle of the hen. In order to maintain egg weight homogeneity, a reduction in the amino acid content is realized. Furthermore, alterations in the environment such as heat and feed intake undermine lipid content in the organism. Heat stress initiates lipid peroxidation in cell membranes due to the release of hormones corticosterone and catecholamines.

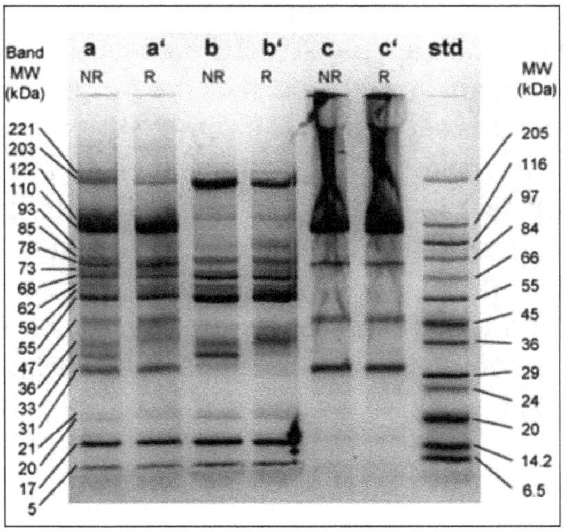

MW (kDa)	Relative band volume (%)	SD (%)	Protein name
221	2.9	1.3	Apolevitellin VIaa
203	8.7	3.4	α- livetin/apovitellenin VIb
122	7.7	2.5	Apolevitellin Vab
110	21.4	8.3	Apolevitellin 3+ 4c
93	0.6	0.3	Apolevitellin Vba
85	1.6	0.7	Apolevitellin Vb
78	4.5	1.8	Apolevitellin 5+6c
73	1.5	0.7	α- livetin
68	3.6	1.4	Apovitellenin IVb
62	1.0	0.4	Apovitellenin IIIb
59	1.3	0.6	Phosvitin
55	10.7	1.3	α- livetin/apovitellenin IIIb
47	4.8	1.8	Apolevitellin 7c

36	2.9	0.8	β- livetin
33	4.8	1.1	β- livetin
31	7.6	1.6	Apovitellenin 8c
21	0.3	0.1	Apovitellenin IIaa
20	1.2	0.5	Apovitellenin IIb
17	9.6	2.1	Apovitellenin Ib
5	3.3	0.6	Apolipoprotein CIId

Low-Density Lipoprotein (LDL)

LDL proteins are predominant in yolk plasma with an 85% protein composition. Its structure is characterized by a micelle nanostructure containing triglycerides and cholesterol. Emulsification properties of LDL are an important application for the food industry. Factors such as heat treatment, ionic strength, particle dispersion and defatting induced protein changes the structure affecting its functionality. For instance, amphipathic side chain structure makes the protein interact with hydrophobic and hydrophilic interfaces such as W/O or O/W. Apolipoproteins in LDL micelle adsorb faster than low molecular weight proteins, helped by its structure flexibility. In contrast, granules protein has shown an emulsification property dependent of pH. Specifically, at pH 4, its emulsification capacity is reduced as a result of protein dimer formation. Due to pH changes and an ionic strength increase, lipoproteins tend to minimize the interaction of granules proteins in an emulsion. The delivery mechanism is among other potential applications of LDL when combined with polysaccharides.

High-Density Lipoprotein (HDL)

HDL is mainly composed of protein, lipids, cholesterols, and minor lipids. Its structure functionality includes antioxidant activity and protective effects against pathogens. Lipid moiety in HDL influences its electron donating properties which can reduce the generation of reactive oxygen species (ROS). Mechanisms proposed to include the reduction of lipid hydroperoxides to non-reactive species through the electron transfer of methionine amino acid, interfering with lipid oxidation propagation.

Phosvitin

Phosvitin is a highly phosphorylated molecule with 124 of 217 amino acids binds to phosphate through covalent bonds, being serine the predominant amino acid. This characteristic yields a high mineral binding capacity, interacting with 95% of the iron present in egg yolk. The addition of ascorbic acid release the phosvitin bonded iron, thereby increasing the lipid peroxidation in egg yolk. On the other hand, its chemical properties derive from the emulsifying functional property. When in complete protein moiety, emulsifying properties are conferred by the interaction of the protein charged Ne and Ce termini. Further, glycosylated phosvitin has shown to improve the visco-elastic layer.

Livetin

Livetin is a globular water-soluble glycoprotein which makes up 30% of the total egg yolk plasma proteins. The protein is present in three forms, namely, a-livetin, b-livetin, and g-livetin. g-livetin is primarily immunoglobulin Y (IgY) which is an ideal substitute for mammalian IgG. The reported molecular weights of a-livetin, b-livetin, and g-livetin are 80,000, 45,000, and 170,000 respectively.

α- livetin has been reported to be the primary allergen responsible for the bird egg syndrome, and the protein is partially heat labile inhalant. The reactivity of IgE towards a-livetin was reported to reduce by almost 90% when it was heated for 30 minutes at 90 C. Only a partial cross-reactivity was observed between a-livetin and conalbumin. Martin et al. reported that although the molecular weights and tyrosine: tryptophan ratios of a-livetin and serum albumin were similar; they were not identical proteins because of the solubility. However, newer studies reported that although there was some precipitation of a-livetin at lower concentrations of $(NH_4)_2SO_4$, most of it was not precipitated by 50% saturation. Moreover, the peptide patterns and immunological results suggested that both a-livetin and serum albumin were the same protein.

β- Livetin contains 7% hexose. This protein is distinct from ovalbumin, although the molecular weights of both the proteins are very similar. Because the immunological patterns of b-livetin were identical to serum protein, it was considered an a2-glycoprotein, from its carbohydrate content and electrophoretic mobility. The sedimentation coefficient of 3S of b-livetin was similar to human serum, although the sialic content was lower in b-livetin as compared to human serum proteins.

The ϒ-livetin or IgY is derived from IgG of hen's serum, although it differs in from mammalian IgG in many of its chemical and structural properties. Yolk IgY consists of Asn-linked oligosaccharides like IgG. However, the oligosaccharide composition is different in both the immunoglobulins. The molecular weight of the heavy chains of IgY is greater than mammalian IgG (Kovacs-Nolan and Mine, 2004). Along with compositional differences, IgG and IgY also have functional differences. For instance, the isoelectric point of IgY is lower, and it is incapable of association with the mammalian complement, Protein G, Protein A, or rheumatoid factors. IgY also shows lesser binding capabilities with bacterial and human Fc receptors.

In conclusion Hen's egg has been considered as one of the most nutritious source of food as it can sustain both life and growth. The proteins present in the egg are nutritionally complete with a great balance of essential amino acids. Although the egg proteins are present in all parts of the eggs, but the major concentration lies in the egg white (50%) and egg yolk (40%), while the remaining proteins are distributed in the egg shell and egg shell membrane. Each protein component of the egg white and egg yolk is responsible for imparting a specific physical and chemical characteristic towards the entire functionality of an egg. Moreover, environmental conditions such as ionic strength, pH, and temperature treatments can modulate the functional properties of these proteins. Therefore, a greater understanding of the egg proteins could help in the development of functional foods, as egg proteins, particularly egg white proteins, have gained a lot of research interest in the recent years. Food industries have also shown a lot of interest in egg proteins to explore the various functional properties of eggs, which could provide them many commercial benefits.

Meat Protein

Meat is a very efficient deliverer of protein. Because the muscles of animals and humans share the same components, eating animal tissue is an easy way to get this necessary nutrient.

Proteins are made up of amino acids. Amino acids determine the structure and function of proteins. Among other things, amino acids help build cells and repair tissue, form antibodies, and carry oxygen throughout the body.

There are twenty-two known amino acids, eight of which are called essential, meaning that our bodies can't manufacture them and must get them from the foods we eat. The table below shows the essential amino acids, the function of the proteins they're found in, and where you can get them in your diet.

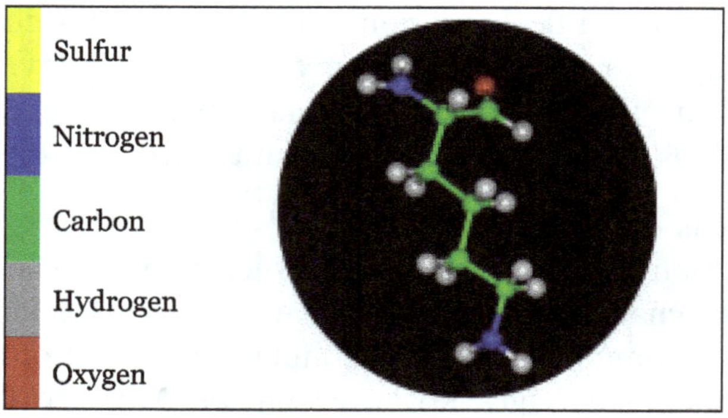

Figure: Isoleucine

Protein Function	Animal Sources	Plant Sources
Blood-sugar regulation	Beef	Almonds
Growth and repair of muscle tissue	Dairy	Lentils
Hemoglobin development	Eggs	Seeds
Energy regulation	Fish	Soy
	Poultry	Wheat

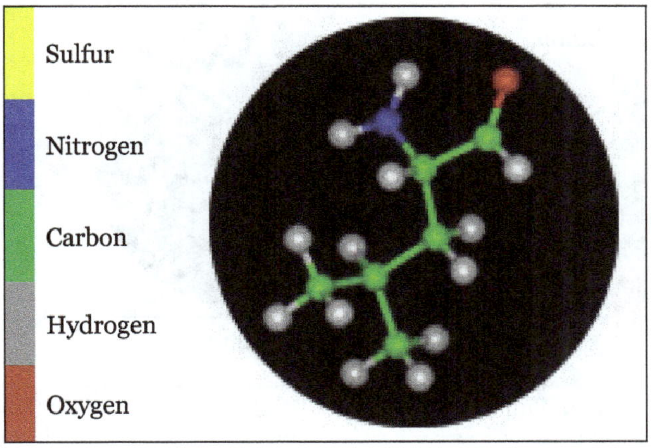

Figure: Leucine.

Protein Function	Animal Sources	Plant Sources
Blood-sugar regulation	Beef	Almonds
Growth and repair of muscle tissue	Dairy	Brown Rice
	Eggs	Lentils
Hemoglobin development	Fish	Seeds
Energy regulation	Poultry	Soy
		Wheat

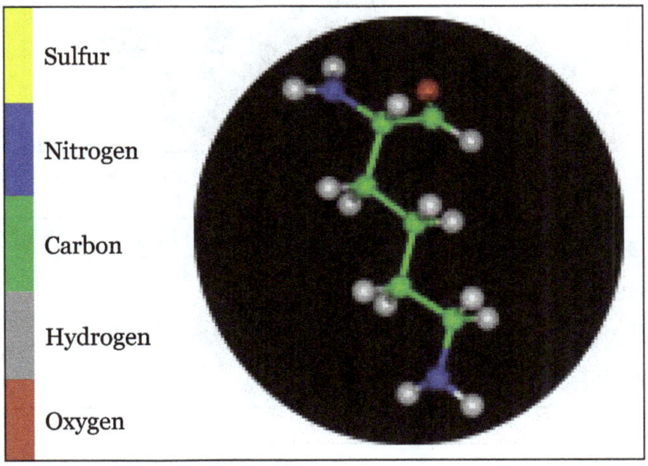

Figure: Lysine

Protein Function	Animal Sources	Plant Sources
Development and regulation of collagen, antibodies, hormones, and enzymes	Beef	Lima
	Dairy	Beans
Promotes calcium absorption	Eggs	Potatoes
Growth and repair of muscle tissue	Fish	Soy
Lowers serum triglycerides		Yeast

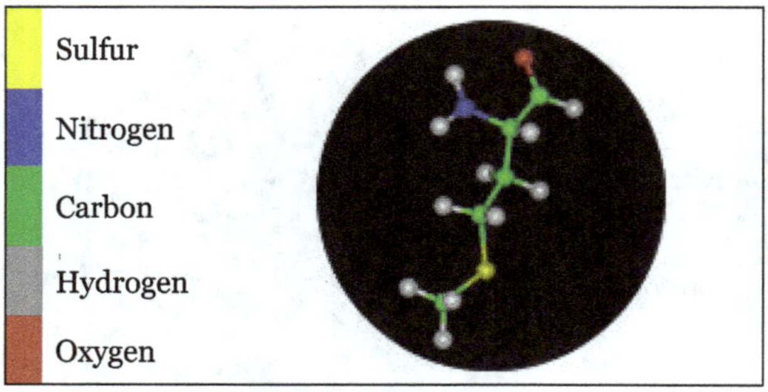

Figure: Methionine

Protein Function	Animal Sources	Plant Sources
May prevent arterial fat buildup May act as an antioxidant Promotes collagen synthesis	Beef Dairy Eggs Fish	Beans Garlic Lentils Onions Soybeans

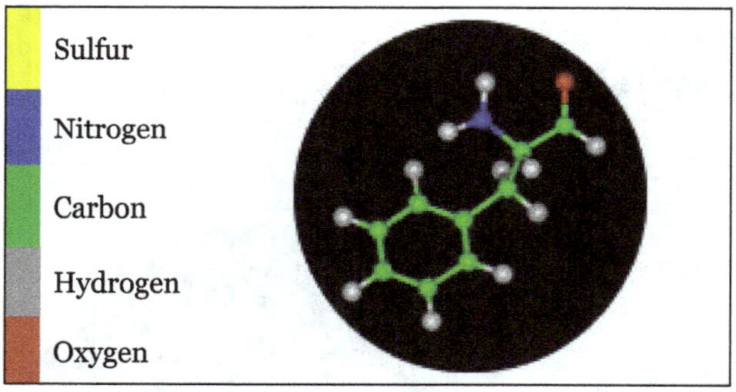

Figure: Phenylalanine

Protein Function	Animal Sources	Plant Sources
Neurotransmitter function increases blood levels of norepinephrine, epinephrine, dopamine	Dairy	Almonds Avocados Peanuts Seeds

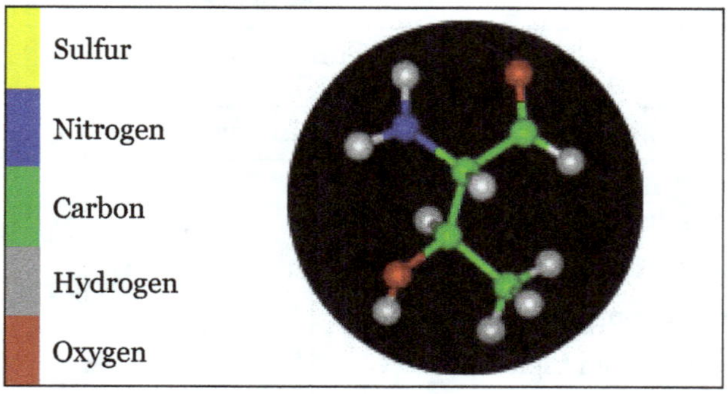

Figure: Threonine

Protein Function	Animal Sources	Plant Sources
Antibody production	Beef Dairy Eggs Poultry	Beans Nuts Seeds

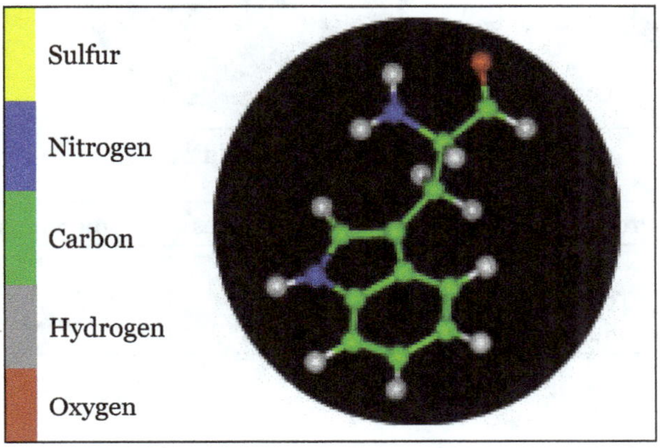

Figure: Tryptophan

Protein Function	Animal Sources	Plant Sources
Precursor for serotonin (aids sleep and combats anxiety) Niacin production	Beef Dairy Fish Poultry	Barley Brown Rice Peanuts Soybeans

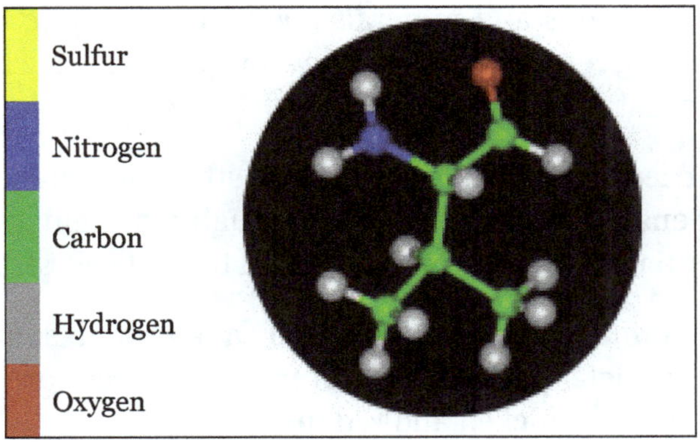

Figure: Valine

Protein Function	Animal Sources	Plant Sources
Growth and repair of muscle tissue Energy regulation Niacin production	Beef Dairy Eggs Poultry	Grains Mushrooms Nuts Soy

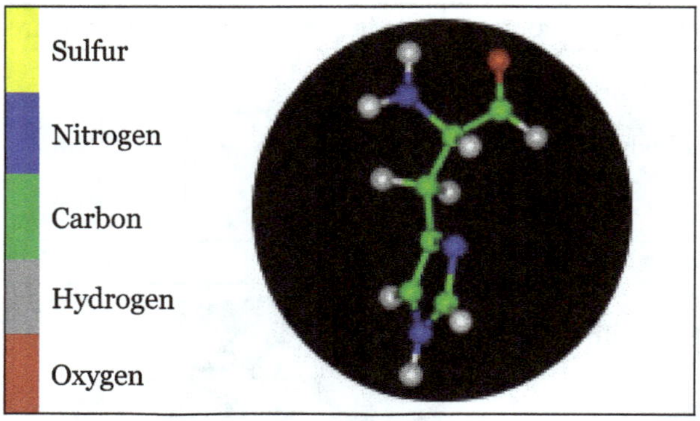

Figure: Histidine

Protein Function	Animal Sources	Plant Sources
Growth Tissue repair Histamine development	Pork Poultry Cheese	Rice Wheat

Plant Based Protein

Plant protein is simply a meaningful food source of protein which is from plants. This group can include pulses, tofu, soya, tempeh, seitan, nuts, seeds, certain grains and even peas. Pulses are a large group of plants, which include chickpeas, lentils, beans (such as black, kidney and adzuki beans) and split peas. Plant proteins are highly nutritious – not only as good sources of protein, but also because they provide other nutrients such as fibre, vitamins and minerals. Our intake of fibre tends to be too low, however by incorporating certain plant proteins into your diet, such as pulses, peas and nuts, you can easily boost your fibre intake.

Protein is a vital nutrient responsible for the growth, maintenance and repair of our bodies. So, we must ensure we eat enough high-quality protein every day to keep our bodies healthy. Essentially, protein is fundamental to the basic structure of our body.

There are 9 essential amino acids, and when you eat a protein source containing all of these it is called a 'complete' protein. Animal protein sources are complete, and they include fish, poultry such as chicken and red meat.

Plant sources of protein, with the exception of soya and quinoa, are 'incomplete'. This is because plant protein sources tend to lack at least 1 of the 9 essential amino acids. So how can you ensure that you consume all of the essential amino acids when eating plant proteins? The answer is protein combining.

Put simply, protein combining means eating a selection of incomplete plant protein sources, to ensure you consume all of the essential amino acids. As a general rule of thumb, pulses and grains lack different essential amino acids. So, eating a pulse and a grain provides an overall complete protein source. With this in mind, it's easy to get all the essential amino acids your body needs. For example, a serving of rice and peas or bread and hummus would give you a complete protein source. And remember, you needn't eat your combined proteins in just one meal – they can be eaten at different points during the day or even the week.

The plant-based diet is rather simple and easy to get your head around as it's centered on foods derived from plant sources. Plant-based diets cheer on the eating of fruits, vegetables, whole grains, legumes, seeds and nuts, meaning these foods comprise the majority of what you eat. To give you a helping hand, our frozen vegetables are a simple yet delicious place to start if you're looking to slowly add more plants into your lifestyle, without making the full move.

This is a classic vegan or vegetarian diet. It's not a plant-based diet only, it is far more flexible and doesn't boycott dairy, meat, seafood and eggs altogether. Their easy-going and inclusive approaches make this diet an attractive one – nobody likes rules, after all! And what's more, flexitarian diets promote consuming a wide variety of plant foods, so there are of course numerous nutritional benefits to adopting this way of eating.

We currently struggle to keep up with this figure, however with a plant-based diet heavily relying on fruit and vegetables; you're likely to find it easier to consume the recommended amount. Likewise, as beans and pulses are greatly encouraged, you're expected to have an increased intake of fibre, vitamins and minerals – ideal as most of us are also not consuming enough fibre! To give you a snapshot of how humble vegetables house an array of nutritional benefits, peas provide protein, fibre, folic acid and vitamin C. It's natural to think that a plant-based diet can lead to a lack of protein, but this is far from the truth – plants provide protein too.

Soy Protein

Soy protein refers to the protein that is found in soybeans that is often used to replace animal proteins in an individual's diet. The soybean is a legume that contains no cholesterol and is low in saturated fat. Soybeans are the only vegetable food that contains all eight essential amino acids. Soybeans are also a good source of fiber, iron, calcium, zinc, and B vitamins.

Benefits of Soy for Health Promotion

Pregnancy

Use of soy products during pregnancy can be encouraged because expectant women are likely to receive the same health benefits as other women. Fortified milk and fortified soymilk are the only reliable dietary sources of vitamin D. All other dairy products contain little or no vitamin D. While many women will obtain enough vitamin

D from exposure to sunlight, soymilk may be an alternative for those who are overly sensitive to the sun or for those who simply are not able to be or do not enjoy being outdoors. Soymilk may also be an alternative for women who do not like regular milk.

Cardiac

Consumption of soy protein in place of animal protein has been found to reduce serum concentrations of total cholesterol, low-density lipoproteins (LDLs), and trigylcerides. The precise mechanism of action is not known, though several theories exist. One theory proposes that cholesterol absorption is impaired or altered. Another theory postulates that phytoestrogens (plant compounds that have hormone-like effects; isoflavones are the phytoestrogens found in soy products) bind to estrogen receptors and produce similar effects including lowering LDLs and increasing high-density lipoproteins, vasomotor tone changes, and arterial wall function. Individuals with elevated cholesterol seem to receive the greatest benefit.

Individuals need to consume about 25 grams of soy protein or more each day to obtain results. Twenty-five grams of soy protein equals 1¼ cups of tofu, 1–2 cups of soymilk, or an ounce of soy flour. Individuals are encouraged to read food labels in order to verify a particular food's soy content. The U.S. Food and Drug Administration (FDA) approved the health claim for the relationship between soy product consumption and reduced risk of coronary heart disease in 1999, based on the result of human clinical intervention trials.

Obesity and Diabetes

Soy protein contributed to the control of hyperglycemia and reduced body weight, hyperlipidemia, and hyperinsulinemia. These characteristics may be useful to both non-diabetic and diabetic persons in the control of obesity and blood sugar.

Cancer Prevention

Genistein, one of the phytochemicals found in soy, can reduce the risk of cancer. To date, prevention of breast cancer has received the most attention, and more recent attention has focused on prostate cancer. Genistein blocks cancer development by preventing tumors from creating blood vessels that would provide nourishment for growth. One serving a day (e.g., 1 cup of soymilk, ½ cup of tofu or soybeans) is effective for cancer prevention.

Menopausal Symptoms

Phytoestrogens are currently being researched to determine their usefulness in acting like synthetic estrogen to protect women from bone loss and maintain a healthy heart. Soy protein has been found to positively influence bone and calcium balance in postmenopausal women. Results were especially significant for women who were not receiving hormone replacement therapy. These same results were not seen in young, healthy women who were still menstruating.

Benefits of Soy for Special Populations

Vegetarians and Vegans

Vegetarians are individuals who, for various reasons, do not eat meat. Vegans, in comparison, are individuals who do not eat any products from animals, including eggs, milk, and cheese. Vitamin B_{12} is only found in animal products and, therefore, may be lacking in the diet of vegans. Use of soymilk is one way to obtain this essential vitamin. Cereals and meat substitutes are other options.

Infants with Special Conditions

Infants born with lactase deficiency or galactosemia, benefit from the use of soy-based formulas. Parents who wish to put their newborn on a vegetarian diet may choose to use a soy-based formula. In addition, infants who are recovering from episodes of diarrhea (and are normally given breast-milk substitutes) may have soy formula recommended to facilitate their recovery. Soy-based breast milk substitutes (formulas) include Prosobee (Mead Johnson) and Isomil (Ross). While soy-based formulas meet an infant's growth and development needs, they do not offer any advantage over milk-based formulas.

Infants who are not able to tolerate lactose formulas (those based on cow's milk, casein/whey-based formulas; e.g., Similac, Enfamil, Carnation) may be prescribed soy-based formulas if they are not breastfed. Each year, about 20%–25% of infants are converted to soy protein formulas. The development of lactose-free cow's milk protein-based formulas has made it unnecessary to switch infants to soy-based formula, though the practice is still common. The use of soy-based formula is effective in only about 20%–50% of infants because the soy protein eventually triggers a reaction in susceptible infants. In this instance, predigested protein formulas can be used (e.g., Nutramigen, Alimentum). According to the ADA, soy-based formulas are not recommended for preterm infants weighing less than 1,000 grams and for infants with low birth weight as a means for preventing or managing colic or gastroenteritis.

Preschool Children

In a recent study, ingesting soy-based formula or soymilk was associated with peanut allergy in a geographically diverse sample of 13,971 preschool children. The association of peanut allergy with the intake of soy products could be related to cross-sensitization through a common substance.

Pea Protein

Pea protein is an extract from split peas, and food manufacturers are adding this protein to a variety of foods like energy bars, meal-replacement shakes, veggie burgers and even cereals. You can also find it as a powder to add when making smoothies.

With protein getting a lot of attention right now, pea protein offers a healthy option. Traditional approaches to boosting protein might have involved larger meat portions, yet evidence is strong that excess red and processed meats increase risk of cancer and other chronic diseases.

Growing interest in vegetarian and plant-based diets has likely prompted the increased availability of pea and other plant-based proteins. Pea protein also appeals to people who are lactose-intolerant or do not include dairy-based protein. But compared to getting protein from foods that bring a bevy of other valuable nutrients, it's not the answer for everyone.

Pea Protein Versus other Plant Proteins

Proteins are made of amino acids and there are nine amino acids that are essential in our diets. Unlike animal sources of protein, protein from plant foods is often low in one or more of these nine amino acids that makes a "complete" protein. As long as you eat a variety of protein sources throughout the day, it's not necessary to consume complete proteins in each meal.

Like the legumes from which it's made, pea protein contains all the essential amino acids but it is low in one called methionine. That means it should be used as only one of many different protein sources, not the major choice throughout the day.

Pea protein is not all the same. Protein and other nutrient content vary based on the brand and whether it is a concentrate or isolate (isolates typically have more protein). Even when supplying equal amounts of protein, the amount of fiber differs. Some are a good source of fiber yet most contain little. This protein is relatively low in fat yet at least one. Compared to protein-fortified products with protein isolated from hemp seed, rice and most other grains, pea protein contains a better balance of essential amino acids.

Compared to protein-fortified products with protein isolated from hemp seed, rice and most other grains, pea protein contains a better balance of essential amino acids. The less desirable aspect of pea protein is that it can have a gritty texture. So it seems to work best in smoothies with a variety of other ingredients, or in protein-enriched products using recipes that overcome that problem.

Pea Protein in the Big Picture

It is good to see people thinking about ways to meet protein needs beyond big meat portions, and including protein in meals throughout the day. But it's important to recognize that just because the grams of protein listed on a bar or drink look good, protein doesn't turn a food lacking in nutrients into a healthy meal.

Consider what else you get from foods that supply protein. The standard size serving of pea protein powder as listed on labels often provides about 21 grams of protein. That's the amount in about 3 ounces of meat, fish or poultry (the size of a deck of cards).

However, in extracting the protein, some of dry peas' other nutrients may be removed. Split peas provide important amounts of magnesium, folate, and potassium, but labels provide no indication of how much is retained in pea protein powder. A serving of pea protein powder does often remain a good source of iron. But isolated pea protein also is missing the pea's carbohydrate compounds that can support anti-inflammatory gut bacteria.

Foods that contain smaller amounts of protein can add up to meet your protein needs and provide other nutrients and phytochemicals. For example, blenderizing a smoothie with soy milk or tofu, or including a handful of nuts in a snack or mixed into salad also supplies magnesium, potassium, polyphenols, and vitamin E.

Brown Rice Protein

Brown Rice is the name in reference to the characteristic brown colour of the bran on the grain, which distinguishes it from white rice. Brown Rice falls under the category of whole grain. Well, whole grain is grain in its natural, fullest form that contains all the nutrients, carbs, vitamins, minerals, fibres and antioxidants.

Brown Rice, unlike the white rice, is unpolished, meaning it has not been hulled and contains all the 3 parts of the grain, the outer fibre-filled layer called the bran, the nutrient-rich core called the germ, and a starchy middle layer called the endosperm.

Brown Rice protein is a protein supplement made from brown rice. The protein is extracted from Brown Rice by treating Brown Rice with enzymes through a special conversion process that causes the separation between carbs and protein. The enzymes are considered vegan and the processing of rice in this technique is considered a 'raw food technique'. Once it is extracted, the protein is converted into a high-quality useful protein powder.

Reason for Considering Brown Rice Protein

It's very essential for us to understand that without a proper protein intake, we'll find ourselves struggling to lose weight, fight fatigue, and suffer from mood swings and many other health issues.

There are endless dairy and non-vegetarian protein sources. But the concern here is with vegetarians and vegans, who do not get sufficient protein from their diet, as vegetarian and vegan sources that provide sufficient and good quality protein are limited.

Brown rice protein has come as an answer to all your worries. It's a protein you can try even if you're not a vegan or vegetarian or don't otherwise follow a restricted diet. It is a good way to give your body the protein it needs while maintaining your dietary goals in following ways:

- Brown Rice Protein is Hypoallergenic: Some individuals are so allergic to egg, milk and soy-based protein that, they refrain themselves from using any sort of protein powder fearing allergic reactions. Good news is that there are no concerns with allergies when it comes to Brown Rice Protein. Brown Rice Protein is best suitable for almost any user. Anyone can eat and reap the benefits of Brown Rice Protein. Besides, Brown Rice protein powder is free from gluten (the wheat protein) that some manufacturers add to protein powders.

- Faster Absorption: The main appeal of Brown Rice Protein is the easy digestibility. Different protein sources are digested and metabolized at various rates. Brown Rice Protein gets to work quickly making it ideal for post-workout recovery.

- Better Taste: Unlike some vegan protein sources which may have strong and distinctive flavours that may be difficult for some users, Rice Protein Powder has a very subtle and familiar taste that makes it suitable to be used in a variety of recipes to improve their nutritional profile.

- Excellent Amino Profile for Muscle Recovery: The amino acids in protein are like little building blocks that help muscles recover and rebuild so that they become stronger than before.

  Brown Rice Protein, although is not a complete protein (some amino acids are missing), it contains high amounts of many essential amino acids. The missing amino acids can be gained by means of a complementary protein source.

- Helps Promote Balanced Blood Sugar: Blood sugar will spike in response to meals, causing the pancreas to secrete the hormone, insulin to facilitate the storage of circulating nutrients.

  Usually, high-carb diets will lead to large insulin spikes which may trigger fat-storage and lead to insulin resistance.

  Combining a whole protein like Brown Rice Protein, which is a low-glycemic index food (with an average GI rating of 55 or less), helps to balance out the effect that carbs have on blood sugar and insulin to help cut down on the associated body fat storage.

- Promotes Weight Loss: You have learnt that high protein diets, regardless of protein sources, support weight loss by speeding up metabolism and decreasing the food intake. Protein supplements like Brown Rice protein have a 'thermic effect', meaning that they create heat in the body through the process of digestion. Since proteins take a lot of energy to digest, you burn calories after eating a meal high in proteins. Peptides in Brown Rice Protein are most effective at reducing weight gain. You can build your weight loss strategy around this lean source of protein and see effective results.
- Reduces Cholesterol: Brown Rice Protein is a perfect choice in achieving your goal of cholesterol regulation. Studies show that the peptides found in Brown Rice Protein, in addition to increasing weight loss, help your liver to synthesis the cholesterol created by the liver itself and by other cells of the body.
- Improves Liver Function: Brown Rice protein is a powerful anti-oxidant. Antioxidants help prevent specific types of cell damage, especially damage caused by oxidation (free radical formation caused by oxygen molecules travelling freely in the body) which can lead to liver damage.

  Researchers have found that the benefits of Brown Rice Protein include hepaprotective effects that defend the liver from damage. Peptides in Brown Rice Protein can help the liver synthesize decreased cholesterol.
- Chickpea Protein: Chickpeas, also known as garbanzo beans, are a type of legume that is full of protein, fiber, and complex carbohydrates. They are nutrient-dense, meaning they have lots of useful nutrients but are relatively low in calories. You'll find the versatile chickpea in many Mediterranean and Indian dishes, and it is a handy plant-based source of protein.

  Chickpea Protein is a natural high protein source, rich in BCAAs and produced to the highest standards. Chickpeas are ideal for inclusion in a range of applications such as nutrition, dairy alternatives and bakery. The product has a mild pulse flavour and is made with a gentle process to ensure great product quality.

Chickpea Protein Isolates have Higher Digestibility

To fully understand the concept of digestibility, first let's have a little sneak peek into the basics. If you are eating 10g of protein, it doesn't mean your body is actually absorbing and using 10g of proteins. For your body to absorb protein, it needs to be broken down into smaller groups, so that your body can utilize it. It is similar to how you can't put and chew a complete roti in your mouth; you would need to break it down into smaller pieces and then chew it. Similarly, in order to absorb the nutrients from our food, our digestion system releases enzymes to break down the big nutrient groups into smaller ones, for easier absorption and digestion.

Protease is an enzyme, released by our pancreas into the smaller intestine, which breaks down the proteins into smaller blocks and in turn, helps our body to absorb and use the proteins throughout our body. Albumin, a globular protein found in chickpeas, is a protease inhibitor. It is like an annoying sibling who won't let you work in peace as long as s/he is in the room. But when your sibling is out of the room, then you can easily and efficiently do your work. During the isolation of proteins from chickpeas, most of the albumin gets removed. Also, chickpea proteins get partially denatured during protein isolation (it means longer chains break down into smaller units) and thus become more accessible to digestive enzymes in our bodies. Both these actions make the chickpea protein isolates more digestible. This higher digestibility of protein isolates makes chickpeas the perfect ingredient for protein-rich foods.

Chickpea Protein Hydrolysates are Soluble over a Wide Range of pH

The water molecule is polar-covalently bonded; it means that it has a slight positive and a negative charge and it tends to bond with other polar, ionized molecules. And if you add another molecule that lacks polar covalent bonds (for e.g., fat) into the water, it won't interact with the water molecules and will remain insoluble.

During the enzymatic treatment, the molecular size of chickpea protein gets smaller and exposed ionizable amino and carboxyl groups increase in number. Now since hydrolysate has more electrically charged functional groups (amino and carboxyl), more hydrolysate particles will attract and bind with water molecules. That's why the chickpea protein hydrolysates are more soluble than isolates and hence, a suitable ingredient in liquid foods and beverages.

The Nutritional Profile of Chickpea is Excellent

Chickpeas have a good balance of amino acids. They also are known for being a good source of saponins – a naturally occurring compound that has shown to lower the cholesterol. Hence, the addition of chickpea protein concentrate in a formulation will help the product developers to increase the nutritional quality of a food product.

Protein Digestion and Absorption

When you eat food the body's digestive system breaks down the protein into the individual amino acids, which are absorbed and used by cells to build other proteins and a few other macromolecules, such as DNA. Eggs are a good dietary source of protein and will be used as our example to describe the path of proteins in the processes of digestion and absorption. One egg, whether raw, hard-boiled, scrambled, or fried, supplies about six grams of protein.

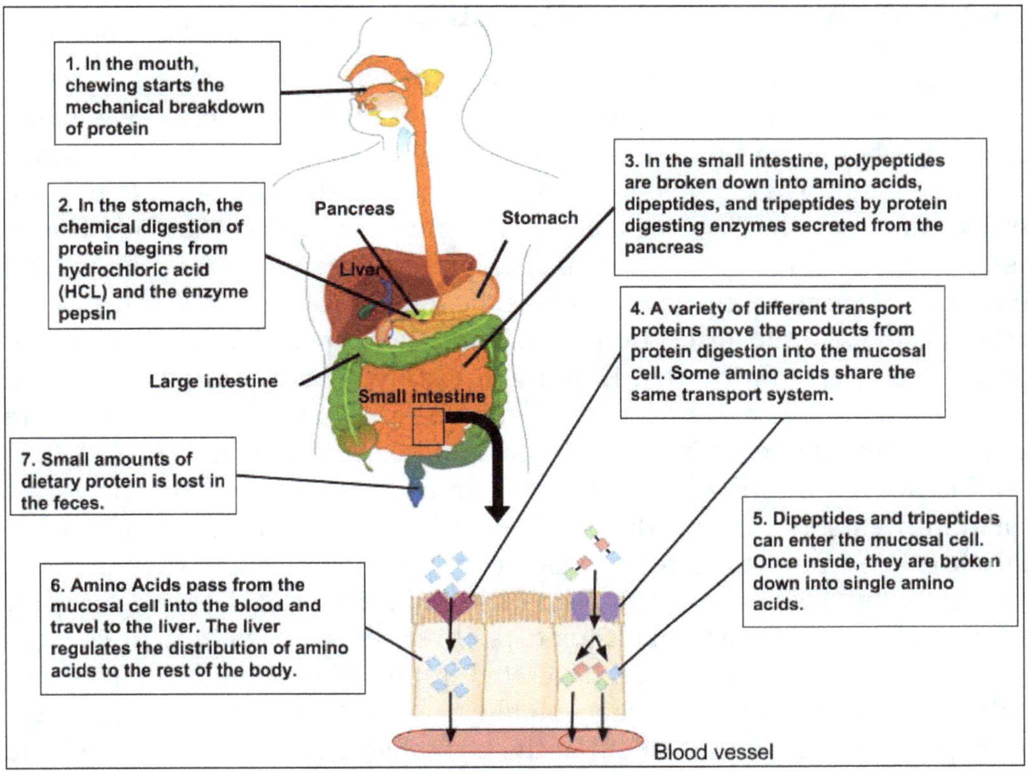

Figure: Digestion and absorption of Protein.

From the Mouth to the Stomach

Unless you are eating it raw, the first step in egg digestion (or any other protein food) involves chewing. The teeth begin the mechanical breakdown of the large egg pieces into smaller pieces that can be swallowed. The salivary glands provide some saliva to aid swallowing and the passage of the partially mashed egg through the esophagus. The mashed egg pieces enter the stomach through the esophageal sphincter. The stomach releases gastric juices containing hydrochloric acid and the enzyme, pepsin, which initiate the breakdown of the protein. The acidity of the stomach facilitates the unfolding of the proteins that still retain part of their three-dimensional structure after cooking and helps break down the protein aggregates formed during cooking. Pepsin, which is secreted by the cells that line the stomach, dismantles the protein chains into smaller and smaller fragments. Egg proteins are large globular molecules and their chemical breakdown requires time and mixing. The powerful mechanical stomach contractions churn the partially digested protein into a more uniform mixture called chyme. Protein digestion in the stomach takes a longer time than carbohydrate digestion, but a shorter time than fat digestion. Eating a high-protein meal increases the amount of time required to sufficiently break down the meal in the stomach. Food remains in the stomach longer, making you feel full longer.

From the Stomach to the Small Intestine

The stomach empties the chyme containing the broken down egg pieces into the small intestine, where the majority of protein digestion occurs. The pancreas secretes digestive juice that contains more enzymes that further break down the protein fragments. The two major pancreatic enzymes that digest proteins are chymotrypsin and trypsin. The cells that line the small intestine release additional enzymes that finally break apart the smaller protein fragments into the individual amino acids. The muscle contractions of the small intestine mix and propel the digested proteins to the absorption sites. In the lower parts of the small intestine, the amino acids are transported from the intestinal lumen through the intestinal cells to the blood. This movement of individual amino acids requires special transport proteins and the cellular energy molecule, adenosine triphosphate (ATP). Once the amino acids are in the blood, they are transported to the liver. As with other macronutrients, the liver is the checkpoint for amino acid distribution and any further breakdown of amino acids, which is very minimal. Recall that amino acids contain nitrogen, so further catabolism of amino acids releases nitrogen-containing ammonia. Because ammonia is toxic, the liver transforms it into urea, which is then transported to the kidney and excreted in the urine. Urea is a molecule that contains two nitrogen and is highly soluble in water. This makes it a good choice for transporting excess nitrogen out of the body. Because amino acids are building blocks that the body reserves in order to synthesize other proteins, more than 90 percent of the protein ingested does not get broken down further than the amino acid monomers.

Amino Acids are Recycled

Just as some plastics can be recycled to make new products, amino acids are recycled to make new proteins. All cells in the body continually break down proteins and build new ones, a process referred to as protein turnover. Every day over 250 grams of protein in your body are dismantled and 250 grams of new protein are built. To form these new proteins, amino acids from food and those from protein destruction are placed into a “pool.” Though it is not a literal pool, when an amino acid is required to build another protein it can be acquired from the additional amino acids that exist within the body. Amino acids are used not only to build proteins, but also to build other biological molecules containing nitrogen, such as DNA, RNA, and to some extent to produce energy. It is critical to maintain amino acid levels within this cellular pool by consuming high-quality proteins in the diet, or the amino acids needed for building new proteins will be obtained by increasing protein destruction from other tissues within the body, especially muscle. This amino acid pool is less than one percent of total body-protein content. Thus, the body does not store protein as it does with carbohydrates (as glycogen in the muscles and liver) and lipids (as triglycerides in adipose tissue).

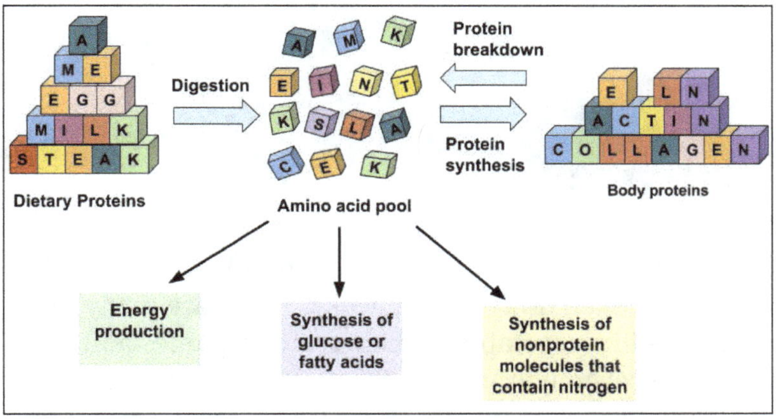

Figure: Options for amino acid use in the human body.

Amino acids in the cellular pool come from dietary protein and from the destruction of cellular proteins. The amino acids in this pool need to be replenished because amino acids are outsourced to make new proteins, energy, and other biological molecules.

References

- The-role-of-proteins-in-foods-cooking-and-denaturation, humannutrition: pressbooks-dev.oer. hawaii.edu, Retrieved 05, April 2020
- Health-talk-pea-protein-is-everywhere-is-it-healthy: aicr.org, Retrieved 16, March 2020
- Everything-you-need-to-know-about-brown-rice-protein, health: asitisnutrition.com, Retrieved 29, June 2020
- Chickpeas-nutrition-facts-calories-and-health-benefits-4118486: verywellfit.com, Retrieved 30, April 2020
- Chickpea-protein, products: aturaproteins.com, Retrieved 11, May 2020
- What-makes-chickpea-protein-the-perfect-ingredient-for-your-new-product: nutritionmeets-foodscience.com, Retrieved 27, July 2020

Carbohydrates

Carbohydrate is a large group of organic compounds that mainly include sugars and starch which are broken down into glucose. There are many foods that contain healthy carbohydrates like vegetables, whole fruits, legumes and nuts. This chapter discusses in detail the carbohydrates, their sources and functions in the body.

Carbohydrates are polyhydroxylated aldehydes or ketones and their derivatives. The word "carbohydrate" includes polymers and other compounds synthesized from polyhydroxylated aldehydes and ketones. They can be synthesized in the laboratory or in living cells. Simple carbohydrates or the entire carbohydrate family may also be called saccharides. In general carbohydrates have the empirical formula $(CH_2O)_n$. The term generated from carbon and hydrate; though some also contain nitrogen, phosphorus, or sulfur. Chemically, carbohydrates are molecules that are composed of carbon, along with hydrogen and oxygen - usually in the same ratio as that found in water (H_2O).

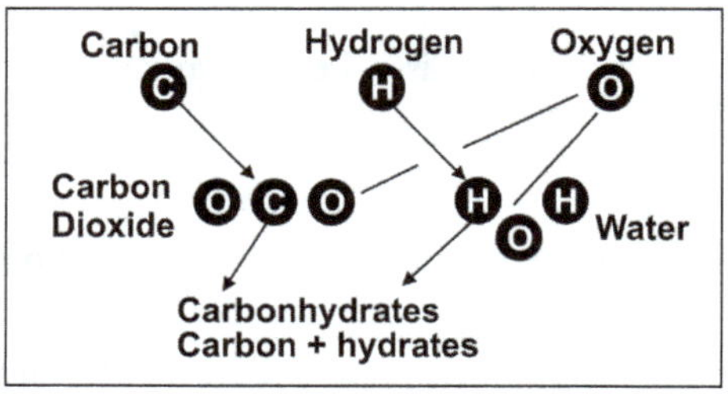

They originate as products of photosynthesis, an endothermic reductive condensation of carbon dioxide requiring light energy and the pigment chlorophyll.

$$nCO_2 + nH_2O + energy \rightarrow C_nH_{2n}O_n + nO_2$$

Typical carbohydrates are composed of strings or chains of monosaccharides - that is, chains of individual sugars.

Importance of Carbohydrates

Carbohydrates are of great importance in biology. The unique reaction, which makes life possible on the Earth, namely the assimilation of the green plants, produces sugar, from which originate, not only all carbohydrates but, directly or indirectly, all other components of living organisms. The carbohydrates are a major source of metabolic energy, both for plants and for animals that depend on plants for food. Aside from the sugars and starch that meet this vital nutritional role, carbohydrates also serve as a structural material (cellulose), a component of the energy transport compound ATP, recognition sites on cell surfaces, and one of three essential components of DNA and RNA.

Metabolic/Nutritional

The important role of carbohydrates, generally, in the metabolism of living organisms, is well known. The biological breakdown of carbohydrates (often spoken of as "combustion") supplies the principal part of the energy that every organism needs for various processes. Carbohydrates and their metabolism has been the subject of biochemical and medical research for a long time.

Carbohydrates play a major role in promoting health fitness, form a major part of food and help a great deal in building body strength, by generating energy. They are one among the three prominent macronutrients that serve as excellent energy providers, the other two being fats and proteins. Carbohydrate intake can take place in different forms like sugar, starch, fibers etc., which are a dietary staple in most parts of the world, and the oxidation of carbohydrates is the central energy-yielding pathway in most non-photosynthetic organisms.

The functions of carbohydrates are multiple and it is owing to this fact that it becomes all the more necessary to incorporate carbohydrates in our meal. For instant for energy generation, sugars and starch act as the perfect fuel that enables us to carry out our physical activities efficiently and effectively. Fiber does wonders in keeping your bowel function going smooth. Carbohydrates add on to the taste and appearance of food item, thus making the dish tempting and mouthwatering. They are sometimes used as flavors and sweeteners. Carbohydrates aid in regulating blood glucose and also do good to our body by breaking down fatty acids, thus preventing ketosis. Talking about the importance of carbohydrates, apart from its direct benefits, there is also an added advantage of carbohydrate consumption and that is that carbohydrates are found in different foods, which if eaten, also pave way for consuming other essential nutrients. Therefore, it is preferable to go in for distinctive carbohydrate food sources.

Structural

The structural diversity possible by linking the different, common sugar is immense: theoretically far greater than that of proteins, which largely consist of 22 amino acids linked by a single type of peptide bond. Linkages between sugars can occur through a glycoside linkage between the anomeric, first carbon of a sugar in either α or β configuration with any of a variety of hydroxyl groups on the adjacent sugar. In fact, many possible combinations of sugars do not seem to exist.

Insoluble carbohydrate polymers serve as structural and protective elements in the cell walls of bacteria and plants and in the connective tissues of animals. Plant cell walls are complex arrangements of cellulose, hemicellulose and lignin. This contributes significantly to the overall digestibility of the fiber. The proportion of each component depends on species and age of the plant. Cellulose is the primary structural component of plants. It is found primarily in the cells walls and is a primary fiber component of animal feeds.

Communication

Glycosaminoglycans as polymers of derivatives of carbohydrates are of critical importance in intercellular communication in organisms. This ubiquitous class of linear polyanions interacts with a wide variety of proteins, including growth factors and chemokines, which regulate important physiological processes. The presence of glycosaminoglycans on cell membranes and in the extracellular matrix also has resulted in their exploitation by infectious pathogens to gain access and entry into animal cells. Other carbohydrate polymers lubricate skeletal joints and participate in recognition and adhesion between cells.

More complex carbohydrate polymers covalently attached to proteins or lipids act as signals that determine the intracellular location or metabolic fate of these hybrid molecules, called glycoconjugates. Glycoconjugates carry various important functions of cell. Glycoproteins act as receptors and integral membrane proteins in membranes, cytoskeletal proteins in cytoplasm, extracellular proteins such as antibodies, hormones, collagen (found outside the cell), enzymes (RNase, DNase, lipases, cholinesterase, phosphatase, pepsinogen, glycosyltransferases) etc. Functions and locations of glycolipids within the cell are diverse—take for example: GAGs: sub maxillary secretions, human gastric mucin, RBC membrane sialoglycoprotein, and membrane protein, secretory proteins without enzymatic functions, immunoglobins, and enzymes.

Biosynthesis of Other Compounds

Carbohydrates are source of carbon for biosynthesis of other compounds. Most people know that the body uses carbohydrates for energy. For example, the simple carbohydrate glucose (dextrose) gets oxidized by liver cells. In exchange, the cells produce adenosine triphosphate (ATP), the main energy-providing compound in the cell. However, carbohydrates are used in a number of ways by plants, animals and bacteria, not just for energy.

In carbohydrate anabolism, simple organic acids can be converted into monosaccharides such as glucose and then used to assemble polysaccharides such as starch. In living cells, glucose is oxidized to give carbon dioxide and energy. The energy produced is in the form of ATP and heat. This reaction is just like the combustion:

$$Glucose + O_2 \rightarrow CO_2 + energy$$

During photosynthesis in plants, glucose can be produced from CO_2 and energy:

$$CO_2 + energy \rightarrow glucose + O_2$$

Here, the energy consumed is in the form of sunlight. This reaction is the reverse of the combustion reaction.

Classification

Carbohydrates are called saccharides or, if they are relatively small, sugars. Classifications of carbohydrates are outlined in the following table.

Complexity	Simple Carbohydrates monosaccharides			Complex Carbohydrates disaccharides, oligosaccharides & polysaccharides		
Size	Tetrose C4 sugars	Pentose C5 sugars	Hexose C6 sugars	Heptose C7 sugars	Octose C8 sugars	Nonose C9 sugars
C=O Function	Aldose: sugars having an aldehyde function or an acetal equivalent.					
C=O Function	Ketose: sugars having a ketone function or an acetal equivalent.					

The compounds carbohydrates have common same functional groups, glyceraldehydes and glucose are classified as aldoses and ribulose and dihydroxyacetone as ketoses. All of these compounds are alcohols with many hydroxyl groups. They are polyhydroxylated and either aldehydes or ketones.

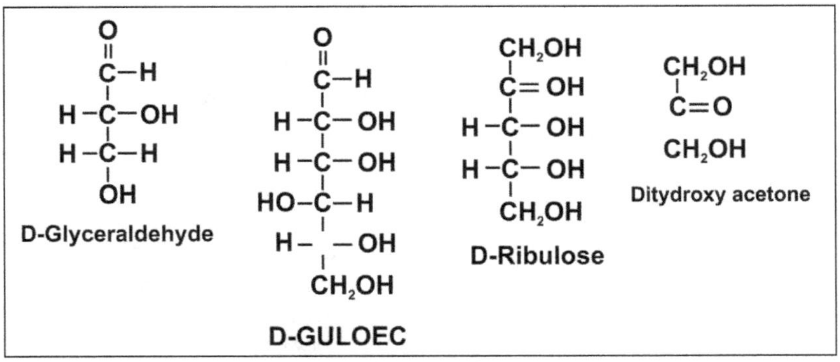

Figure: Aldose and Ketose.

Monosaccharides

The simplest and smallest unit of the carbohydrates is the monosaccharide, (mono = one, saccharide = sugar) from which disaccharides, oligosaccharides, and polysaccharides are constructed. Monosaccharides are either aldehydes or ketones, with one or more hydroxyl groups; the six-carbon monosaccharides glucose (an aldohexose) and fructose (a keto hexose) have five hydroxyl groups. The carbon atoms, to which hydroxyl groups are attached, are often chiral centers, and stereoisomerism is common among monosaccharides.

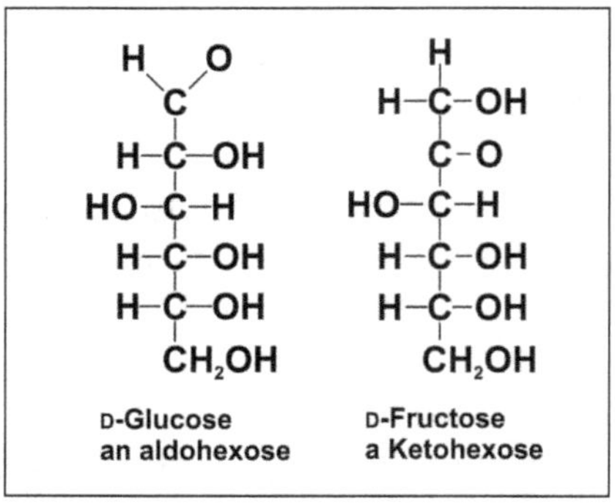

Simple monosaccharides with four, five, six, and seven carbon atoms are called tetroses, pentoses, hexoses, and heptoses, respectively. Because these molecules have multiple asymmetric carbons, they exist as diastereoisomers, isomers that are not mirror images of each other, as well as enantiomers. In regard to these monosaccharides, the symbols D and L designate the absolute configuration of the asymmetric carbon farthest from the aldehyde or keto group. D-Ribose, the carbohydrate component of RNA, is a five carbon aldose. D-Glucose, D-mannose, and D-galactose are abundant six-carbon aldoses. It may be noted that D-glucose and D-mannose differ in configuration only at C-2. Sugars differing in configuration at a single asymmetric center are called epimers. Thus, D-glucose and D-mannose are epimeric at C-2; D-glucose and D-galactose are epimers with respect to C-4.

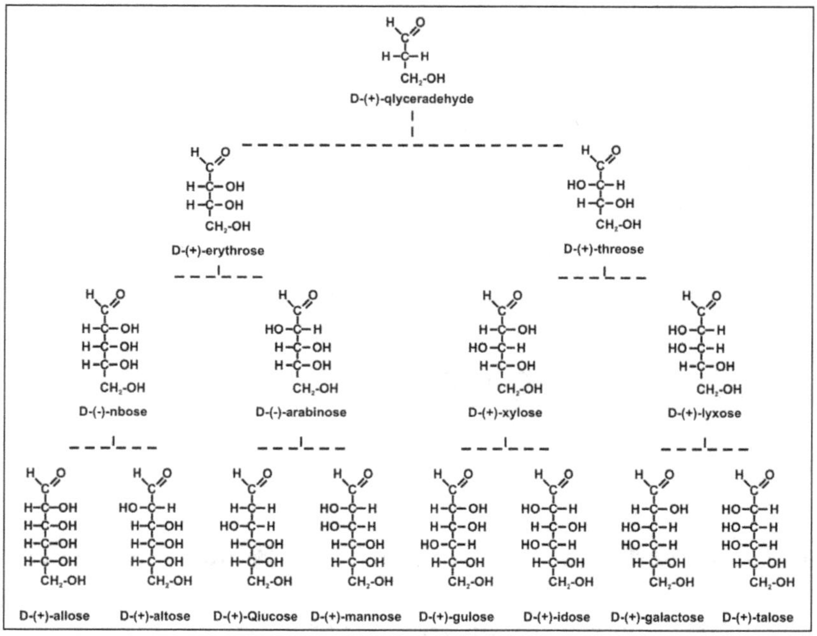

Figure: Epimers

Disaccharides

A disaccharide consists of two monosaccharides joined by an O-glycosidic bond.

Disaccharides can be homo- and heterodisaccharide. Three most abundant disaccharides are sucrose, lactose, and maltose. In sucrose the anomeric carbon atoms of a glucose unit and a fructose unit are joined. Lactose, the disaccharide of milk, consists of galactose joined to glucose by a β (1→4) glycosidic linkage. In maltose, α (1→4) glycosidic linkage joins two glucose units. Sucrose and lactose are heterosaccharides and maltose is homosaccharide.

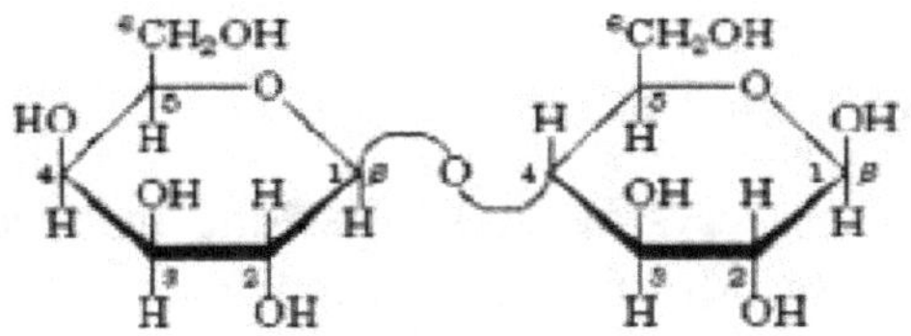

Lactose (β form)
β-D-galactopyranosyl-(1→4)-β-D-glucopyranose
Gal(β1→4)Glc

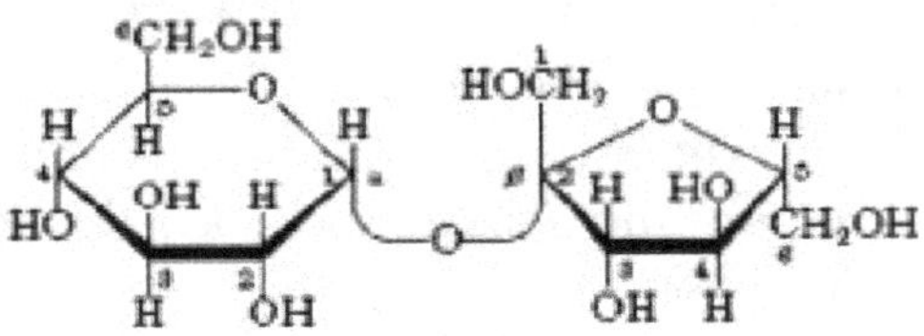

Sucrose
α-D-glucopyranosyl β-D-fructofuranoside
Glc(α1↔2β)Fru

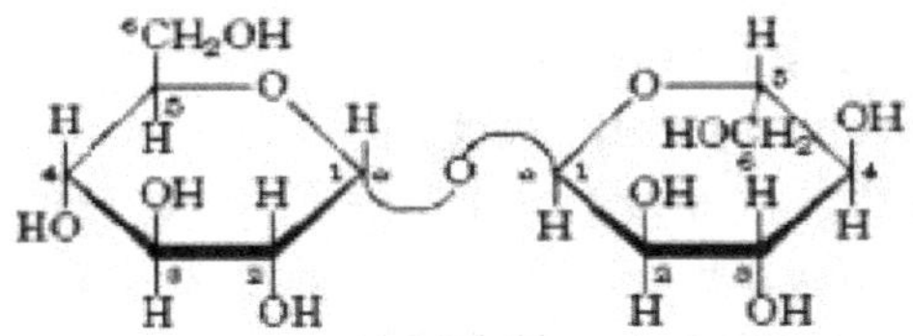

Trehalose
α-D-glucopyranosyl α-D-glucopyranoside
Glc(α1↔1α)Glc

Oligosaccharide

An oligosaccharide is a saccharide polymer containing a small number (typically three to ten) of component sugars, and is also known as simple sugars. They are generally found either O- or N-linked to compatible amino acid side chains in proteins or to lipid moieties. They (homo-and hetero-oligosaccharides) are also liberated as intermediate products of saccharification by action of glycosidases on polysaccharides.

Polysaccharides

Polysaccharides are relatively complex carbohydrates. They are polymers made up of many monosaccharides joined together by glycosidic bonds. They are, therefore, very large, often branched, macromolecules. They tend to be amorphous, insoluble in water, and have no sweet taste. When all the monosaccharides in a polysaccharide are of the same type, the polysaccharide is called a homopolysaccharide and when more than one type of monosaccharide is present, they are called heteropolysaccharides. Examples include storage polysaccharides such as starch and glycogen and structural polysaccharides such as cellulose, and chitin. Xylan a hemicellulose is a heteropolysaccharide. Polysaccharides have a general formula of $C_n (H_2O)_{n-1}$ where n can be any number between 200 and 2500. Considering that the repeating units in the polymer backbone are often six-carbon monosaccharides, the general formula can also be represented as (C6H10O5)n where n={40...3000}.

Families of Monosaccharides

Monosaccharides are colorless, crystalline solids that are freely soluble in water but insoluble in nonpolar solvents. Most have a sweet taste. The backbone of monosaccharides is an unbranched carbon chain in which all the carbon atoms are linked by single bonds. One of the carbon atoms is double-bonded to an oxygen atom to form a carbonyl group; each of the other carbon atoms has a hydroxyl group. If the carbonyl group is at an end of the carbon chain, the monosaccharide is an aldehyde and is called an aldose; if the carbonyl group is at any other position, the monosaccharide is a ketone and is called a ketose. The simplest monosaccharides are the two three-carbon trioses: glyceraldehyde, an aldose, and dihydroxyacetone, a ketose.

Structure of Monosaccharide

Structures of monosaccharides are defined by Fischer projection, where all horizontal bonds project toward the viewer, while vertical bonds project away from the viewer. Therefore, a Fischer projection cannot be rotated by $(2_n+1) \times 90°$ in the plane of the page or the screen, as the orientation of bonds relative to one another can change, converting a molecule to its enantiomer.

Examples of monosaccharide include glucose (dextrose), fructose, galactose, and ribose. Monosaccharides are the building blocks of disaccharides like sucrose (common sugar) and polysaccharides (such as cellulose and starch and hemicellulose). Further, each carbon atom that supports a hydroxyl group (except for the first and last) is chiral, giving rise to a number of isomeric forms, all with the same chemical formula. Galactose and glucose are both aldohexoses, but they have different chemical and physical properties.

With few exceptions (e.g., deoxyribose or dexyglucose), monosaccharides have the chemical formula $(CH_2O)_n$+m with the chemical structure $H (CHOH)_nC{=}O(CHOH)_mH$. If n or m is zero, it is an aldehyde and is termed an aldose; otherwise it is a ketone and is termed a ketose. Examples of some aldo and keto sugars are presented in table. Monosaccharides contain a ketone or aldehyde functional group, and hydroxyl groups on most or all of the non-carbonyl carbon atoms. Most monosaccharides form cyclic structures, which predominate in aqueous solution, by forming hemiacetals or hemiketals (depending on whether they are aldoses or ketoses) between an alcohol and the carbonyl group of the same sugar. Glucose, for example, readily forms a hemiacetal linkage between its carbon-1 and the hydroxyl group of its carbon-5. Since such a reaction introduces an additional stereogenic center, two anomers are formed (α-anomer and β-anomer) from each distinct straight-chain monosaccharide.

Table: Monosaccharides

Monosaccharides	Aldo form	Keto form
Trioses	Glyceraldehydes	Dihydroxyacetone
Tetroses	Erythrose and Threose	Erythrulose
Pentoses	Arabinose, Lyxose, Ribose and Xylose	Ribulose and Xylulose
Hexoses	Allose, Altrose, Galactose, Glucose, Gulose, Idose, Mannose and Talose	Fructose, Psicose, Sorbose and Tagatose
Heptoses	NA	Mannoheptulose, Sedoheptulose
Octoses	NA	2-Keto-3-deoxymanno-octonate
Nonoses	NA	Sialose

The cyclic structure of monosaccharides is represented by Haworth projection, where the α-anomer has the OH- of the anomeric carbon under the ring structure, and the β-isomer, has the OH- of the anomeric carbon on top of the ring structure.

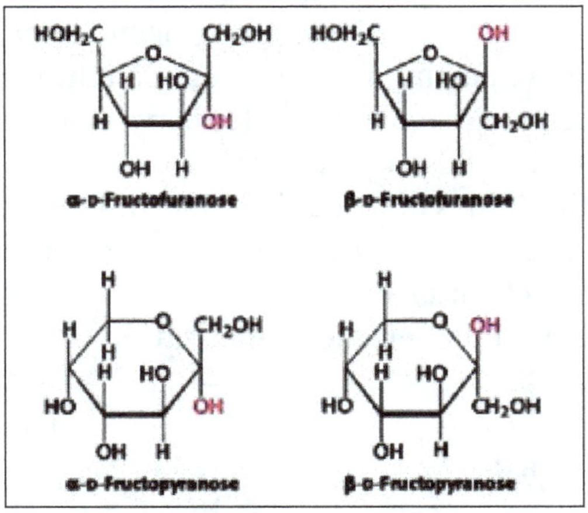

Figure: Cyclic form.

Haworth Projection: A Haworth projection is a common way of representing the cyclic structure of monosaccharides with a simple three-dimensional perspective. The Haworth projection was named after the English chemist Sir Walter N. Haworth. A Haworth projection has the following characteristics:

- Carbon is the implicit type of atom. In the example on the right, the atoms numbered from 1 to 6 are all carbon atoms. Carbon 1 is known as the Anomeric Carbon.

- Hydrogen atoms on carbon are implicit. In the example, atoms 1 to 6 have extra hydrogen atoms not depicted.

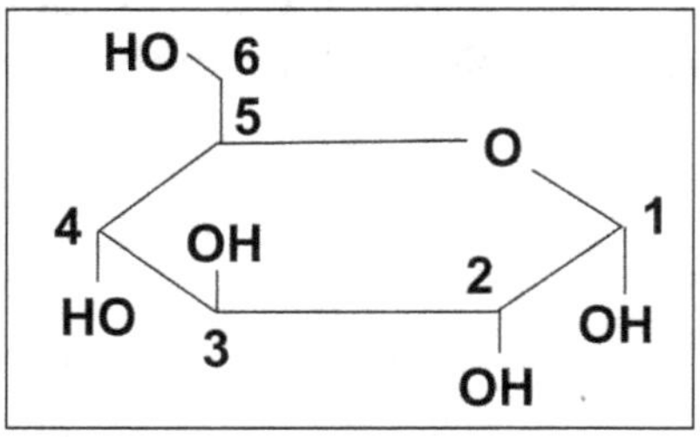

A thicker line indicates atoms that are closer to the observer. In the following figure, atoms 2 and 3 (and their corresponding OH groups) are the closest to the observer, atoms 1 and 4 are further from the observer and finally the remaining atoms (5, etc.) are the furthest.

There is another way of representation of cyclic structure of saccharides; one is chair and another is boat conformation. In chair conformation, the α-anomer has the OH- of the anomeric carbon in an axial position, whereas the β-isomer has the OH- of the anomeric carbon in equatorial position The lowest-energy chair conformation, 6 of the 12 hydrogens are in axial positions their C-H bonds are parallel to each other and appear to stick up and down from the ring structure, the other 6 are in equatorial positions.

On the other hand, boat conformation has a higher energy than the chair form due to steric strain resulting from the two axial 1, 4-hydrogen atoms. The torsional strain in the boat conformation has a maximum value because all the carbon bonds are eclipsed. The boat and envelope forms are transition states between the twist forms and the twist and chair forms respectively, and are impossible to isolate. The twist-boat conformation is less stable than the chair conformation. The difference in energy between the chair and the twist-boat conformation of monosaccharides can be measured indirectly by taking the difference in activation energy for the conversion of the chair to the twist-boat conformation and that of the reverse isomerization.

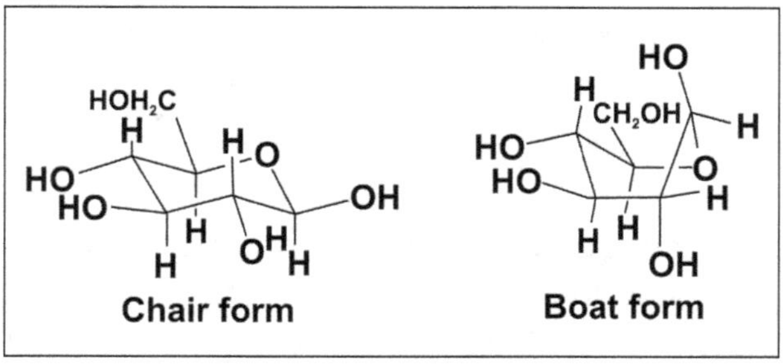

Figure: Chair and boat form.

Axial & equatorial position: The axial hydrogen is those sigma bonds that are parallel to an imaginary axis running through the ring structure. The equatorial hydrogens are those whose sigma bonds are perpendicular to that axis.

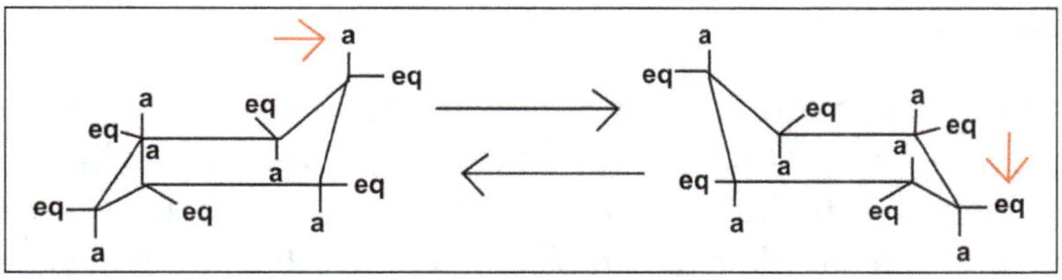

In the figures given not all of the hydrogens attached to the ring carbons in cyclohexane are equivalent. Replacing all but one of the 12 hydrogens with deuterium leaving one position as regular hydrogen can prove this. Because the ring flip occurs so rapidly at room temperature, there will be only one nuclear magnetic resonance (NMR) signal for the one hydrogen. Deuterium atoms do not have a spin state that would generate an NMR signal. However when we slow the molecular motion down by lowering the temperature of the sample to an extremely low temperature so the ring flip occurs much less rapidly, we observe two separate NMR signals with slightly different chemical shifts. This would indicate that the hydrogen has changed positions as the ring underwent flipping so that the two positions are non-equivalent. These two non-equivalent hydrogen positions are called the axial and equatorial positions. The axial bonds run vertical to the molecule. The equatorial bonds run approximately horizontal to the molecule. During the ring flip process the axial hydrogens become equatorial and the equatorial hydrogens become axial.

Isomerism

Isomers are defined as molecule with the same chemical formula and often with the same kinds of chemical bonds between atoms, but in which the atoms are arranged differently (analogous to a chemical anagram). That is to say, they have different structural formulae. Many isomers share similar if not identical properties in most chemical contexts. Isomerism can be of two types: Structural isomerism and Stereoisomerism.

Chirality

A carbon is chiral if it is sp3 hybridized and it has 4 different groups attached to it. Molecule is chiral if it is not superimposable on its mirror image. This means that none of its conformations (out of the infinite number of them) has a plane of symmetry through it. Remember, there are as many conformations in a molecule as there are rotations about single bonds.

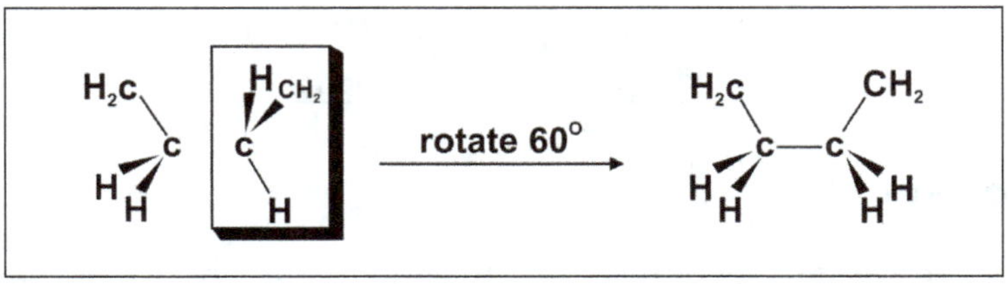

Chiral Carbon Centers

All chiral molecules have non-superimposable mirror images. And as a general rule of thumb, chiral molecules must have one or more chiral centers -- that is, carbons that have four non-identical substituents around it. (There are, of course, exceptions to this rule). A classic case of a simple chiral molecule is the following halogenated methane derivative to it. Chiral carbons result in stereoisomers.

Structural Isomerism

In structural isomers, the atoms and functional groups are joined together in different ways. This group includes chain isomerism, position isomerism and functional group isomerism. This is also termed as constitutional isomerism.

- Chain isomerism: Here hydrocarbon chains have variable amounts of branching. In carbon-chain isomerism, the difference between the isomers is the length of the carbon chain. For example, if the compound contains four carbon atoms, they can be arranged with two different chain lengths as below:

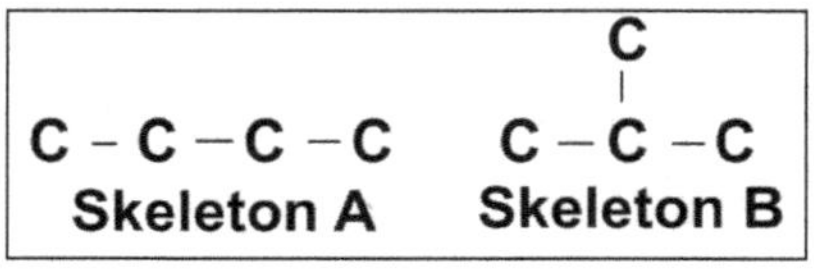

- Positional isomerism: This deals with the position of a functional group on a chain. Positional isomers have the same functional group in different locations on the carbon skeleton. For example, there are two isomers of molecular formula C3H8O. In one isomer (propan-1-ol) the –OH group is bonded to an end carbon atom; in the other (propan-2-ol) it is bonded to the middle carbon atom.

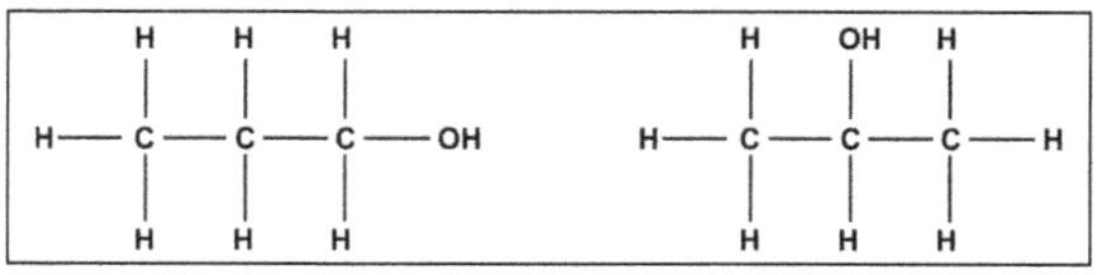

- Functional-group isomerism: Here one functional group is split up into different ones. The isomers are members of different homologous series and, therefore, have different functional groups. For example, there are two isomers of molecular formula C_2H_6O. One isomer is the alcohol, ethanol, CH_3CH_2OH; the other is the ether, methoxymethane, CH_3OCH_3.

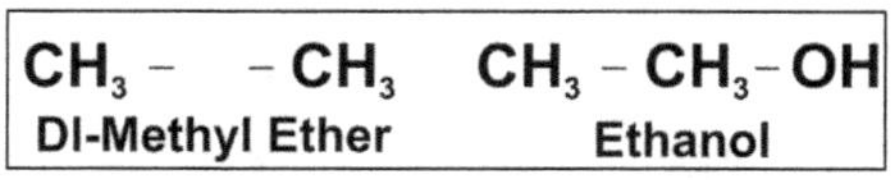

Stereoisomerism

The stereoisomers have same chemical formula and connectivity of atoms, but different arrangements of those atoms. This is also termed as spatial isomerism. This class includes enantiomers and diastereomers. Diastereomerism is of two types: conformational isomerism (conformers) and cis-trans isomerism. Conformers can be referred to as having a diastereomeric relationship; the isomers over all are not diastereomers, since bonds in conformers can be rotated to make them mirror images.

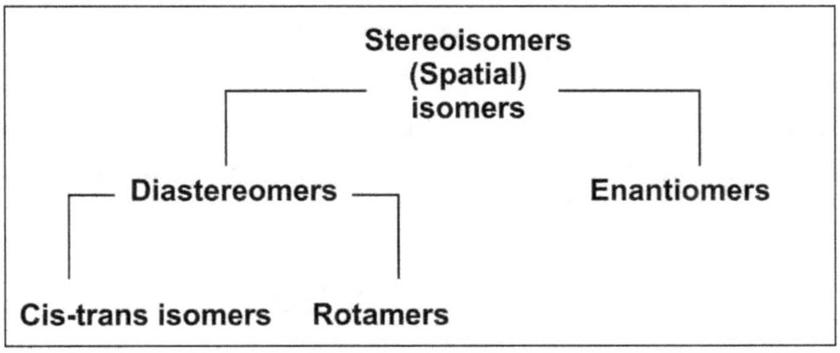

Enantiomers: Enantiomers are mirror images of chiral molecules. Enantiomers are not superimposable on each other. Only chiral molecules will have a non-superimposable mirror image. If two molecules are enantiomers, all of the chiral centers in it must have opposite configurations.

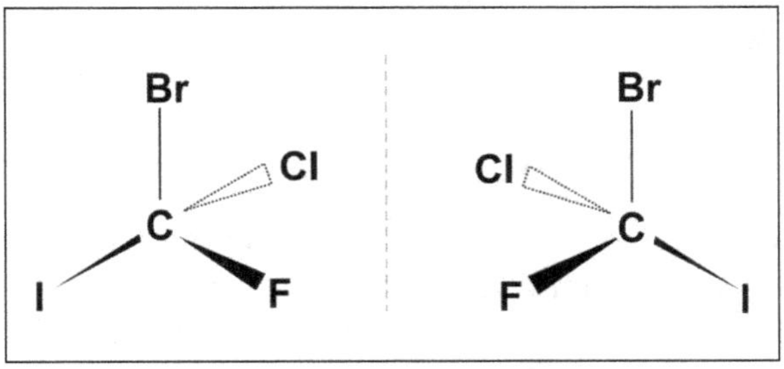

The above carbon atom has four non-identical substituents around it, making this carbon a chiral center, and as proof of its chirality the molecule has a non-superimposable mirror image. To distinguish between enantiomers, chemists use the R and S classification system. Stereocenters, (sometimes called chiral centers or stereogenic centers) are carbons that have four non-identical substituents on them, and are designated as either of R stereochemistry or S stereochemistry. If a molecule has one stereocenter of R configuration, then in the mirror image of that molecule, the stereocenter would be of S configuration, and vice versa.

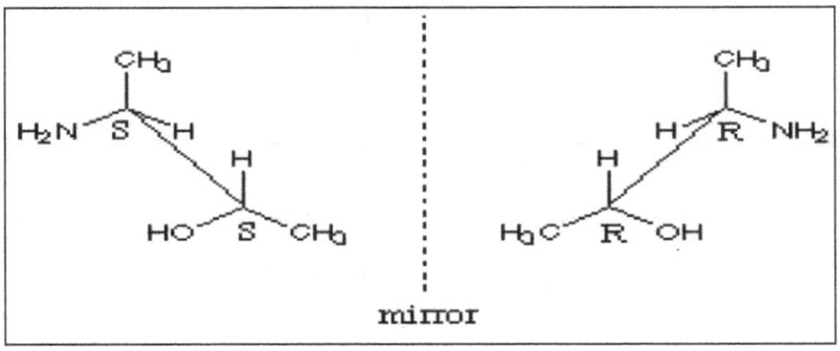

Enantiomers have identical physical properties (b.p., m.p., density, etc.) with several exceptions such as enantiomers have opposite specific rotations; they are distinguishable by NMR spectroscopy in chiral media (but not achiral), they may exhibit different chemical properties, such as very different rates of reaction.

Given the importance of stereochemistry in reactions between biomolecules, biochemists must name and represent the structure of each biomolecule so that its stereochemistry is unambiguous. For compounds with more than one chiral center, the most useful system of nomenclature is the RS system. In this system, each group attached to a chiral carbon is assigned a priority. The priorities of some common substituents are:

$$OOCH_2 > OOH > ONH_2 > OCOOH > OCHO > OCH_2OH > OCH_3 > OH$$

For naming in the RS system, the chiral atom is viewed with the group of lowest priority pointing away from the viewer. If the priority of the other three groups (1 to 3) decreases in clockwise order, the configuration is; if in counterclockwise order, the configuration is (S). In this way each chiral carbon is designated either (R) or (S), and the inclusion of these designations in the name of the compound provides an unambiguous description of the stereochemistry at each chiral center.

Mutarotation

The term for interconversion between the two anomers is called mutarotation. The two different anomers are two distinct chemical structures, and thus have different physical and chemical properties, notably optical rotation. For example, α-D-glucose has an optical rotation of +112 degrees and its anomer, β-D-glucose, has an optical rotation of +19 degrees.

Isomeric forms of monosaccharides that differ only in their configuration about the hemiacetal or hemiketal carbon atom are called anomers. The hemiacetal (or carbonyl) carbon atom is called the anomeric carbon. The α and β anomers of D-glucose interconvert in aqueous solution by a process called mutarotation.

α-D-glucose	H_2O	**equilibrated solution**	H_2O	**β-D-glucose**
$C_6H_{12}O_6$	⇌	$[\alpha]=+52.7°$	⇌	$C_6H_{12}O_6$
m.p. 146°		36% α + 64% β		m.p. 150°
$[\alpha]=+112°$				$[\alpha]=+19°$

The figure is self-explanatory and shows that this mixture consists of about one-third α-D-glucose, two-thirds β-D-glucose, and very small amounts of the linear and five-membered ring (glucofuranose) forms.

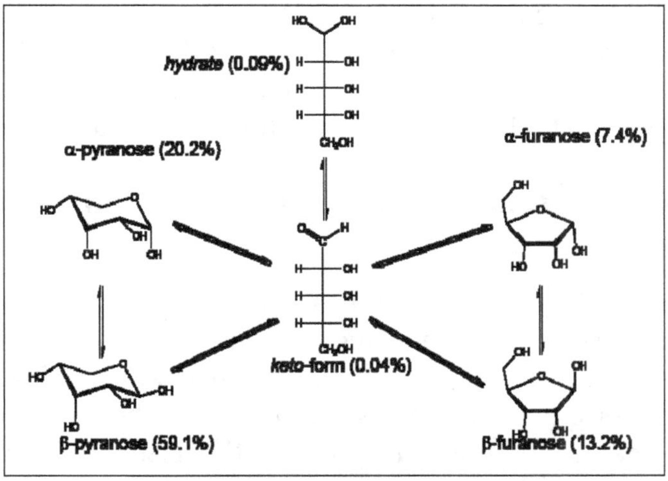

Figure: Mutarotate forms of glucose.

Anomers

In sugar chemistry, an anomer is a special type of epimer. It is a stereoisomer (diastereomer, more exactly) of a saccharide (in the cyclic form) that differs only in its configuration at the hemiacetal (or hemiketal) carbon, also called the anomeric carbon. If the structure is analogous to one with the hydroxyl group on the anomeric carbon in the axial position of glucose, then the sugar is an alpha anomer. If, however, that hydroxyl is in the equatorial position, then the sugar is a beta anomer. For example, α-D-glucopyranose and β-Dglucopyranose, the two cyclic forms of glucose, are anomers. For -L- the α and β are contrary wise. The anomeric effect helps stabilize the α-anomer.

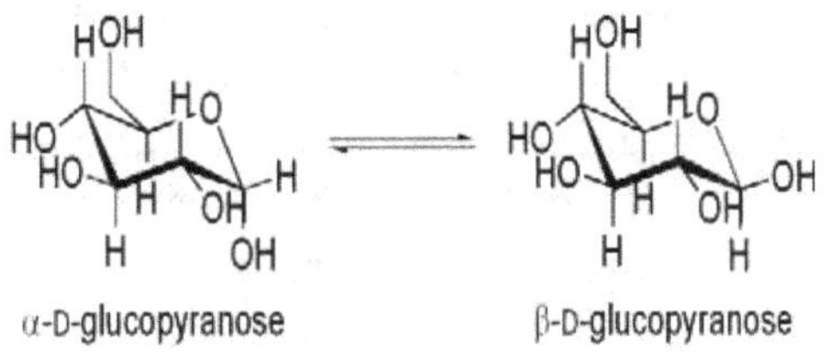

[The α- and β-anomers of D- glucopyranose]

Configuration of Glucose

There are four chiral centers in glucose, which indicate possibility of sixteen stereoisomers that would exist as eight diastereomeric pairs of enantiomers. German chemists Emil Fischer in 1891 devised a method of representing the configuration of each chiral center in an unambiguous manner. Fischer established a network of related aldose configurations termed as D-family through an arbitrary choice for (+)-glucose. Consequently, the mirror images of these configurations were designated the L-family of aldoses.

The last chiral center in an aldose chain (farthest from the aldehyde group) was chosen by Fischer as the D / L designator site. If the hydroxyl group in the projection formula pointed to the right, it was defined as a member of the D-family and a left directed hydroxyl group (the mirror image) then represented the L-family. The sign of a compound's specific rotation (an experimental number) does not correlate with its configuration (D or L) and optical rotation can be measured by with a polarimeter.

Three-dimensional Structure is Described by Configuration and Conformation

The covalent bonds and functional groups of a biomolecule are, of course, central to its function, but so also is the arrangement of the molecule's constituent atoms in three-dimensional space—its stereochemistry. A carbon-containing compound commonly exists as stereoisomers, molecules with the same chemical bonds but different stereochemistry— that is, different configuration, the fixed spatial arrangement of atoms. Interactions between biomolecules are invariably stereospecific, requiring specific stereochemistry in the interacting molecules.

Configuration is conferred by the presence of either (1) double bonds, around which there is no freedom of rotation, or (2) chiral centers, around which substituent groups are arranged in a specific sequence. The identifying characteristic of configurational isomers is that they cannot be interconverted without temporarily breaking one or more covalent bonds. A binding site (on an enzyme, for example) that is complementary to one of these molecules would not be a suitable binding site for the other, which explains why the two compounds have distinct biological roles despite their similar chemistry.

In the second type of configurational isomer, four different substituents bonded to a tetrahedral carbon atom may be arranged two different ways in space—that is, have two configurations —yielding two stereoisomers with similar or identical chemical properties but differing in certain physical and biological properties. A carbon atom with four different substituents is said to be asymmetric, and asymmetric carbons are called chiral centers. A molecule with only one chiral carbon can have two stereoisomers; when two or more (n) chiral carbons are present, there can be 2n stereoisomers. Some stereoisomers are enantiomers and others, pairs of stereoisomers that are not mirror images of each other are called diastereomer.

Distinct from configuration is molecular conformation, the spatial arrangement of substituent groups that, without breaking any bonds, are free to assume different positions in space because of the freedom of rotation about single bonds. In the simple hydrocarbon ethane, for example, there is nearly complete freedom of rotation around the COC bond. Many different, interconvertible conformations of ethane are possible, depending on the degree of rotation. Two conformations are of special interest: the staggered, which is more stable than all others and thus predominates, and the eclipsed, which are least stable. We cannot isolate either of these conformational forms, because they are freely interconvertible. However, when one or more of the hydrogen atoms on each carbon is replaced by a functional group that is either very large or electrically charged, freedom of rotation around the COC bond is hindered. This limits the number of stable conformations of the ethane derivative.

Interactions between Biomolecules are Stereospecific

Biological interactions between molecules are stereospecific: the "fit" in such interactions must be stereochemically correct. The three-dimensional structure of biomolecules large and small—the combination of configuration and conformation—is of the utmost importance in their biological interactions: reactant with enzyme, hormone with its receptor on a cell surface, antigen with its specific antibody. The study of biomolecular stereochemistry with precise physical methods is an important part of modern research on cell structure and biochemical function. In living organisms, chiral molecules are usually present in only one of their chiral forms. For example, the amino acids in proteins occur only as their L isomers; glucose occurs only as its D isomer. In contrast, when a compound with an asymmetric carbon atom is chemically synthesized in the laboratory, the reaction usually produces all possible chiral forms: a mixture of the D and L forms, for example. Living cells produce only one chiral form of biomolecules because the enzymes that synthesize them are also chiral.

Stereospecificity, the ability to distinguish between stereoisomers, is a property of enzymes and other proteins and a characteristic feature of the molecular logic of living cells. If the binding site on a protein is complementary to one isomer of a chiral compound, it will not be complementary to the other isomer, for the same reason that a left glove does not fit a right hand.

Optical Activity

Optical activity is the ability of a chiral molecule to rotate the plane of plane-polarized light. It is measured using a polarimeter, which consists of a light source, polarizing lens, sample tube and analyzing lens. When light passes through a sample that can rotate plane polarized light, the light appears to dim to the eye because it no longer passes straight through the polarizing filters. The amount of rotation is quantified as the number of degrees that the analyzing lens must be rotated by so that it appears as if no dimming, of the light has occurred.

Louis Pasteur encountered the phenomenon of optical activity in 1843, during his investigation of the crystalline sediment that accumulated in wine casks (a form of tartaric acid called paratartaric acid—also called racemic acid). He used fine forceps to separate two types of crystals identical in shape but mirror images of each other. Both types proved to have all the chemical properties of tartaric acid, but in solution one type rotated polarized light to the left (levorotatory), the other to the right (dextro rotatory). Pasteur later described the experiment and its interpretation.

In isomeric bodies, the elements and the proportions in which they are combined are the same, only the arrangement of the atoms is different. We know, on the one hand, that the molecular arrangements of the two tartaric acids are asymmetric, and, on the other hand, that these arrangements are absolutely identical, excepting that they exhibit asymmetry in opposite directions. Are the atoms of the dextro acid grouped in the form of a right-handed spiral, or are they placed at the apex of an irregular tetrahedron, or are they disposed according to this or that asymmetric arrangement?

X-ray crystallographic studies in 1951 confirmed that the levorotatory and dextrorotatory forms of tartaric acid are mirror images of each other at the molecular level and established the absolute configuration of each.

Measurement of Optical Activity

When rotation is quantified using a polarimeter it is known as an observed rotation, because rotation is affected by path length (l), or the distance for which the light travels through a sample and concentration (c), of the sample present to rotate the light. When these effects are eliminated a standard for comparison of all molecules is obtained, the specific rotation, [α], when concentration is expressed as sample in grams /100ml solution:

$$[\alpha] = 100a \ / \ cl$$

Specific rotation is a physical property like the boiling point of a sample. Enantiomers will rotate the plane of polarization in exactly equal amounts (same magnitude) but in opposite directions. Dextrorotary designated as (+), clockwise rotation (to the right) Levorotary designated as (-), anti-clockwise rotation (to the left).

If only one enantiomer is present a sample is considered to be optically pure. When a sample consists of a mixture of enantiomers, the effect of each enantiomer cancels out, molecule for molecule. For example, a 50:50 mixture of two enantiomers or a racemic mixture will not rotate plane polarized light and is optically inactive. A mixture that contains one enantiomer excess, however, will display a net plane of polarization in the direction characteristic of the enantiomer that is in excess.

Determination of Optical Purity

The optical purity or the enantiomeric excess (ee %) of a sample can be determined as follows:

Optical purity = % enantiomeric excess = % enantiomer1 - % enantiomer2

$$= 100 \ [\alpha]mixture \ / \ [\alpha]pure\ sample$$

$$ee\ \% = 100 \ ([R]-[S]) \ / \ ([R]+[S])$$

Where [R] = concentration of the R-isomer [S] = concentration of the S-isomer.

Structure, Occurrence and Biological Importance of Monosaccharides

Glucose

Systemic name: D-Glucose

Molecular formula: $C_6H_{12}O_6$

Glucose (Glc), a monosaccharide (or simple sugar), is an important carbohydrate in biology. The living cell uses it as a source of energy and metabolic intermediate. Glucose is one of the main products of photosynthesis and starts cellular respiration in both prokaryotes and eukaryotes. The name comes from the Greek word 'glykys', which means "sweet", plus the suffix "-ose" which denotes a sugar.

Two stereoisomers of the aldohexose sugars are known as glucose, only one of which (D-glucose) is biologically active. This form (D-glucose) is often referred to as dextrose monohydrate, or, especially in the food industry, simply dextrose (from dextrorotatory glucose). The mirror-image of the molecule, L-glucose, cannot be metabolized by cells in the biochemical process known as glycolysis.

Function: Enzyme-regulated addition of glucose to proteins by glycosylation is often essential to their function:

- As an energy source - Glucose is a ubiquitous fuel in biology. It is used as an energy source in most organisms, from bacteria to humans. Use of glucose may be by either aerobic or anaerobic respiration (fermentation). Carbohydrates are the human body's key source of energy, through aerobic respiration, providing approximately 3.75 kilocalories (16 kilojoules) of food energy per gram. Breakdown of carbohydrates (e.g. starch) yields mono- and disaccharides, most of which is glucose. Through glycolysis and later in the reactions of the Citric acid cycle (TCA), glucose is oxidized to eventually form CO_2 and water, yielding energy, mostly in the form of ATP. The insulin reaction and other mechanisms, regulate the concentration of glucose in the blood.
- Use of glucose as an energy source in cells is via aerobic or anaerobic respiration. Both of them start with the early steps of the glycolysis metabolic pathway. The first step of this is the phosphorylation of glucose by hexokinase to prepare it for later breakdown to provide energy.

As a precursor: Glucose is used as a precursor for the synthesis of several important substances. Starch solution Starch, cellulose, and glycogen are common glucose polymers (polysaccharides). Lactose, the predominant sugar in milk, is a glucose-galactose disaccharide. In sucrose, another important disaccharide, glucose is joined to fructose.

Galactose

Systemic name: D-Galactose

Molecular formula: $C_6H_{12}O_6$

Galactose (Gal) is a type of sugar, which is less sweet than glucose and not very water-soluble. Galactose is more commonly found in the disaccharide, lactose or milk sugar. It is found as the monosaccharide in peas. Galactose is classified as a monosaccharide, an aldose, a hexose, and is a reducing sugar. It is considered a nutritive sweetener because it has food energy. A genetic defect of not being able to utilize galactose is called Galactosemia. The disorder is caused by a deficiency in one or more enzymes required to metabolize galactose. Since galactose is in milk as part of lactose, it builds up in the blood and urine. Undiagnosed it may lead to mental retardation, failure to grow, formation of cataracts, and in severe cases death by liver damage.

Fructose

Systemic name: D-Fructose

Molecular formula: $C_6H_{12}O_6$

Fructose (or laevulose) is a simple reducing sugar (monosaccharide) found in many foods and is one of the three most important blood sugars along with glucose and galactose. Honey, tree fruits, berries, melons, and some root vegetables, such as beets, sweet potatoes, parsnips, and onions, contain fructose, usually in combination with sucrose and glucose. Fructose is also derived from the digestion of sucrose, a disaccharide consisting of glucose and fructose that is broken down by glycoside hydrolase enzymes during digestion. Fructose is the sweetest naturally occurring sugar, estimated to be twice as sweet as sucrose.

Fructose is often recommended for, and consumed by, people with diabetes mellitus or hyperglycemia, because it has a very low glycemic index (GI) relative to cane sugar (sucrose). The low GI is due to the unique and lengthy metabolic pathway of fructose, which involves phosphorylation and a multi-step enzymatic process in the liver.

2 Deoxy-D-glucose

Systemic name: 2 Deoxy-D-arabino-hexose

Molecular formula: $C_6H_{12}O_5$

2-Deoxy-D-glucose is a glucose molecule, which has the 2-hydroxyl group, replaced by hydrogen, so that it cannot undergo further glycolysis. It is also called as non-metabolizable form of glucose. The sugar is responsible for inhibiting glycosylating of proteins if used in culture medium.

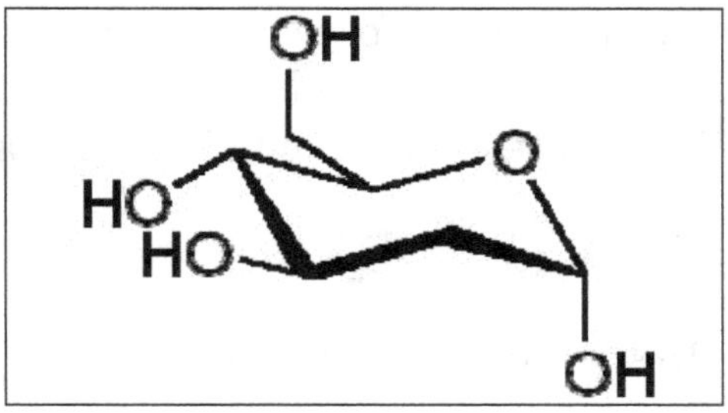

Xylose

Systemic name: D-Xylose

Molecular formula: $C_5H_{10}O_5$

Xylose or wood sugar is an aldopentose – a monosaccharide containing five carbon atoms and including an aldehyde functional group. It has chemical formula C5H10O5. Xylose is found in the embryos of most edible plants.

Function:

- Xylose is an antibacterial and antifungal, particularly with gram-negative organisms and Candida sp.
- Absorption rate of Xylose is decreased in some patients with intestinal disorders, including those with colitis and diabetes, suggesting that when absorption problems are corrected, these conditions might also reverse themselves.
- Unlike sucrose or artificial sweeteners, xylose promotes the growth of "friendly flora" in the intestines, thus increasing the manufacture and absorption of all nutrients and strengthening the immune system to help fight off any type of illness.

Ribose

Systemic name: D-ribose

Molecular formula: $C_5H_{10}O_5$

Ribose, primarily seen as D-ribose, is an aldopentose — a monosaccharide containing five carbon atoms, and including an aldehyde functional group in its linear form. It has the chemical formula $C_5H_{10}O_5$, and was discovered in 1905 by Phoebus Levene.

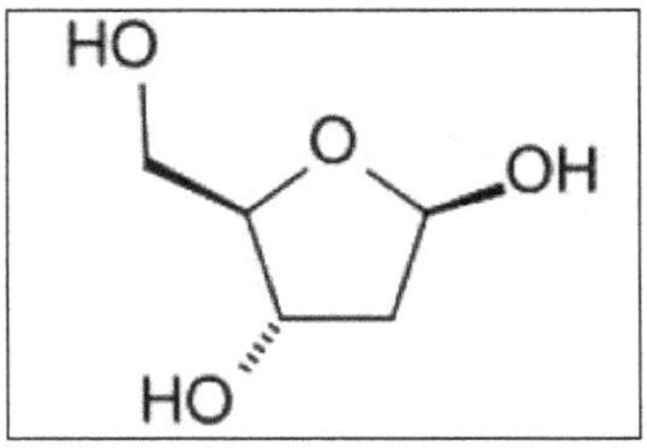

As a component of the RNA that is used for genetic transcription, ribose is critical to living creatures. It is related to deoxyribose, which is a component of DNA. It is also a component of ATP, NADH, and several other chemicals that are critical to metabolism.

Deoxyribose

Systemic name: 2 -Deoxy-D-erythro-pentoseD-ribose

Molecular formula: $C_5H_{10}O_4$

Deoxyribose, also known as D-Deoxyribose and 2-deoxyribose, is an aldopentose — a monosaccharide containing five carbon atoms, and including an aldehyde functional group in its linear structure. It is a deoxy sugar derived from the pentose sugar ribose by the replacement of the hydroxyl group at the 2 position with hydrogen, leading to the net loss of an oxygen atom.

Ribose forms a five-member ring composed of four carbon atoms and one oxygen atom. Hydroxyl groups are attached to three of the carbons. The other carbon and a hydroxyl group are attached to one of the carbon atoms adjacent to the oxygen. In deoxyribose, the carbon furthest from the attached carbon is stripped of the oxygen atom in what would be a hydroxyl group in ribose. Due to the common C3' and C4' stereochemistry of D-ribose and D-arabinose, D-2-deoxyribose is also D-2-deoxyarabinose.

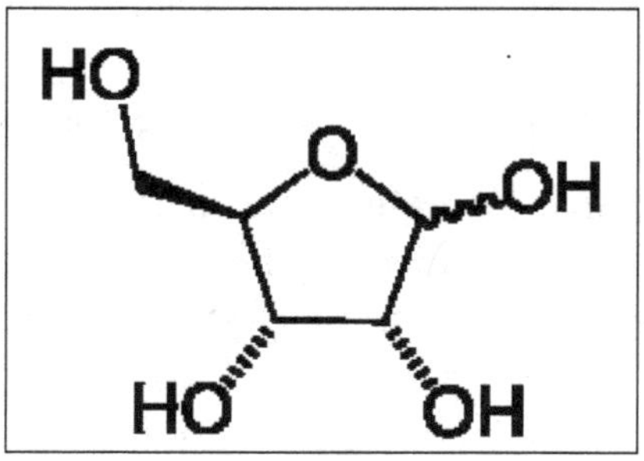

Biological Importance

Ribose and 2-deoxyribose derivatives have an important role in biology. Among the most important derivatives are those with phosphate groups attached at the 5 position. Mono-, di-, and triphosphate forms are important, as well as 3-5 cyclic monophosphates. Purines and pyrimidines form an important class of compounds with ribose and deoxyribose. When these purine and pyrimidine derivatives are coupled to a ribose sugar, they are called nucleosides. In these compounds, the convention is to put a ′ (pronounced "prime") after the carbon numbers of the sugar, so that in nucleoside derivatives a name might include, for instance, the term "5′-monophosphate", meaning that the phosphate group is attached to the fifth carbon of the sugar, and not to the base. The bases are attached to the 1′ ribose carbon in the common nucleosides. Phosphorylated nucleosides are called nucleotides.

One of the common bases is adenine (a purine derivative); coupled to ribose it is called adenosine; coupled to deoxyribose it is called deoxyadenosine. The 5′-triphosphate derivative of adenosine, commonly called ATP, for adenosine triphosphate, is an important energy transport molecule in cells.

2-Deoxyribose and ribose nucleotides are often found in unbranched 5′-3′ polymers. In these structures, the 3′carbon of one monomer unit is linked to a phosphate that is attached to the 5′carbon of the next unit, and so on. These polymer chains often contain many millions of monomer units. Since long polymers have physical properties distinctly different from those of small molecules, they are called macromolecules. The sugar-phosphate-sugar chain is called the backbone of the polymer. One end of the backbone has a free 5′phosphate, and the other end has a free 3′OH group. The backbone structure is independent of which particular bases are attached to the individual sugars.

Genetic material in earthly life often contains poly 5′-3′, 2′-deoxyribose nucleotides, in structures called chromosomes, where each monomer is one of the nucleotides deoxyadenine, thymine, guanine or cytosine. This material is commonly called deoxyribonucleic acid, or simply DNA for short. DNA in chromosomes forms very long helical structures containing two molecules with the backbones running in opposite directions on the outside of the helix and held together by hydrogen bonds between complementary nucleotide bases lying between the helical backbones. The lack of the 2′ hydroxyl group in DNA appears to allow the backbone the flexibility to assume the full conformation of the long double-helix, which involves not only the basic helix, but additional coiling necessary to fit these very long molecules into the very small volume of a cell nucleus In contrast, very similar molecules, containing ribose instead of deoxyribose, and known generically as RNA, are known to form only relatively short double-helical complementary base paired structures. These are well known, for instance, in ribosomal RNA molecules and in transfer RNA (tRNA), where so-called hairpin structures from palindromic sequences within one molecule.

Structure, Occurrence and Biological Importance of Disaccharide

Sucrose

Systematic name: D-glucopyranosyl-(1→2)-β-D-fructofuranoside

Molecular formula: $C_{12}H_{22}O_{11}$

Sucrose (common name: table sugar, also called saccharose) is a disaccharide (glucose + fructose) best known for its role in human nutrition and is formed by plants but not by other organisms such as animals. Sucrose is an easily assimilated macronutrient that provides a quick source of energy to the body, provoking a rapid rise in blood glucose upon ingestion. However, pure sucrose is not normally part of a human diet balanced for good nutrition, although it may be included sparingly to make certain foods more palatable. Sucrose, as a pure carbohydrate, has an energy content of 3.94 kilocalories per gram (or 17 kilojoules per gram). When a large amount of foods that contain a high percentage of sucrose is consumed, beneficial nutrients can be displaced from the diet, which can contribute to an increased risk for chronic disease such as defect in glucose metabolism or diabetes mettlitus.

Cellobiose

Systemic name: 4-O- β-D-glucopyranosyl-D-glucose

Molecular formula $C_{12}H_{22}O_{11}$

Cellobiose is a disaccharide derived from the condensation of two glucose molecules linked in a β (1→4) bond. It can be hydrolyzed by bacteria or cationic ion exchange resins to give glucose. Cellobiose has eight free alcohol (COH) groups and three ether linkages, which give rise to strong inter- and intra-molecular hydrogen bonds.

Trehalose

Systemic name: α-D-glucopyranosyl- α-D-glucopyranoside

Molecular formula: $C_{12}H_{22}O_{11}$

Trehalose, also known as mycose, is a natural alpha-linked disaccharide formed by an α, α1, 1-glucoside bond between two α-glucose units. It can be synthesized by fungi, plants, and invertebrate animals. It is implicated in anhydrobiosis — the ability of plants and animals to withstand prolonged periods of desiccation. It has high water retention capabilities and is used in food and cosmetics. The sugar forms a gel phase as cells dehydrate, which prevents disruption of internal cell organelles by effectively splinting them in position. Rehydration then allows normal cellular activity to be resumed without the major, lethal damage that would normally follow a dehydration/rehydration cycle. Trehalose has the added advantage of being an antioxidant. Trehalose can be found in nature, animals, plants, and microorganisms. In animals, trehalose is prevalent in shrimp, and also in insects, including grasshoppers, locusts, butterflies, and bees, in which blood sugar are trehalose. The trehalose is then broken down into glucose by the catabolic enzyme trehalase for use. In plants, the presence of trehalose is seen in sunflower seeds, selaginella mosses, and sea algae. Within the fungus family, it is prevalent in mushrooms shiitake (Lentinula edodes), maitake (Grifola fondosa), nameko (Pholiota nameko), and Judas's ear (Auricularia auricula-judae) contain 1% to 17% percent of trehalose in dry weight form. Trehalose is found in such microorganisms as baker's yeast and wine yeast. When tardigrades (water bears) dry out, the glucose in their bodies changes to trehalose when they enter a state called cryptobiosis - a state wherein they appear dead. However, when they receive water, they revive and return to their metabolic state. Larva of sleeping chironomid (polypedihum vanderplanki) and artemia (sea monkeys, brine shrimp) can withstand dehydration, because they store trehalose within their cells. In the plant kingdom, selaginella mosses that grow in desert and mountainous areas, although they may be cracked and dried out, will turn green again and revive after a rain, because of the function of Trehalose. Dried shitake mushrooms spring back into shape in water because they contain trehalose.

Trehalose is metabolized by a number of bacteria, including Streptococcus mutans, the common oral bacteria responsible for dental plaque. The enzyme trehalase, a glycoside hydrolase, breaks trehalose into two glucose molecules, which can then be readily absorbed in the gut. Trehalose is the major carbohydrate energy storage molecule used by insects for flight to be used as glucose for the rapid energy requirement of flight.

Lactose

Systemic name: 4-O- β-D-galactopyranosyl-D-glucose

Molecular formula: $C_{12}H_{22}O_{11}$

Lactose (also referred to as milk sugar) is a sugar, which is found most notably in milk. Lactose makes up around 2–8% of milk (by weight). The name comes from the Latin word for milk, plus the -ose ending used to name sugars. Lactose is the only significant sugar or carbohydrate of animal origin. Lactose is a disaccharide that consists of β-Dgalactose and β-D-glucose fragments bonded through a β (1→4) glycosidic linkage.

An enzyme, lactase, is essential for digestion of lactose, and a majority of adults in this country do not have lactase, which digests milk sugar, or lactose. Thus, it is very difficult for them to digest milk and may contribute to gaseousness, cramping, and diarrhea.

Maltose

Systemic name: 4-O-α -D-glucopyranosyl-D-glucose

Molecular formula: $C_{12}H_{22}O_{11}$

Maltose, or malt sugar, is a disaccharide formed from two units of glucose joined with an α(1→4) linkage. It is the second member of an important biochemical series of glucose chains. The addition of another glucose unit yields maltotriose; further additions will produce dextrins (also called maltodextrins) and eventually starch. Maltose can be broken down into two glucose molecules by hydrolysis. In living organisms, the enzyme maltase can achieve this very rapidly. In the laboratory, heating with a strong acid for several minutes will produce the same result. The production of maltose from germinating cereals, such as barley, is an important part of the brewing process. When barley is malted, it is brought into a condition in which the concentration of maltose producing amylases has been maximized. Mashing is the process by which these amylases convert the cereal's starches into maltose. Metabolism of maltose by yeast during fermentation then leads to the production of ethanol and carbon dioxide.

Structure, Occurrence and Biological Importance of Trisaccharides

Raffinose

Systemic name: β-D-Fructofuranosyl-O-α-D-galactopyrnosyl-(1→6)- α-Dglucopyranoside

Molecular formula: $C_{18}H_{32}O_{11}$

Raffinose is a trisaccharide composed of galactose, fructose, and glucose. It can be found in beans, cabbage, brussels sprouts, broccoli, asparagus, other vegetables, and whole grains. Raffinose can be hydrolyzed to D-galactose and sucrose by the enzyme αgalactosidase (α-GAL), an enzyme not found in humans. α-GAL also hydrolyzes other αgalactosides such as stachyose, verbascose, and galactinol, if present. The enzyme does not cleave β-linked galactose, as in lactose. The raffinose families of oligosaccharides (RFOs) are alpha-galactosyl derivatives of sucrose, and the most common are the trisaccharide raffinose, the tetrasaccharide stachyose, and the pentasaccharide verbascose. RFOs are almost ubiquitous in the plant kingdom, being found in a large variety of seeds from many different families, and they rank second only to sucrose in abundance as soluble carbohydrates. Raffinose is also used as a base substance for sucralose.

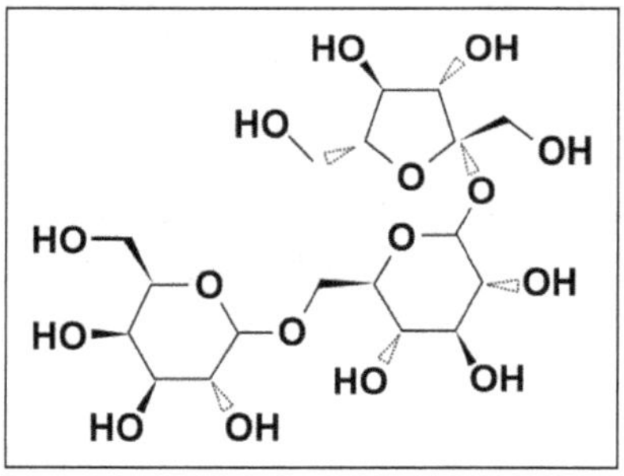

Humans and other monogastric animals (pigs and poultry) do not possess the α-GAL enzyme to break down RFOs and these oligosaccharides pass undigested through the stomach and upper intestine. In the lower intestine, they are fermented by gas-producing bacteria which do possess the α-GAL enzyme and make carbon dioxide, methane, and/or hydrogen -- leading to the flatulence commonly associated with eating beans and other vegetables. α-GAL is present in digestive aids such as the product Beano.

Acarbose

Systemic name: O-4,6-Dideoxy-4[[[1S-(1α,4α,5β,6α)]-4,5,6-trihydroxy-3-(hydroxy methyl)-2-cyclohexen-1yl] amino]-α-D-glucopyranosyl-(1→4)-O- α-Dglucopyranosyl-(1→4)-D-glucose

Molecular formula: $C_{25}H_{43}NO_{18}$

Acarbose is an anti-diabetic drug used to treat type 2 diabetes mellitus and, in some countries, prediabetes. It is an inhibitor of alpha glucosidase, an enteric enzyme that releases glucose from larger carbohydrates.

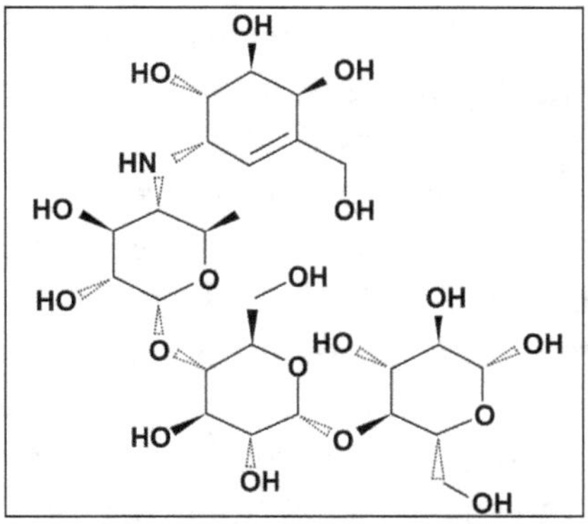

Melezitose

Systemic name: O- α -D-glucopyranosyl-(1→3) - β-D- fructofuranosyl- α-Dglucopyranoside.

Molecular formula: $C_{18}H_{32}O_{16}$

Melezitose, also spelled melicitose, is a non-reducing trisaccharide sugar that is produced from lice such as Cinara pilicornis by an enzyme reaction. This is beneficial to the insects, as it reduces the stress of osmosis by reducing their own water potential. The melezitose is part of the honeydew of the honey produced by bees, and acts as an attractant for ants. This is useful to the lice as they have a symbiotic relationship with ants. Melezitose can be partially hydrolyzed to glucose and turanose, the latter of which is an isomer of sucrose.

Since acarbose prevents the degradation of complex carbohydrates into glucose, the carbohydrates will remain in the intestine. In the colon, bacteria will digest the complex carbohydrates, thereby causing gastrointestinal side effects such as flatulence (78% of patients) and diarrhea (14% of patients).

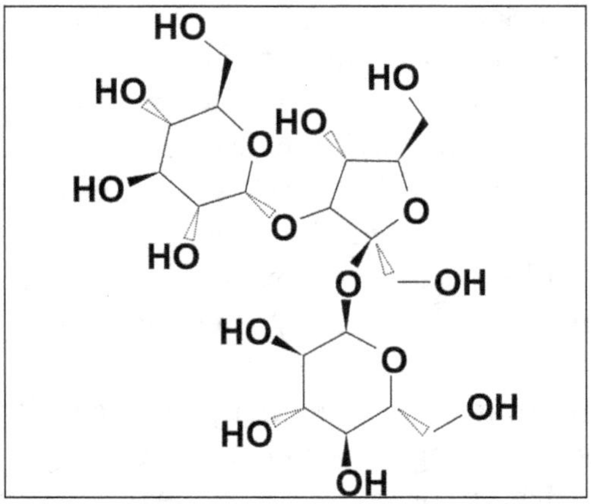

Structure, Occurrence and Biological Importance of Polysaccharides

Carbohydrate composed of ten or more monosaccharide units joined together by glycosidic linkages are classified as polysaccharides. Most of the carbohydrates found in nature occur as polysaccharides, polymers of high molecular weight; which on hydrolysis yield monosaccharides or products related to monosaccharides, most frequently D-glucose. Others monosaccharides obtained are D-mannose, D- and L-galactose, L-arabinose, Dglucuronic acid, D- and L-galactose, L-arabinose. D-glucuronic acid, D-glucosamine, etc. Polysaccharides, also called glycans, differ from each other in the identity of their recurring monosaccharide units, in the length of their chains, in the types of bonds linking the units, and in the degree of branching. Polysaccharides can be classified-as homopolysaccharidcs and heleropolysciccharide depending on the variety of sugar moieties joined to the sugar chain. Some are linear polymers and others are branched. Some typical polysaccharides are starches, glycogens celluloses, agar, gum chitin, etc.

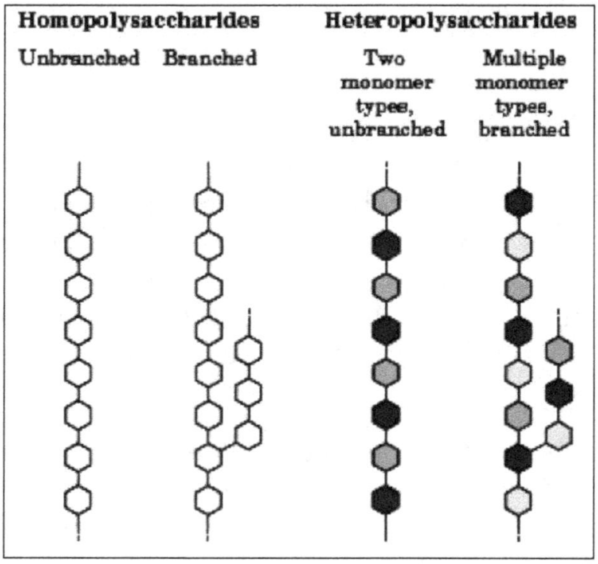

Some homopolysaccharides serve as storage forms of monosaccharides used as fuels; starch and glycogen are homopolysaccharides of this type. Other homopolysaccharides (cellulose and chitin) serve as structural elements in plant cell walls and animal exoskeletons. Heteropolysaccharides provide extracellular support for organisms of all kingdoms. The rigid layer of the bacterial cell envelope (the peptidoglycan) is a heteropolysaccharide built from two alternating monosaccharide units. In animal tissues, several heteropolysaccharides occupy the extracellular space forming a matrix that holds individual cells together and provides protection, shape, and support to cells, tissues, or organs. Hyaluronic acid accounts for the toughness and flexibility of cartilage and tendon, is among this group of extracellular polysaccharides. Other heteropolysaccharides, sometimes in very large aggregates with proteins (proteoglycans), account for the high viscosity and lubricating properties of some extracellular secretions.

Unlike proteins, polysaccharides generally do not have definite molecular weights, due to consequence of the mechanisms of assembly of the two types of polymers. Proteins are synthesized on a template (messenger RNA) of defined sequence and length, by enzymes that copy the template exactly. For polysaccharide synthesis, with no template; the program for polysaccharide synthesis is intrinsic to the enzymes that catalyze the polymerization of monomeric units. For each type of monosaccharide to be added to the growing polymer there is a separate enzyme, which acts only when the enzyme that inserts the preceding subunit has acted. The alternating action of several enzymes produces a polymer with a precise repeating sequence, but the exact length varies from molecule to molecule, within a general size class.

Homopolysaccharides

A homopolysaccharide is made up of a single kind of mono-saccharide. Starches, glycogens, and celluloses, which are made up of only glucose residues, are example of homopolysaccharides.

Starch

The starches occur widespread as reserve carbohydrate in tubers such as potatoes, in many fruits, grains and seeds. In the grains, the starch is arranged in concentric layers. When starch grains are treated with boiling water, the substance in the center passes into solution, but the greater part of the grain is not soluble. This insoluble portion swells as it absorbs water and the whole mass becomes starch paste. Both the soluble portion and the insoluble portion are heterogeneous mixtures. The soluble fraction is referred to as amylose, and the insoluble fraction as amylopectin. Most starches contain 80-90 per cent amylopectin and 10—20 per cent amylose. Amylose and amylopectin can be separated by taking advantage of the difference in solubility in water. Both amylose and amylopectin are polymers of glucose and upon hydrolysis with acid they give D-glucose as the product.

Structure of amylose: Amylose is an unbranched long chain polymer in which the glucose residues are linked through α-1, 4- glycosidic linkages. The amylose structure may be regarded as a repeated maltose structure with a free sugar group (acetal group) at one end. This is also known as the reducing end (nth residue), whereas, the opposite end (first residue) is referred to as the non-reducing end. Any particular preparation of amylose usually consists of a mixture of populations of molecules, which differ widely in chain length (number of glucose residues per chain).

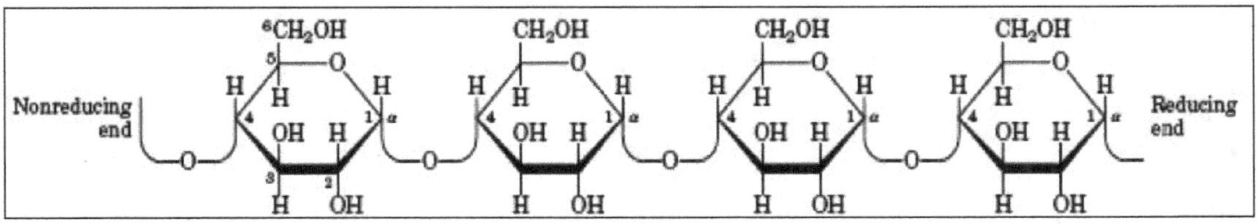

Figure: Amylose.

Structure of amylopectin: Amylopectin is also made of chains of glucose residues, but the chains are highly branched. The glucose residue situated at the branching point is substituted not only on carbon 4 but also on carbon 6. Both amylose and amylopectin give characteristic colour reactions with iodine. Amylose produces a blueblack colour, whereas, amylopectin gives a purple colour.

Saccharification of starch by amylases: Amylases are enzymes of plant and animal origin and they hydrolyze starch. There are two kinds of amylases, alpha-amylases and beta amylases. Alpha-amylases are endo enzymes, act on amylose and amylopectin in a random fashion. Initially more central linkages are cleaved and smaller polysaccharide chains are formed. As the reaction proceeds, these are further hydrolyzed to maltose and glucose.

α-amylases hydrolyze amylose and amylopectin in an orderly fashion. It acts from one end of the polymer and cleaves off two glucose residues at a time, as a maltose unit. As the reaction proceeds, amylose is completely hydrolyzed to maltose. However, with the amylopectin, the reaction stops as a branch point is approached. The terminal parts of the branches are digested away as maltose units in an orderly fashion and the central core is left behind as the enzyme is blocked at 1-6 glycosidic linkages or branch points. The polysaccharide fragment that remains after such incomplete hydrolysis is called a dextrin.

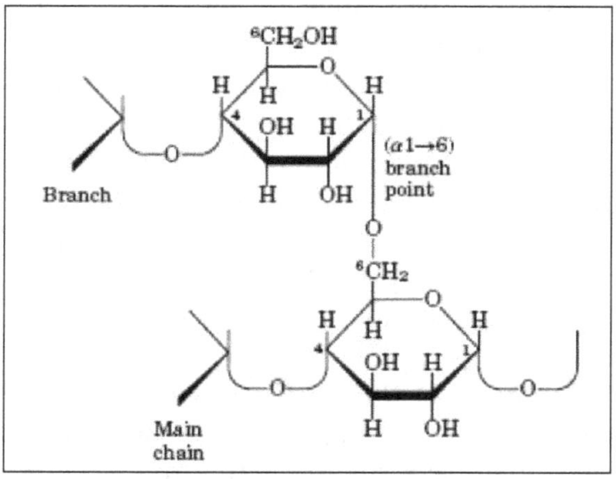

Dextrins formed from amylopectin by β-amylase are highly branched and give a red colour with iodine. Dextrins of relatively small molecular size do not give a colour with iodine. The colour produced by reaction with iodine is used as an indication of the degree of branching of starch. Starch is readily hydrolyzed by dilute mineral acid with ultimate formation of glucose in quantitative yield. The course of hydrolysis may be followed by the gradual change in colour produced by iodine: blue-black-purple-red-colorless.

Celluloses

Cellulose is the most abundant organic compound in nature and it is the chief constituent of the fibrous parts of plants. The purest form of cellulose is usually obtained from cotton. Cellulose is a polymer made up of glucose residues. Upon hydrolysis, cellulose yields D-glucose as the product. Cellulose molecules are not branched and consist essentially of long chains with glucose residues linked in repeating sequence of cellobiose structures. The glucose residues are linked together through β-l, 4-glycosidic linkages. The celluloses obtained from different sources differ in molecular size though they are all made up of glucose. Cellulose is found in plants as micro fibrils (2-20 nm diameter and 100 - 40 000 nm long). These form the structurally strong framework in the cell walls.

Structural unit: Cellulose is a linear polymer of β-(1→ 4) D-glucopyranose units in $^4C_1$ conformation. The fully equatorial conformation of β-linked glucopyranose residues stabilizes the chair structure, minimizing its flexibility (for example, relative to the slightly more flexible α-linked glucopyranose residues in amylose). Cellulose preparations may contain trace amounts (~ 0.3%) of arabinoxylans.

Molecular structure: Cellulose is an insoluble molecule consisting of between 2000 - 14000 residues with some preparations being somewhat shorter. It forms crystals (cellulose Iα) where intra-molecular ($O_3-H \rightarrow O_5'$ and $O_6 \rightarrow H-O_2'$) and intra-strand ($O_6-H \rightarrow O_3'$) hydrogen bonds holds the network flat allowing the more hydrophobic ribbon faces to stack. Each residue is oriented 180° to the next. Although individual strand of cellulose are intrinsically no less hydrophilic, or no more hydrophobic, than some other soluble polysaccharides (such as amylose) this tendency to form crystals utilizing extensive intra and intermolecular hydrogen bonding makes it completely insoluble in normal aqueous solutions. It is thought that water molecules catalyze the formation of the natural cellulose crystals by helping to align the chains through hydrogen-bonded bridging. Part of a cellulose preparation is amorphous between these crystalline sections. The overall structure is of aggregated particles with extensive pores capable of holding relatively large amounts of water by capillarity. The natural crystal is made up from metastable Cellulose I with all the cellulose strands parallel and no inter-sheet hydrogen bonding. This cellulose I (natural cellulose) contains two coexisting phases' cellulose Iα (triclinic) and cellulose Iβ (monoclinic) in varying proportions dependent on its origin.

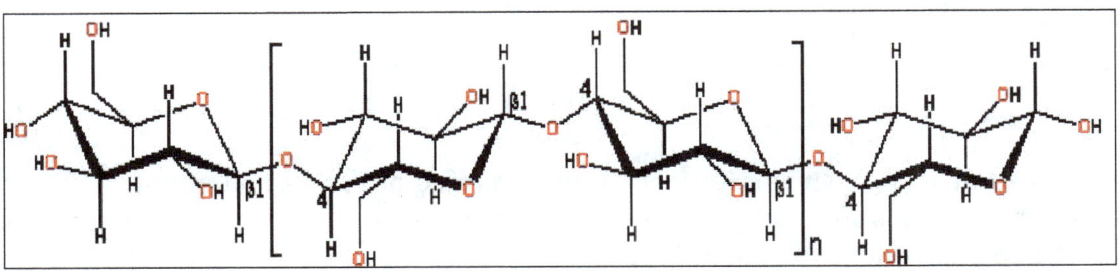

Function: Cellulose is the structural component of the primary cell wall of green plants, many forms of algae and the oomycetes. Some species of bacteria secrete it to form biofilms.

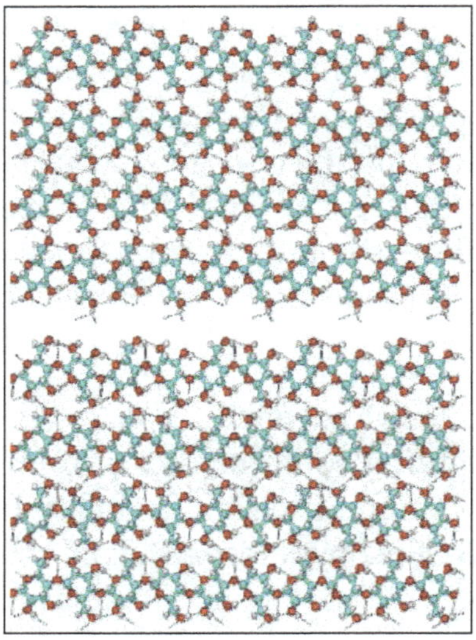

Figure: Organization of glucose chains in cellulose.

Glycogen

Glycogen is the reserve carbohydrate in the animals and it is found in significant amounts in the liver and muscle. Glycogen is made up of D-glucose residues. Upon hydrolysis, it yields D-glucose as the product. Glycogen is a highly branched chain polysaccharide and it resembles amylopectin in structure. Thus glucose residues are linked together through α-l, 4- glycosidic linkages except at the branch points. The branch is linked to the main chain through α-l, 6-glycosidic linkages. It is very similar to the structure of amylopectin. The average molecular weights of glycogen preparations vary from 270,000 to 100,000,000. A single preparation usually consists of a mixture of populations of molecules that differ in molecular weight. In the structure of glycogen, O represents glucose residues. The arrows indicate the α-1→6 glycosidic linkage. All the other glycosidic linkage are α-1,4 . The asterisks indicate the non—reducing end groups and r.e. strands for reducing end group.

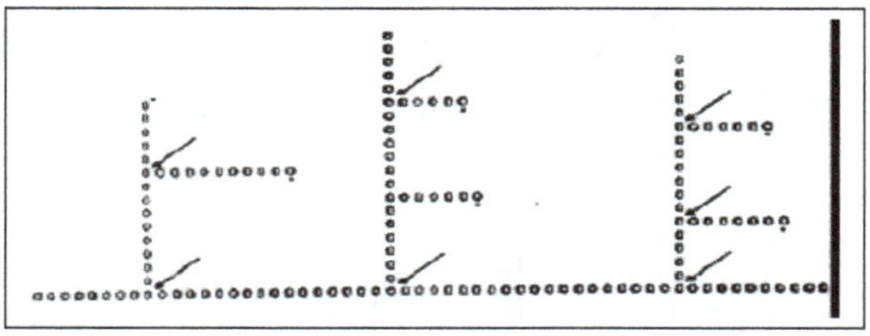

In a wide range of organisms, excess glucose is stored not as monomer but converted to polymeric forms for storage—glycogen in vertebrates and many microorganisms, starch in plants. With two minor differences, glycogen has almost the same structure as amylopectin (a constituent of starch). The glycogen molecule is roughly twice as large as amylopectin and branching frequency—that also controls the mobilization of stored polysaccharide. Glycogen has roughly twice as many branches (branching occurs on an average after every 8-12 residues unlike amylopectin where it is after every 24-30 residues). There is an advantage to branched polysaccharides such as amylopectin and glycogen. During times of shortage, enzymes attack one end of the polymer chain and cut off glucose molecules, one at a time. The more the branches, more will be the points at which the enzyme attacks the polysaccharide. Thus, a highly branched polysaccharide is better suited for the rapid release of glucose than a linear polymer.

In vertebrates, glycogen is found primarily in the liver and skeletal muscle but can also be made by the brain, uterus, and the vagina. However, muscle glycogen is not generally available to other tissues, because muscle lacks the enzyme glucose-6-phosphatase. Glycogen may represent up to 10% of the weight of liver and 1% to 2% of the weight of muscle. Stores of glycogen in the liver are considered the main buffer of blood glucose levels. If this much glucose was dissolved in the cytosol of a hepatocyte, its concentration would be about 0.4 M, enough to dominate the osmotic properties of the cell. When stored as a long polymer (glycogen), however, the same mass of glucose has a concentration of only 0.01 μM. Glycogen is stored in large cytosolic granules. The elementary particle of glycogen, the β particle, about 21 nm in diameter, consists of up to 55,000 glucose residues with about 2,000 non-reducing ends. The major site of daily glucose consumption (75%) is the brain via aerobic pathways. Most of the remainder of it is utilized by erythrocytes, skeletal muscle, and heart muscle. Due to disbalance in glucose utilization diabetics may experience.

Glycogen degradation and synthesis are relatively simple biochemical processes. Glycogen synthesis differs from glycogen breakdown. Unlike breakdown, synthesis is endergonic, meaning that glycogen is not synthesized without the input of energy. Energy for glycogen synthesis comes from UTP, which reacts with glucose-1-phosphate, forming UDP-glucose, in reaction catalyzed by UDP-glucose pyrophosphorylase. Glycogen is synthesized from monomers of UDP-glucose by the enzyme Glycogen synthase, which progressively lengthens the glycogen chain. As glycogen synthase can only lengthen an existing chain, the protein glycogenin is needed to initiate the synthesis of glycogen. Glycogen degradation consists of three steps:

- The release of glucose 1-phosphate from glycogen.
- The remodeling of the glycogen substrate to permit further degradation.
- The conversion of glucose 1-phosphate into glucose 6-phosphate for further metabolism.

It is cleaved from the non-reducing ends of the chain by the enzyme glycogen phosphorylase to produce monomers of glucose-1-phosphate that is then converted to glucose 6-phosphate. A special debranching enzyme is needed to remove the α (1-6) branches in branched glycogen and reshape the chain into linear polymer. Debranching enzyme has two independent active sites, consisting of residues in different segments of a single polypeptide chain, that catalyze α(1-6) glucosidase and transferase (transglycosylase) reactions.

The transferase of the debranching enzyme transfers three glucose residues from a

4-residue limit branch to the end of another branch, diminishing the limit branch to a single glucose residue. The α(1-6) glucosidase moiety of the debranching enzyme then catalyzes hydrolysis of the α(1-6) linkage, yielding free glucose. This is a minor fraction of glucose released from glycogen. The major product of glycogen breakdown is glucose-1-phosphate, arising from phosphorylase activity, which is subsequently converted, to glucose-6- phosphate. The G6P monomers produced have three possible fates:

- G6P can continue on the glycolysis pathway and be used as fuel.
- G6P can enter the pentose phosphate pathway via the enzyme glucose-6-phosphate dehydrogenase to produce NADPH and 5-carbon sugars.
- In the liver and kidney, G6P can be dephosphorylated back to glucose by the enzyme glucose 6-phosphatase. This is the final step in the gluconeogenesis pathway.

Chitin

Chitin is a linear homopolysacchande composed of N-acetyl- D-glucosamine residues in βlinkage. The only chemical difference from cellulose is the replacement of a hydroxyl group at C-2 with an acetylated amino group. Chitin forms extended fibers similar to those of cellulose, and structure of glycogen. Chitin like cellulose is indigestible by vertebrate animals. It is the main component of the cell walls of fungi, the exoskeletons of arthropods, such as crustaceans (like the crab, lobster and shrimp) and the insects, including ants, beetles and butterflies, the radula of mollusks and the beaks of the cephalopods, including squid and octopuses. Chitin is probably the second most abundant polysaccharide next to cellulose, in nature.

Chitin is used in water purification, and as an additive to thicken and stabilize foods and pharmaceuticals. It also acts as a binder in dyes, fabrics, and adhesives. Industrial separation membranes and ion-exchange resins can be made from chitin. Processes to size and strengthen paper employ chitin. Its properties as a flexible and strong material make it favorable as surgical thread. Its biodegradability means it wears away with time as the wound heals. Moreover, the polysaccharide has some unusual properties that accelerate healing of wounds in humans. Most recent studies point out that chitin is a good inductor for defense mechanisms in plants. It is being tested as a fertilizer that can help plants develop healthy immune responses, and have a much better yield and life expectancy.

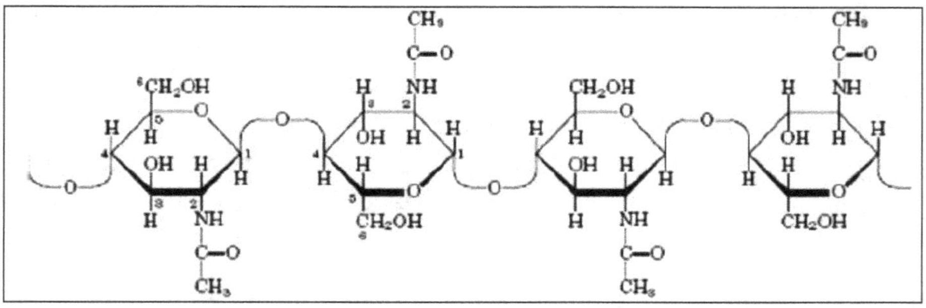

Heteropolysaccharides

A heteropolysaccharide is made up of two or more different monosaccharides, or monosaccharide derivatives.

Agar

Agar (agar-agar, kanten, agal-agal, Ceylon agar, china grass) is a gelatinous substance chiefly used as a solid substrate to culture medium for microbiological work. It is an unbranched polysaccharide obtained from the cell membranes of some species of red algae or seaweed. Chemically, agar is a polymer made up of subunits of the sugar galactose. Agar polysaccharides serve as the primary structural support for the algae's cell walls. Agar is a heterogeneous mixture of two classes of polysaccharide: agaropectin and agarose. Although both polysaccharide classes share the same galactose-based backbone, agaropectin is heavily modified with acidic side-groups, such as sulfate and pyruvate. Agarose is composed of agarobiose repeating disaccharide units alternating with 1, 3-linked-β-Dgalactopyranose and 1, 4-linked-3, 6-anhydro-α-L-galactopyranose. The agaropectin seems to have the same backbone as the agarose, but contains considerable amount of acid groups such as sulfate, pyruvate and glucuronate groups.

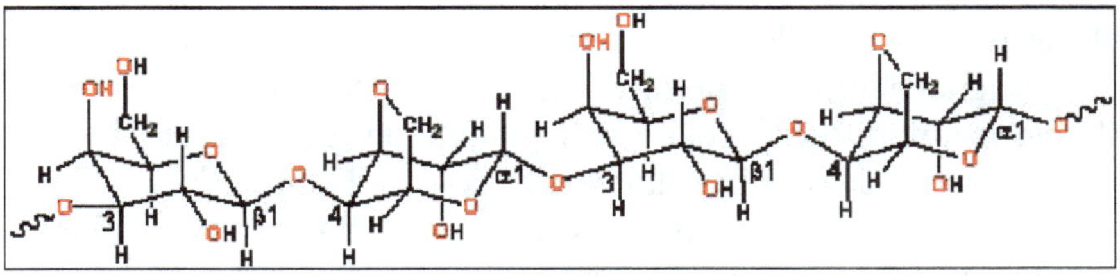

Property: Agar is insoluble in cold water but dissolves to give random coils in boiling water. Gelation is reported to follow a phase separation process (although these findings are disputed) and association on cooling (~ 35°C), forming gels with up to 99.5% water and remaining solid up to about 85°C. It is derived primarily from Gracilaria species.

Uses: Agar has a major use in microbiological media as it is not easy for microorganisms to metabolize and forms clear, stable and firm gels, but in the food area it is used in icings, glazes, processed cheese, jelly sweets and marshmallows. It may be used in tropical countries and by vegetarians as a substitute for gelatin. Agar is used to form a surface for the growth of bacterial colonies. Another commercial use of agar is for the capsules in which some vitamins and drugs are packaged; the dried agar material dissolves readily in the stomach and is metabolically inert.

Agarose

Certain marine red algae, including some of the seaweeds, have cell walls that contain agar, a mixture of sulfated heteropolysaccharide made up of D-galactose and an Lgalactose derivative ether-linked between C-3 and C-6. The two major components of agar are the unbranched polymer agarose (Mr ~ 120,000) and a branched component, agaropectin. The remarkable gel-forming property of agarose makes it useful in the biochemistry. When a suspension of agarose in water is heated and cooled, the agarose forms a double helix; two molecules in parallel orientation twist together with a helix repeat of three residues; water molecules are trapped in the central cavity. These structures in turn associate with each other to form a gel, a three-dimensional matrix that traps large amounts of water. Exterior hydroxyl groups allow aggregation of up to 10,000 of these helices to form suprafibers. Agarose gels are used as inert supports for the electrophoretic separation of nucleic acids, an essential part of the DNA sequencing process.

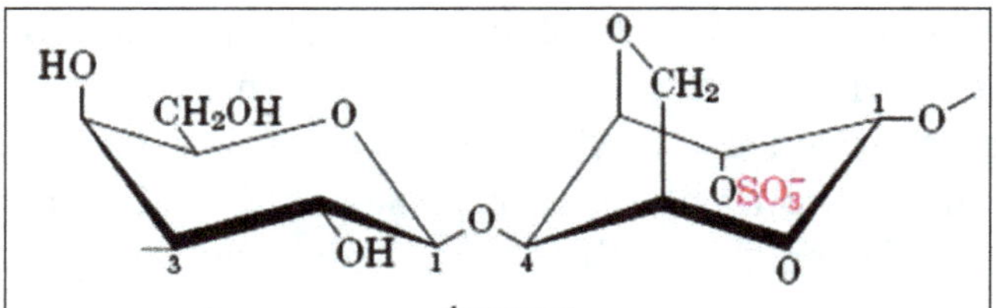

Agarose
3)D-Gal(β1→4)3,6-anhydro-L-Gal2S(α1 repeats

Xylan

Lignocelluloses in plant kingdom are composed of cellulose, hemicellulose and lignin. 15- 30% of the lignocellulose is hemicellulose, where xylan is the main component. They are almost as ubiquitous as cellulose in plant-cell walls and contain predominantly beta-Dxylose units linked as in cellulose. Xylan is a heteropolysaccharide found in plant cell walls and some algae. It is found in almost all parts of the plant, in the cell walls of some green algae, especially macrophytic siphonous genera, where it replaces cellulose.

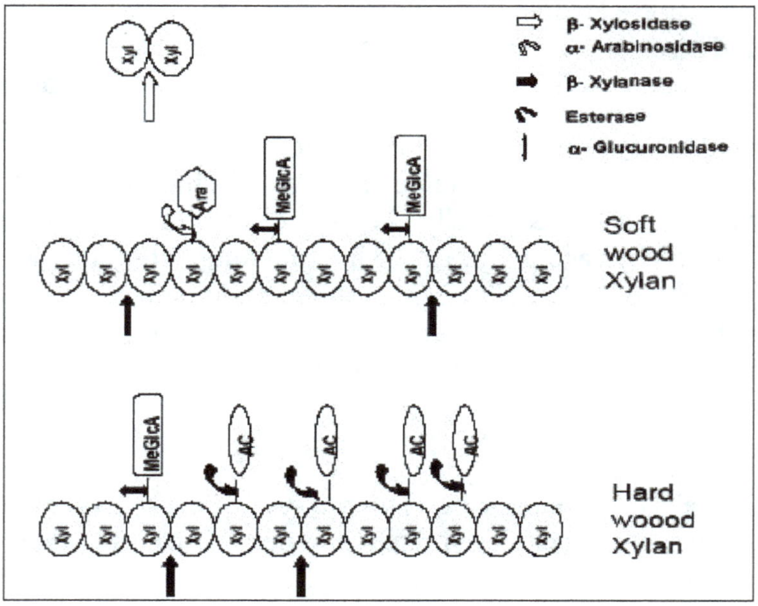

Similarly, it replaces the inner fibrillar cell-wall layer of cellulose in some red algae. Xylans are polysaccarides mainly having backbone of 1,4 beta-linked xylose. The backbone is branched with sugars like glucose, arabinose, acetylated sugars and esters through alpha linkage. Xylans are of little commercial importance, but being associated with cellulose, forms a part of sugar hydrolysis project to be converted to alcohol and other value added products. In tune with the emergent need for production of ethanol from sugars xylan as hemicellulose forms the main component, which supports complete utilization of cellulose through enzymatic saccharification.

Alginate

Alginates are produced by brown seaweeds (Phaeophyceae, mainly Laminaria). Alginates are linear unbranched polymers containing β-(1-4)-linked D-mannuronic acid (M) and α-(1- 4)-linked L-guluronic acid (G) residues. Although these residues are epimers (Dmannuronic acid residues being enzymatically converted to L-guluronic acid after polymerizationa) and only differ at C5, they possess very different conformations; Dmannuronic acid being 4C1 with diequatorial links between them and L-guluronic acid being 1C4 with diaxial links between them. Bacterial alginates are additionally O-acetylated on the 2 and/or 3 positions of the D-mannuronic acid residues. The bacterial O-acetylase may be used to O-acetylate the algal alginates, so increasing their water binding.

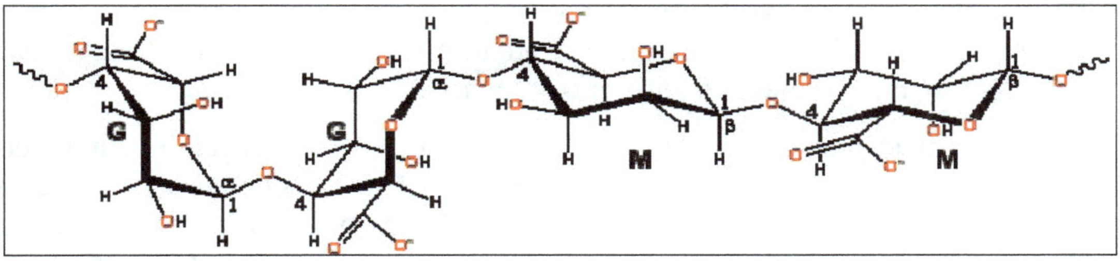

Molecular Structure

Alginates are not random copolymers but, according to the source algae, consist of blocks of similar and strictly alternating residues (that is, MMMMMM, GGGGGG and GMGMGMGM), each of which have different conformational preferences and behavior. As examples, the M/G ratio of alginate from Macrocystis pyrifera is about 1.6 whereas that from Laminaria hyperborea is about 0.45.

Functionality

The primary functions of the alginates are as thermally stable cold setting gelling agents in the presence of calcium ions; gelling at far lower concentrations than gelatin. Such gels can be heat treated without melting, although they may eventually degrade.

Alginate's solubility and water-holding capacity depend on pH (precipitating below about pH 3.5), molecular weight (lower molecular weight calcium alginate chains with less than 500 residues showing increasing water binding with increasing size), ionic strength (low ionic strength increasing the extended nature of the chains) and the nature of the ions present. Generally alginates show high water absorption and may be used as low viscosity emulsifiers and shear-thinning thickeners. They can be used to stabilize phase separation in low fat fat-substitutes.

Food Contains Healthy Carbohydrates

Carbohydrates are an essential component of the diet, and many high-carb foods offer excellent health benefits.

High-Carb Vegetables

Adding these healthful, high-carb vegetables to a meal will boost its carbohydrate content.

- Sweet Potatoes: Sweet potatoes are a delicious favorite to include in a range of meals. One medium, baked sweet potato with the skin on has 23.61 grams (g) of carbohydrates. Sweet potatoes are an excellent source of potassium and vitamins A and C. Some of the carbohydrate molecules in purple sweet potato may also have antioxidant and antitumor benefits.
- Beets: Beetroots, or beets, are a sweet, purple root vegetable that people can eat either raw or cooked. One cup of raw beets has 13 g of carbs. Beets are rich in potassium, calcium, folate, and vitamin A. They also provide people with naturally occurring inorganic nitrates that can benefit heart health.
- Corn: Corn is a popular vegetable that people can enjoy year-round as a side dish, on the cob, or in a salad. A measure of 100 g of corn contains 25 g of carbohydrates and 3.36 g of protein. It also provides a good amount of vitamin C. Corn is beneficial for blood sugar levels and high blood pressure.

High-Carb Grains

Grains and pseudo grains, which are the seeds of broadleaf plants, are great sources of carbohydrates. Whole-grain varieties provide protein and fiber and offer plenty of additional healthful benefits.

Grains are versatile and can form the main part of many meals. Rather than eating white rice and white bread, people can incorporate the following healthful high-carb grains into their diet:

- Quinoa: Quinoa is a nutritious pseudo grain. It tastes similar to other types of grain, and people can prepare and eat it in the same way. One cup of quinoa contains 39.41 g of carbohydrates, 8.14 g of protein, and only 1.61 g of sugar. Quinoa is also rich in minerals, including magnesium, potassium, and phosphorus. As quinoa is high in both fiber and protein, it may help people lose weight. Quinoa may help control blood sugar levels too.
- Brown Rice: Brown rice is a common side dish and a healthful alternative to white rice. One cup of cooked brown rice has 36 g of carbohydrates. This grain is also rich in antioxidants.
- Oats: Oats are one of the most healthful and versatile whole grains. Different varieties are available, including rolled, steel cut, and quick oats. A cup of old-fashioned rolled oats will provide 27 g of carbohydrates, in addition to 5 g of protein and 4 g of fiber.

High-Carb Fruits

Fruits are an excellent source of healthful carbohydrates, particularly those below:

- Bananas: Bananas are widely available and make for a convenient snack. One medium banana has 26.95 g of carbs. Like sweet potatoes, they are also rich in potassium and vitamins A and C. As a result of their potassium content, bananas are good for heart health and lowering blood pressure.
- Apples: Apples are crunchy fruits that it is possible to buy year-round in grocery stores. They come in many varieties. One medium apple contains 25.13 g of carbohydrates. It also provides vitamins A and C, potassium, and fiber. According to a study involving older women, apples may lower the risk of disease-related mortality, including cancer mortality.
- Mangos: Mangos are a sweet tropical fruit. One cup of chopped mangos has 24.72 g of carbohydrates. Mangos are also high in vitamins A and C, potassium, and fiber. Try adding mango chunks to breakfast cereals or smoothies. Mango is also great eaten alone as a snack. They are ready to eat when they yield slightly to gentle pressure.

High-Carb Dried Fruits

A range of healthful dried fruits can help people achieve their daily carbohydrate needs. People can try eating the following dried fruits alone as a snack or adding them to a trail mix or meal:

- Dates: There are many varieties of date, and they are naturally sweet enough to be used as a sweet snack or dessert. There are 17.99 g of carbohydrates in one pitted Medjool date. This fruit is also rich in fiber, calcium, phosphorus, potassium, and vitamin A.

- Raisins: Raisins are dried grapes that work as a standalone snack or can add flavor and texture to cereal bars, salads, yogurts, or granola. One cup of raisins packs in 129.48 g of carbohydrates. They also contain minerals, including potassium, magnesium, phosphorus, and calcium. Raisins are a good source of antioxidants too.
- Goji Berries: People refer to goji berries as a superfood due to their high antioxidant content. One cup has 32 g of carbohydrates and 5 g of protein. Goji berries are also a great source of vitamin A.

High-Carb Pulses

Pulses, such as beans and lentils, are high in carbohydrates, protein, and fiber. They are a great addition to any diet and can help people feel fuller for longer. Try the following healthful, high-carb pulses:

- Kidney Beans: Kidney beans belong to the legume family. They are one of the most common beans to include in the diet. One cup of kidney beans has 21 g of carbohydrates. They are also a good source of protein and fiber, with 6.99 g and 8.1 g per cup respectively. These beans also contain potassium and iron. The consumption of white or dark kidney beans may improve inflammation in the colon.
- Garbanzo Beans: Garbanzo beans, or chickpeas, are also legumes. They are the primary ingredient of hummus. One cup contains 19.01 g of carbohydrates as well as 5 g of protein. Garbanzo beans are rich in fiber and calcium. Study results suggest that they can improve heart health and digestion.
- Lentils: Lentils are popular high-protein legumes. One cup of boiled lentils provides 39.86 g of carbohydrates along with 17.86 g of protein and 15.6 g of fiber. Lentils are high in phosphorus, potassium, calcium, and folate.

Carbohydrates Function in Body

Carbohydrates are an essential part of our diet. Most importantly, they provide the energy for the most obvious functions of our body, such as moving or thinking, but also for the 'background' functions that most of the time we do not even notice . During digestion, carbohydrates that consist of more than one sugar get broken down into their monosaccharides by digestive enzymes, and then get directly absorbed causing a glycaemic response. The body uses glucose directly as energy source in muscle, brain and other cells. Some of the carbohydrates cannot be broken down and they get either fermented by our gut bacteria or they transit through the gut without being changed. Interestingly, carbohydrates also play an important role in the structure and function of our cells, tissues and organs.

Carbohydrates as Energy Source and their Storage

Carbohydrates broken down to mainly glucose are the preferred source of energy for our body, as cells in our brain, muscle and all other tissues directly use monosaccharides for their energy needs. Depending on the type, a gram of carbohydrates provides different amounts of energy:

- Starches and sugars are the main energy-providing carbohydrates, and supply 4 kilocalories (17 kilojoules) per gram.
- Polyols provide 2.4 kilocalories (10 kilojoules) (erythritol is not digested at all, and thus gives 0 calories).
- Dietary fibre 2 kilocalories (8 kilojoules).

Monosaccharides are directly absorbed by the small intestine into the bloodstream, where they are transported to the cells in need. Several hormones, including insulin and glucagon, are also part of the digestive system. They maintain our blood sugar levels by removing or adding glucose to the blood stream as needed.

If not used directly, the body converts glucose to glycogen, a polysaccharide like starch, which is stored in the liver and the muscles as a readily available source of energy. When needed, for instance, between meals, at night, during spurs of physical activity, or during short fasting periods, our body converts glycogen back to glucose to maintain a constant blood sugar level.

The brain and the red blood cells are especially dependent on glucose as energy source, and can use other forms of energy from fats in extreme circumstances, like in very extended periods of starvation. It is for this reason that our blood glucose must be constantly maintained at an optimum level. Approximately 130 g of glucose are needed per day to cover the energy needs of the adult brain alone.

The Glycaemic Response and Glycaemic Index

When we eat a carbohydrate containing food our blood glucose level rises and then decreases, this process is known as the glycemic response. It reflects the rate of digestion and absorption of glucose, as well as the effects of insulin in normalizing the blood glucose level. A number of factors influence the rate and duration of the glycaemic response:

- The food itself:
  - The type of the sugar(s) that form(s) the carbohydrate; e.g. fructose has a

lower glycemic response than glucose, and sucrose has a lower glycemic response than maltose.

- The structure of the molecule; e.g. a starch with more branches is more easily broken down by enzymes and therefore more readily digestible than others.
- The cooking and processing methods used.
- The amount of other nutrients in the food, such as fat, protein, and fibre.

- The (metabolic) circumstances in every individual:
  - The extent of chewing (mechanical breakdown).
  - The rate of gastric emptying.
  - Transit time through the small intestine (which is partly influenced by the food).
  - Metabolism itself.
  - The time of day the food is ingested.

The impact of different foods (as well as the processing technique of foods) on the glycaemic response is classified relative to a standard, usually white bread or glucose, within two hours after eating. This measurement is called the glycaemic index (GI). A GI of 70 means that the food or drink causes 70% of the blood glucose response which would be observed with the same amount of carbohydrate from pure glucose or white bread; however, most of the time carbohydrates are eaten as a mixture and alongside proteins and fats which all influence the GI.

High GI foods cause a greater blood glucose response than low GI foods. At the same time, foods with a low GI are digested and absorbed more slowly than foods which have a high GI. There is a lot of discussion in the scientific community, but currently insufficient evidence to suggest that a diet based on low GI foods is associated with a reduced risk of developing metabolic diseases such as obesity and type 2 diabetes.

The Glycaemic index of some common foods (using glucose as standard)	
Foods with a very low GI (≤ 40)	Raw apple Lentils Soybeans Kidney beans Cow's milk Carrots (boiled) Barley

Foods with a low GI (41-55)	Noodles and pasta Apple juice Raw oranges/orange juice Dates Raw banana Yoghurt (fruit) Whole grain bread Strawberry jam Sweet corn Chocolate
Foods with an intermediate GI (56-70)	Brown rice Rolled oats Soft drinks Pineapple Honey Sourdough bread
Foods with a high GI (> 70)	White and wholemeal bread Boiled potato Cornflakes French Fries Mashed potatoes White rice Rice crackers

Gut Function and Dietary Fibre

Although our small intestine is unable to digest dietary fibre, fibre helps to ensure good gut function by increasing the physical bulk in the bowel, and thereby stimulating the intestinal transit. Once the indigestible carbohydrates pass into the large intestine, some types of fibre such as gums, pectins and oligosaccharides are broken down by the gut microflora. This increases the overall mass in the bowel and has a beneficial effect on the make-up of our gut microflora. It also leads to formation of bacterial waste products, like the short-chain fatty acids, which are released in the colon with beneficial effects on our health.

Digestion and Absorption of Carbohydrates

From the Mouth to the Stomach

The mechanical and chemical digestion of carbohydrates begins in the mouth. Chewing, also known as mastication, crumbles the carbohydrate foods into smaller and smaller pieces. The salivary glands in the oral cavity secrete saliva that coats the food particles. Saliva contains the enzyme, salivary amylase. This enzyme breaks the bonds between the monomeric sugar units of disaccharides, oligosaccharides, and starches. The salivary amylase breaks down amylose and amylopectin into smaller chains of glucose, called dextrins and maltose. The increased concentration of maltose in the mouth that results from the mechanical and chemical breakdown of starches in whole grains is what enhances their sweetness. Only about five percent of starches are broken down in the mouth. (This is a good thing as more glucose in the mouth would lead to more tooth decay.) When carbohydrates reach the stomach no further chemical breakdown occurs because the amylase enzyme does not function in the acidic conditions of the stomach. But mechanical breakdown is ongoing—the strong peristaltic contractions of the stomach mix the carbohydrates into the more uniform mixture of chyme.

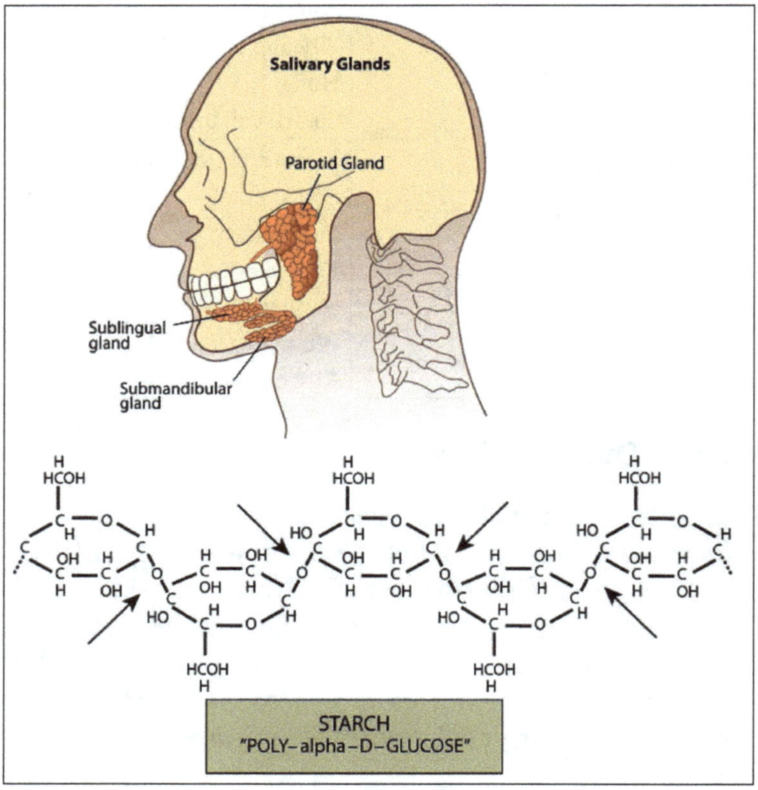

Figure: Salivary Glands in the Mouth.

Salivary glands secrete salivary amylase, which begins the chemical breakdown of carbohydrates by breaking the bonds between monomeric sugar units.

From the Stomach to the Small Intestine

The chyme is gradually expelled into the upper part of the small intestine. Upon entry of the chyme into the small intestine, the pancreas releases pancreatic juice through a duct. This pancreatic juice contains the enzyme, pancreatic amylase, which starts again the breakdown of dextrins into shorter and shorter carbohydrate chains. Additionally, enzymes are secreted by the intestinal cells that line the villi. These enzymes, known collectively as disaccharidase, are sucrase, maltase, and lactase. Sucrase breaks sucrose into glucose and fructose molecules. Maltase breaks the bond between the two glucose units of maltose, and lactase breaks the bond between galactose and glucose. Once carbohydrates are chemically broken down into single sugar units they are then transported into the inside of intestinal cells.

When people do not have enough of the enzyme lactase, lactose is not sufficiently broken down resulting in a condition called lactose intolerance. The undigested lactose moves to the large intestine where bacteria are able to digest it. The bacterial digestion of lactose produces gases leading to symptoms of diarrhea, bloating, and abdominal cramps. Lactose intolerance usually occurs in adults and is associated with race. Most people with lactose intolerance can tolerate some amount of dairy products in their diet. The severity of the symptoms depends on how much lactose is consumed and the degree of lactase deficiency.

Absorption: Going to the Blood Stream

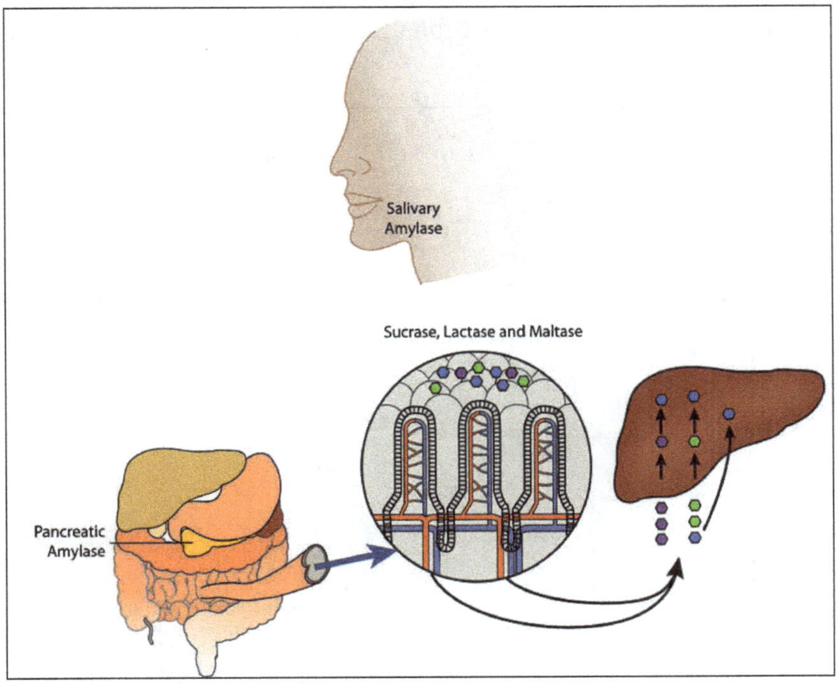

Figure: Carbohydrate Digestion.

The cells in the small intestine have membranes that contain many transport proteins in order to get the monosaccharides and other nutrients into the blood where they can be distributed to the rest of the body. The first organ to receive glucose, fructose, and galactose is the liver. The liver takes them up and converts galactose to glucose, breaks fructose into even smaller carbon-containing units and either stores glucose as glycogen or exports it back to the blood. How much glucose the liver exports to the blood is under hormonal control and you will soon discover that even the glucose itself regulates its concentrations in the blood.

Carbohydrate digestion begins in the mouth and is most extensive in the small intestine. The resultant monosaccharides are absorbed into the bloodstream and transported to the liver.

Maintaining Blood Glucose Levels: The Pancreas and Liver

Glucose levels in the blood are tightly controlled, as having either too much or too little glucose in the blood can have health consequences. Glucose regulates its levels in the blood via a process called negative feedback. An everyday example of negative feedback is in your oven because it contains a thermostat. When you set the temperature to cook a delicious homemade noodle casserole at 375°F the thermostat senses the temperature and sends an electrical signal to turn the elements on and heat up the oven. When the temperature reaches 375°F the thermostat senses the temperature and sends a signal to turn the element off. Similarly, your body senses blood glucose levels and maintains the glucose "temperature" in the target range. The glucose thermostat is located within the cells of the pancreas. After eating a meal containing carbohydrates glucose levels rise in the blood.

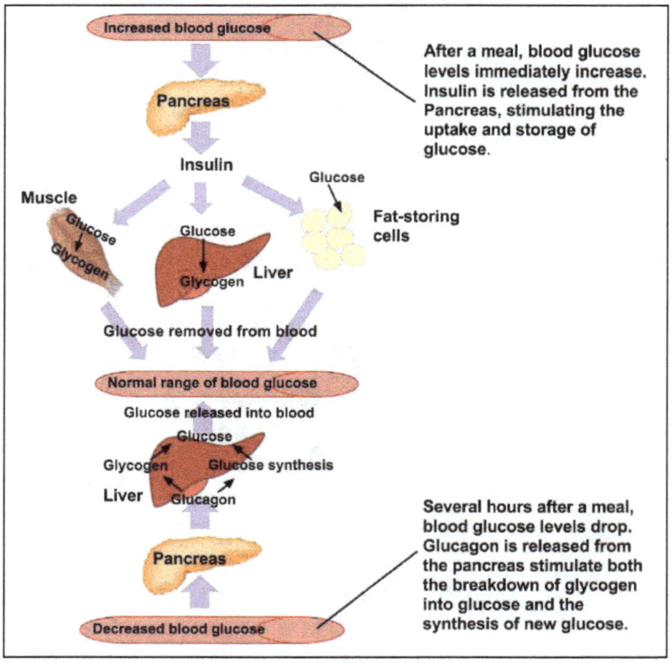

Figure: The Regulation of Glucose.

Insulin-secreting cells in the pancreas sense the increase in blood glucose and release the hormone, insulin, into the blood. Insulin sends a signal to the body's cells to remove glucose from the blood by transporting it into different organ cells around the body and using it to make energy. In the case of muscle tissue and the liver, insulin sends the biological message to store glucose away as glycogen. The presence of insulin in the blood signifies to the body that glucose is available for fuel. As glucose is transported into the cells around the body, the blood glucose levels decrease. Insulin has an opposing hormone called glucagon. Glucagon-secreting cells in the pancreas sense the drop in glucose and, in response, release glucagon into the blood. Glucagon communicates to the cells in the body to stop using all the glucose. More specifically, it signals the liver to break down glycogen and release the stored glucose into the blood, so that glucose levels stay within the target range and all cells get the needed fuel to function properly.

Leftover Carbohydrates: The Large Intestine

Almost all of the carbohydrates, except for dietary fiber and resistant starches, are efficiently digested and absorbed into the body. Some of the remaining indigestible carbohydrates are broken down by enzymes released by bacteria in the large intestine. The products of bacterial digestion of these slow-releasing carbohydrates are short-chain fatty acids and some gases. The short-chain fatty acids are either used by the bacteria to make energy and grow, are eliminated in the feces, or are absorbed into cells of the colon, with a small amount being transported to the liver. Colonic cells use the short-chain fatty acids to support some of their functions. The liver can also metabolize the short-chain fatty acids into cellular energy. The yield of energy from dietary fiber is about 2 kilocalories per gram for humans, but is highly dependent upon the fiber type, with soluble fibers and resistant starches yielding more energy than insoluble fibers. Since dietary fiber is digested much less in the gastrointestinal tract than other carbohydrate types (simple sugars, many starches) the rise in blood glucose after eating them is less, and slower. These physiological attributes of high-fiber foods (i.e. whole grains) are linked to a decrease in weight gain and reduced risk of chronic diseases, such as Type 2 diabetes and cardiovascular disease.

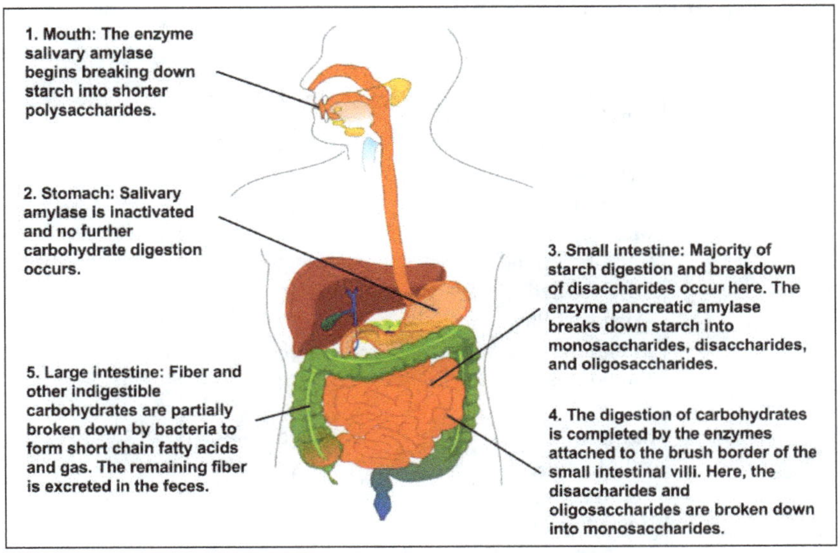

Figure: Carbohydrate Digestion.

A Carbohydrate Feast

You are at a your grandma's house for family dinner and you just consumed kalua pig, white rice, sweet potatoes, mac salad, chicken long rice and a hot sweet bread roll dripping with butter. Less than an hour later you top it off with a slice of haupia pie and then lie down on the couch to watch TV. The "hormone of plenty," insulin, answers the nutrient call. Insulin sends out the physiological message that glucose is abundant in the blood, so that cells can absorb it and either use it or store it. The result of this hormone message is maximization of glycogen stores and all the excess glucose, protein, and lipids are stored as fat.

A typical American Thanksgiving meal contains many foods that are dense in carbohydrates, with the majority of those being simple sugars and starches. These types of carbohydrate foods are rapidly digested and absorbed. Blood glucose levels rise quickly causing a spike in insulin levels. Contrastingly, foods containing high amounts of fiber are like time-release capsules of sugar. A measurement of the effects of a carbohydrate-containing food on blood-glucose levels is called the glycemic response.

Glycemic Index

The glycemic responses of various foods have been measured and then ranked in comparison to a reference food, usually a slice of white bread or just straight glucose, to create a numeric value called the glycemic index (GI). Foods that have a low GI do not raise blood-glucose levels neither as much nor as fast as foods that have a higher GI. A diet of low-GI foods has been shown in epidemiological and clinical trial studies to increase weight loss and reduce the risk of obesity, Type 2 diabetes, and cardiovascular disease.

Table: The glycemic index - Foods in comparison to glucose.

Foods	GI Value
Low GI Foods (< 55)	36
Apple, raw	43
Orange, raw	51
Banana, raw	51
Mango, raw	39
Carrots, boiled	53
Taro, boiled	46
Corn tortilla	37
Spaghetti (whole wheat)	48
Baked beans	34
Soy milk	37
Skim milk	39
Whole milk	41
Yogurt, fruit	14
Yogurt, plain	51
Ice cream	

Medium GI Foods (56–69)	59
Pineapple, raw	65
Cantaloupe	70
Mashed potatoes	69
Whole-wheat bread	55
Brown rice	60
Cheese pizza	63
Sweet potato, boiled	64
Macaroni and cheese	65
Popcorn	
High GI Foods (70 and higher)	**82**
Banana (over-ripe)	72
Corn chips	83
Pretzels	70
White bread	72
White rice	72
Bagel	86
Rice milk	74
Cheerios	73
Raisin Bran	99
Fruit roll-up	78
Gatorade	

The type of carbohydrate within a food affects the GI along with its fat and fiber content. Increased fat and fiber in foods increases the time required for digestion and delays the rate of gastric emptying into the small intestine which, ultimately reduces the GI. Processing and cooking also affects a food's GI by increasing their digestibility. Advancements in the technologies of food processing and the high consumer demand for convenient, precooked foods in the United States has created foods that are digested and absorbed more rapidly, independent of the fiber content. Modern breakfast cereals, breads, pastas, and many prepared foods have a high GI. In contrast, most raw foods have a lower GI. (However, the more ripened a fruit or vegetable is, the higher its GI.)

The GI can be used as a guide for choosing healthier carbohydrate choices but has some limitations. The first is GI does not take into account the amount of carbohydrates in a portion of food, only the type of carbohydrate. Another is that combining low- and high-GI foods changes the GI for the meal. Also, some nutrient-dense foods have higher GIs than less nutritious food. (For instance, oatmeal has a higher GI than chocolate because the fat content of chocolate is higher.) Lastly, meats and fats do not have a GI since they do not contain carbohydrates.

4

Vitamins

A vitamin is an organic molecule that is required in the diet for the normal growth of the body since our body cannot synthesize it. Vitamins are classified as water-soluble and fat-soluble. The topics elaborated in this chapter will help in gaining a better perspective about the types, digestion and absorption of vitamins.

The vitamins are natural and essential nutrients, required in small quantities and play a major role in growth and development, repair and healing wounds, maintaining healthy bones and tissues, for the proper functioning of an immune system, and other biological functions. These essential organic compounds have diverse biochemical functions.

There are thirteen different types of vitamins and all are required for the metabolic processes. The discovery of the vitamins was begun in the year 1912. Based on research and discoveries on vitamins, their sources, functions and deficiency disorders, he is considered as the father of vitamins and vitamin therapy. Similar to minerals, vitamins cannot be synthesized by our body. Therefore, we need to get them from the food we consume or in extreme cases supplements to keep ourselves healthy.

Types of Vitamins

Based on the solubility, vitamins have been classified into two different groups:

Fat-Soluble Vitamin

Fat-soluble vitamins are stored in the fat cells and as the name suggests, these vitamins require fat in order to be absorbed. Vitamin A, D, E and K are fat-soluble vitamins.

Water-Soluble Vitamin

Water-soluble vitamins are not stored in our body as its excess gets excrete through the urine. Therefore, these vitamins need to be replenished constantly. Vitamin B and C are water-soluble vitamins.

Sources of Vitamins

The human body is so designed that it takes what it needs from the food we eat and then it passes out waste as excreta.

These organic substances are abundantly found in both plants and animals source and play a vital role in both growth and development and optimal health. The best sources of fat-soluble vitamins include:

- Vitamin A: Found in potato, carrots, pumpkins, spinach, beef and eggs.
- Vitamin D: Found in fortified milk and other dairy products.
- Vitamin E: Found in fortified cereals, leafy green vegetables, seeds, and nuts.
- Vitamin K: Found in dark green leafy vegetables and in turnip or beet green.

Vitamin C is abundantly found in all citrus fruits. Other sources of Vitamin B and C include:

- Vitamin B1 or Thiamin: Found in pork chops, ham, enriched grains and seeds.
- Vitamin B2 or Riboflavin: Found in whole grains, enriched grains and dairy products.
- Vitamin B3 or Niacin: Found in mushrooms, fish, poultry, and whole grains.
- Vitamin B5 or Pantothenic Acid: Found in chicken, broccoli, legumes and whole grains.
- Vitamin B6 or Pyridoxine: Found in fortified cereals and soy products.
- Vitamin B7 or Biotin: Found in many fruits like fruits and meats.
- Vitamin B9 or Folic Acid: Found in leafy vegetables.
- Vitamin B12: Found in fish, poultry, and meat and dairy products.
- Vitamin C: Found in citrus fruits and juices, such as oranges and grapefruits.

Types of Vitamins

Water-soluble vitamins include eight well-recognized members of the vitamin B complex: thiamine, riboflavin, pyridoxine, pantothenic acid, niacin, biotin, folic acid and vitamin B_{12}; the water-soluble essential nutritional factors: choline, inositol, ascorbic acid; and vitamins with less-defined activity for fish: p-aminobenzoic acid, lipoic acid and citrin. The first eight, though required only in small amounts in the diet, play major roles in growth, physiology and metabolism. Choline, inositol and ascorbic acid are required in appreciable quantities in the diet and sometimes are not referred to as vitamins but as major dietary nutrients.

Table: Water-Soluble vitamin test diet H-440[1/].

Complete test diet (g)		Vitamin mix Mineral mix (mg) (mg)			
Vitamin-free casein	38	Thiamine HCl	5	USP XII No. 2	plus
Gelatin	12	Riboflavin	20	$AlCl_3$	15
Corn oil	6	Pyridoxine HCl	5	$ZnSO_4$	300
Cod liver oil	3	Choline chloride	500	CuCl	10
White dextrin	28	Nicotinic acid	75	$MnSO_4$	80
α -Cellulose mixture [2/]	9	Calcium	50	KI	15
		pantothenate			
α -Cellulose	8	Inositol	200	$CaCl_2$	100
Vitamins	$\frac{1}{9}$	Biotin	0.5	per 100 g of salt mixture	
		Folic acid	1.5		
Mineral mix	4	L-Ascorbic acid	100		
Water	200	Vitamin B_{12} [4/]	0.01		
Total diet as fed	300	Menadione (K)	4		
		a -Tocopherol acetate (E) [3/]	40		

1/ Diet preparation: Dissolve gelatin in cold water. Heat with stirring on water bath to 80°C. Remove from heat. Add with stirring - dextrin, casein, minerals, oils, and vitamins as temperature decreases. Mix well to 40°C. Pour into containers; move to refrigerator to harden. Remove from trays and store in sealed containers in refrigerator until used. Consistency of diet adjusted by amount of water in final mix and length and strength of beating.

2/ Delete two parts α -cellulose and add two parts CMC for preliminary feeding

3/ Dissolve α -tocopherol in oil mix

4/ Add vitamin B_{12} in water during final mixing

Thiamine

Experimental avian polyneuritis, a condition resembling beriberi, was produced by Eijkman in Java in 1886 and the anti-beriberi factor was crystallized and named "vitamine". The term "thiamine" was introduced when the chemical nature of the factor was established. Thiamine was isolated from rice polishing in 1926 and synthesized in 1936.

Chemistry

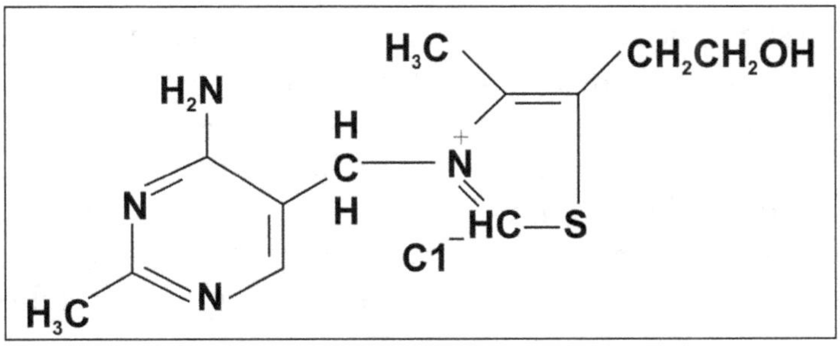

Figure: Thiamine hydrochloride.

Thiamine hydrochloride is a water-soluble, colorless, monoclinic, crystalline compound. It is comparatively stable to dry heat but is rapidly broken down in neutral or alkaline solutions and is split by sulphites into constituent pyrimidine and thiazole moieties. It has a characteristic yeast-like odor. The pyrimide ring is relatively stable, but the thiazole ring is easily opened by hydrolysis. Several derivatives are stable to heat and appear to be more completely soluble in weak alkaline solutions than thiamine itself and still show biological activity in animals. These derivatives include thiamine propyl disulphide, benzoylthiamine disulphide, dibenzoylthiamine, and benzoylthiamine monophosphate. Both thiamine hydrochloride and thiamine mononitrate have been successfully used as the active vitamin in test diets for fish nutrition studies.

Positive Functions

Thiamine functions in all cells as the coenzyme cocarboxylase, thiamine pyrophosphate, which participates in the oxidative decarboxylation of pyruvic acid to acetate for entry into the tricarboxylic acid (TCA) cycle.

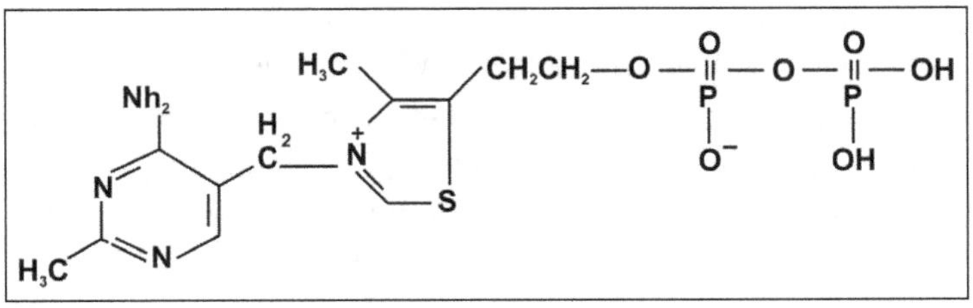

Figure: Thiamine pyrophosphate.

Thiamine pyrophosphate is also a coenzyme of the transketolase system by which direct oxidation of glucose occurs in the cytoplasm of cells via the pentose phosphate pathway. Erythrocyte (RBC) levels of metabolites of this system have been used to indicate thiamine status in experimental animals, including salmon and trout.

Thiamine is essential for good appetite, normal digestion, growth and fertility. It is needed for normal functioning of the nervous tissue and the requirement is determined by the caloric density of the diet.

Deficiency Syndrome

Deficiency signs in salmonids include impaired carbohydrate metabolism, nervous disorders, poor appetite, poor growth, and increased sensitivity to shock. A trunk-winding symptom in eels has been reported, together with hemorrhage at the base of the fins. Skin congestion and subcutaneous hemorrhage occurs in carp fed thiamine-deficient diets. Thiamine deficiency has also been reported in marine flatfish started on clam neck diets stored long enough for thiaminase present to hydrolyze the thiamine in the ration. Typical nervous paralysis occurred with rapid mortality from physical shock.

Table: Vitamin deficiency syndromes.

Vitamin	Symptoms in salmon, trout, carp, catfish
Thiamine	Poor appetite, muscle atrophy, convulsions, instability and loss of equilibrium, oedema, poor growth.
Riboflavin	Corneal vascularization, cloudy lens, hemorrhagic eyes - photophobia, dim vision, incoordination, abnormal pigmentation of iris, striated constrictions of abdominal wall, dark coloration, poor appetite, anemia, poor growth.
Pyridoxine	Nervous disorders, epileptiform fits, hyperirritability, ataxia, anemia, loss of appetite, oedema of peritoneal cavity, colorless serous fluid, rapid postmortem rigor mortis, rapid and gasping breathing, flexing of opercles.
Pantothenic acid	Clubbed gills, prostration, loss of appetite, necrosis and scarring, cellular atrophy, gill exudate, sluggishness, poor growth.
Inositol	Poor growth, distended stomach, increased gastric emptying time, skin lesions.
Biotin	Loss of appetite, lesions in colon, coloration, muscle atrophy, spastic convulsions, fragmentation of erythrocytes, skin lesions, poor growth.
Folic acid	Poor growth, lethargy, fragility of caudal fin, dark coloration, macrocytic anaemia.
Choline	Poor growth, poor food conversion, hemorrhagic kidney and intestine.
Nicotinic acid	Loss of appetite, lesions in colon, jerky or difficult motion, weakness, oedema of stomach and colon, muscle spasms while resting, poor growth.
Vitamin B12	Poor appetite, low hemoglobin, fragmentation of erythrocytes, macrocytic anemia.
Ascorbic acid	Scoliosis, lordosis, impaired collagen formation, altered cartilage, eye lesions, hemorrhagic skin, liver, kidney, intestine, and muscle.
p-Aminobenzoic acid	No abnormal indication in growth appetite, mortality.

Requirements

In determining dietary thiamine requirements of fish, some considerations must be placed upon the composition of dietary ingredients in the ration. Fat content of the diet may affect not only caloric intake but also the thiamine requirement because cocarboxylase participates in the oxidation of that through a-ketoglutarate. Therefore, fish on a high fat diet and low thiamine intake might take longer to develop deficiencies and will give an erroneous requirement.

Sources and Protection

Common sources for thiamine are dried peas, beans, cereal bran, and dried yeast. Fresh glandular tissue is also a good source for thiamine and other members of the vitamin B water-soluble complex, but is seldom used in modern commercial fish diets.

Thiamine can be easily lost by holding diet ingredients too long in storage or by preparing the diet under slightly alkaline conditions or in the presence of sulphide. Wet or frozen diets pose a problem because moisture content increases the chance of enzymatic (thiaminase) hydrolysis and subsequent destruction of thiamine. Obviously, wet or moist diet, preparations containing any fresh fish or shellfish tissue must be used immediately.

Antimetabolites and Inactivation

Acetylcholine is an antagonist to thiamine and pyrithiamine. Oxythiamine and normal butylthiamine are specific antimetabolites. Several thiaminases occur which destroy thiamine. These rupture the thiazole ring at the sulphur bond making the residue inactive. Freshwater fish tissues have high thiaminase activity as do tissues from clams, shrimp and mussels. Thiaminases have also been found in beans and mustard seed and in several micro-organisms. Thiaminase activity is low in most saltwater fish tissues, however, and the enzyme is inactivated by heating or prolonged pasteurization. Thiamine present in fresh Torula yeast is relatively unavailable to fish, but the yeast becomes an excellent thiamine source after rupturing the cells by steam treatment or by dehydration.

Clinical Assessment

Clinical assessment of thiamine status has been made by measuring erythrocyte transketolase activity. Typical saturated levels for thiamine activity in sea salmon range from 15 to 20 g of thiamine/g of wet liver tissue. Fingerling chinook or coho salmon reared in 10 or 15 C water on test diets containing the listed amount or more of thiamine hydrochloride: assayed at 8-10 g of thiamine/g of wet liver tissue. These liver storage levels and normal erythrocyte transketolase activity in the absence of any deficiency sign will indicate an adequate thiamine intake for that fish population.

Riboflavin

Following the recognition that the original water-soluble B consisted of more than one factor, a new growth-promoting factor consisting of yellow-green pigments was isolated in 1879. This new factor was designated G by some and 83 by others. The second water-soluble vitamin discovered was given its specific chemical name riboflavin. Lactoflavin, hepatoflavin, and ovoflavin were also shown to be identical with the pure riboflavin. Riboflavin occurs in the free form only in the eye, whey and urine.

Table: Vitamin requirements for growth1/.

Vitamin (mg/kg dry diet)	Rainbow trout	Brook trout	Brown trout	Atlantic salmon	Chinook salmon	Coho salmon
Thiamine	10-12	10-12	10-12	10-15	10-15	10-15
Riboflavin	20-30	20-30	20-30	5-10	20-25	20-25
Pyridoxine	10-15	10-15	10-15	10-15	15-20	15-20
Pantothenate	40-50	40-50	40-50	*	40-50	40-50
Niacin	120-150	120-150	120-150	*	150-200	150-200
Folacin	6-10	6-10	6-10	5-10	6-10	6-10
Cyanocobalamin	*	*	*	*	0.015-0.02	0.015-0.02
myo-Inositol	200-300	*	*	*	300-400	300-400
Choline	*	*	*	*	600-800	600-800
Biotin	1-1.5	1-1.5	1.5-2	-	1-1.5	1-1.5
Ascorbate	100-150	*	*	*	100-150	50-80
Vitamin A	2 000-2 500 I.U.	*	*	-	*	*
Vitamin E 2/	*	*	*	-	40-50	*
Vitamin K	*	*	*	-	*	*

1/ Fish fed at reference temperature with diets at about protein requirement.

2/ Requirement directly affected by amount and type of unsaturated fat fed.

* Denotes a requirement, the level of which has not been established.

Table: (concluded) vitamin requirements for growth1/.

Vitamin (mg/kg dry diet)	Carp	Channel catfish	Eel	Sea bream	Turbot	Yellowtail
Thiamine	2-3	1-3	2-5	*	2-4	*
Riboflavin	7-10	*	*	*	*	-
Pyridoxine	5-10	*	*	2-5	*	*
Pantothenate	30-40	25-30	*	*	*	*
Niacin	30-50	*	-	*	-	-
Folacin	-	*	*	-	*	-
Cyanocobalamin	-	*	-	*	-	-
myo-Inositol	200-300	*	-	300-500	-	-
Choline	500-600	*	-	*	*	-
Biotin	1-15	*	*	-	*	*
Ascorbate	30-50	30-50	-	*	-	*
Vitamin A	1 000-2 000 I.U.	*	-	-	-	*
Vitamin E	80-100	*	-	-	-	*
Vitamin K	*	*	-	-	-	-

1/ Fish fed at reference temperature with diets at about protein requirement.

2/ Requirement directly affected by amount and type of unsaturated fat fed.

* Denotes a requirement, the level of which has not been established.

Chemistry

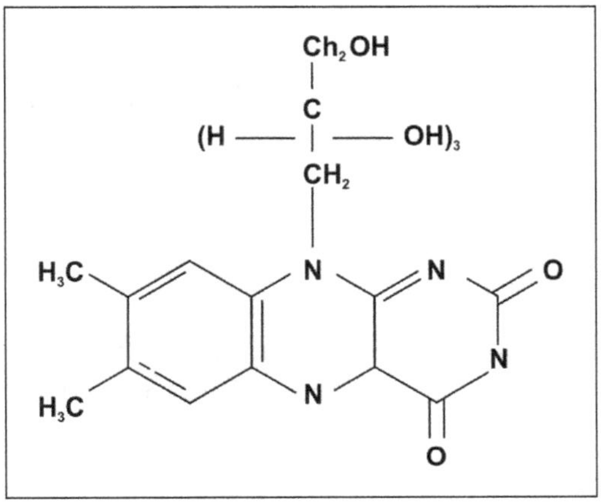

Riboflavin is a yellow-brown crystalline pigment. The vitamin is very slightly soluble in water but soluble in alkali. It is insoluble in most organic solvents. Riboflavin is stable to oxidizing agents in strong mineral acids and in neutral aqueous solution. It is also stable to dry heat but is irreversibly decomposed on irradiation with ultraviolet rays or visible light, breaking down to lumiflavin. Riboflavin phosphate is the chemically active group of Warburg's 'yellow' enzyme.

Positive Functions

Riboflavin functions in the tissues in the form of flavin adenine dinucleotide (FAD) or as flavin mononucleotide (FMN). The flavo-proteins function as enzymes of tissue respiration and are involved in hydrogen transport to catalyze the oxidation of reduced pyridine nucleotides (NADH and NADPH). Thus, they function as coenzymes for many oxidases and redunctases such as cytochrome e reductase, D- and L-amino acid oxidases, xanthine and aldehyde oxidase, succinic dehydrogenase, glucose oxidase and fumaric dehydrogenase. Riboflavin is also involved with pyridoxine in the conversion of tryptophan to nicotinic acid and is most important in the respiration of poorly vascularized tissues such as the cornea of the eye. Riboflavin is involved in the retinal pigment during light adaptation and lack of it causes impaired vision and photophobia in experimental animals, including fish.

Deficiency Syndrome

Tissue riboflavin is exhausted in young salmonids after 10 to 12 weeks on riboflavin-deficient diets in 10-15 °C water systems. Poor appetite and poor diet efficiency are the first signs, followed by photophobia, mono or bilateral cataract's, corneal vascularization, eye hemorrhage, incoordination, and general anemia. Dark pigmentation, coupled with striated constrictions of abdominal wall in salmon has been noted. Skin atrophy has been reported for some fish species and abnormal pigmentation of both skin and iris has been noted. Replacement of riboflavin in the diet reduced the symptoms except when cataracts have developed. This irreversible condition will continue in monolateral cataracts throughout the life of the fish, whereas bilateral cataracts largely result in eventual starvation and death of the afflicted animal. The first specific signs have consistently appeared in and about the eyes of salmonids, carps and catfish.

Requirements

Values for the trout are slightly lower than those reported for salmon. The requirements may vary depending upon the balance of other dietary ingredients, caloric density and environmental conditions under which the fish is raised. The values established under these standard test conditions should serve as tentative-levels which will satisfy biological demands for normal growth, health, and physiological function. Most of these studies have been made on very young fish, often initially feeding fry, with the logical assumption that their vitamin needs would be more than that of larger fish having advanced metabolic enzyme systems capable of synthesizing at least some of these vitamins to partially meet the requirements.

Sources and Protection

Riboflavin is widely distributed in plants and in animal glandular tissues. Milk, liver, kidney, heart, yeast, germinated grains, peanuts, soybeans and eggs are rich sources. Keeping feeds from sunlight or intense artificial light is necessary to minimize loss of the vitamin by conversion to lumiflavin.

Antimetabolites and Inactivation

When the ribose group in the molecule is replaced by other groups, analogues are formed which either have reduced activity or become antimetabolites. Galactoflavin is an antagonist to riboflavin and inhibits growth of rats when the diet contains this compound. Flavin monosulphate inhibits D-amino acid oxidase and appears to act as a competitor and inhibitor for growth of Lactobacillus casei. The hydroxyethyl analogue is an antagonist for riboflavin function in both rats and bacteria and also shows antifungal activity.

Clinical Assessment

Liver tissue of actively feeding sea salmon contains 6-8 g of riboflavin/g of wet tissue. In a freshwater environment, young fish fed test diets in 15 °C water systems showed liver storage of 3.5-4.0 μg/g. Riboflavin content of blood plasma does not change significantly in riboflavin deficiency in experimental animals. However, the erythrocyte riboflavin content has been reported at around 10 μ g/100 ml blood for man on low riboflavin intake and approximately twice that level on high intake. Urinary excretion of riboflavin has been used clinically to indicate dietary status, with 200 μ g/24 it suggesting adequate intake and less than 100 μg indicating low intake. Excretion of 50 μg or less daily is strong indication of extended dietary deficiency.

Pyridoxine

A new factor which could cure dermatitis in rats was reported by Györgi in 1935 and was named vitamin B_6. The name pyridoxine is also attributed to Györgi. The active material was isolated in 1939 and pyridoxine was subsequently synthesized. Pyridoxine deficiency has since been reported in trout and in salmon.

Chemistry

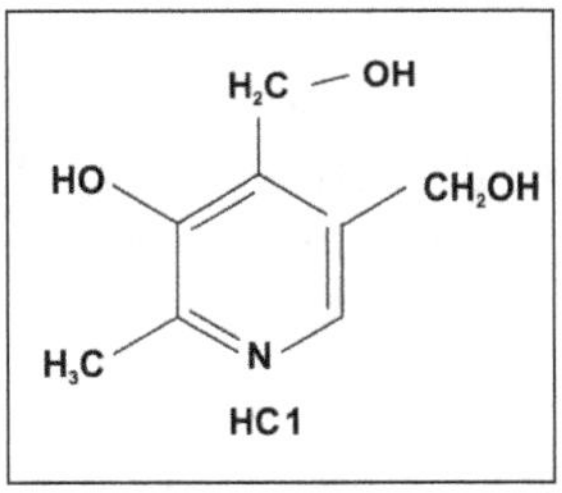

Figure: Pyrodoxine hydrochloride

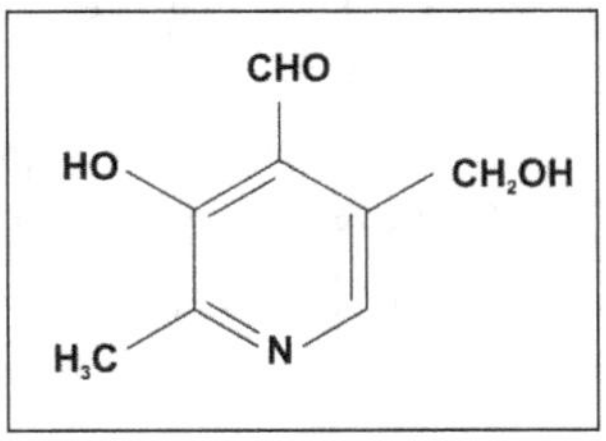

Figure: Pyridoxal

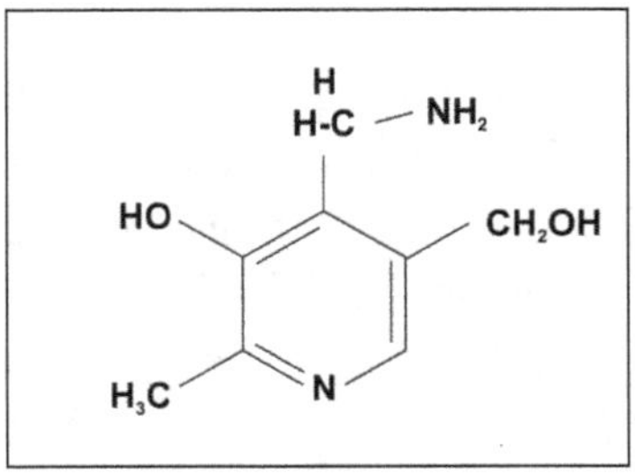

Figure: Pyridoxamine

Compounds which have vitamin B_6 activity include: pyridoxine, pyridoxal and pyridoxamine. Pyridoxine hydrochloride is readily soluble in water and is heat stable in either acid or alkaline solution. It acts as a coenzyme in a number of enzyme systems. Pyridoxine is sensitive to ultraviolet light in neutral or alkaline solutions. Pyridoxamine and pyridoxal in dilute solutions are labile compounds which are rapidly destroyed on exposure to air, heat, or light. Therefore, most vitamin supplementation is in the form of pyridoxine hydrochloride and analysis for pyridoxine activity by microbiological assay of diet ingredients probably measures pyridoxal phosphate and other intermediates as well.

Positive Functions

Pyridoxal phosphate is the coenzyme, codecarboxylase, involved in the decarboxylation of amino acids. It is also the co-factor of the 22 different transaminases present in animal tissues. As codecarboxylase, pyridoxal phosphate has been shown to participate in the decarboxylation of 5-hydroxytryptophan to produce 5-hydroxytryptamine or serotonin. As a co-factor of the enzyme desulphydrase converts cysteine to pyruvic acid. Pyridoxal phosphate is the co-factor for the synthesis of d -amino-levulinate, the latter a precursor of haeme. Many neuro hormones require pyridoxal phosphate as a coenzyme in their synthesis. Pyridoxine is also involved in fat metabolism, especially of the essential fatty acids. It is involved in the synthesis of messenger RNA which determines amino acids sequence in polypeptide synthesis. Pyridoxine plays a most important role in protein metabolism and, as a result, carnivorous fish have stringent requirements for the vitamin in the diet and stores are rapidly exhausted.

Deficiency Syndrome

Since salmonids, ictalurids, and very young cyprinids are carnivorous, with protein requirements for young animals between 40-50 percent of the ration, pyridoxine stores are rapidly exhausted when fish are held on pyridoxine-deficient rations. Acute deficiency signs occur in salmon after 14-21 days on a high protein diet of pyridoxine and the entire population dies within 28 days in 12-15 C water. Deficiency is followed by general nervous disorders, and alteration in control of melanophore contraction. Postmortem rigor mortis occurs very rapidly. Rapid and gasping breathing with flexing of the opercules is a common observation and oedema in the peritoneal cavity with colorless serous fluid occurs in fish on some experimental treatments.

Salmon, trout, carp and yellowtail exhibit premortem rigor a few hours before death. Recovery at late stage deficiency is very unlikely unless fish are injected with pyridoxal phosphate. Handling the animals generally induces more damage than vitamin administration will correct. Recovery among fish still feeding is equally rapid and dramatic upon administration of pyridoxine hydrochloride in the diet. Deficiency signs disappear within a day or two. Erythrocyte and plasma transaminase activities reflect the deficiency state.

Requirements

Supplementing commercial fish diets with pyridoxine is desirable because of the important role the vitamin plays in protein metabolism.

Sources and Protection

Good sources of pyridoxine are yeast, whole cereals, egg yolk, liver and glandular tissues. Pyridoxine compounds in phosphorylated form present in agricultural products are fairly stable but are sensitive to ultraviolet radiation. Some pyridoxal phosphate will be lost on exposure to air. Free forms or pyridoxal and pyridoxamine are rapidly destroyed by air, light and heat when moist.

Antimetabolites and Inactivation

Antagonists may compete for reaction sites of the apoenzyme or may react with pyridoxal phosphate to form inactive compounds. Deoxypyridoxine is a potent pyridoxine antagonist because of competition for apoenzyme sites but is a useful agent to accelerate pyridoxine deficiency in experimental animals. This same compound inhibits tyrosine decarboxylase. Methoxypyridoxine is another antagonist. Oxopyrimidine (2-methyl-4-amino-5-hydroxymethyl-pyrimidine) produces liver damage and inhibits glutamate decarboxylase.

Clinical Assessment

Plasma and erythrocyte transaminase activity in most instances reflects pyridoxine status of fish although high tryptophan load in the diet tends to increase the pyridoxine requirement. Liver storage measured by microbiological assay showed 5-6 V-g of pyridoxine activity/g in fresh sea salmon liver; whereas, fingerling salmon fed a 50 percent protein diet in freshwater had 2-3 mg/g of wet tissue. Assay of diet for pyridoxine by microbiological methods gives a truer representation of total pyridoxine activity including intermediates.

Pantothenic Acid

A chick dermatitis was cured by Elvehjem and Köehn in 1935 using a factor containing b -alanine. The term pantothenic acid was given earlier by Williams to a yeast growth factor which was later recognized as the anti-dermatitis factor. Pantothenic acid was synthesized by Stiller in 1940. Phillips observed clubbed gills in trout fed pantothenic acid-deficient diets in 1945. Rucker detected the same condition in salmon fed low pantothenic acid diets.

Chemistry

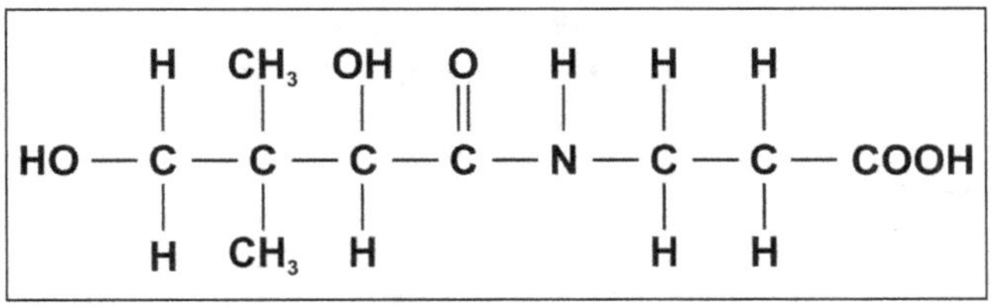

Pantothenic acid may be considered as dihydroxydimethylbutyric acid bonded to b -alanine. The free acid is a yellow, viscous oil and therefore the compound generally used in fish diet preparation is the calcium salt. This salt is a white crystalline powder readily soluble in water, mild acid, and is almost insoluble in organic solvents. It is stable to oxidizing and reducing agents and to autoclaving, but is labile to dry heat, hot alkali, or hot acid. Pantothenol has almost as much activity as pantothenic acid for growth of chicks. Pantothenic acid acetate, benzoate, and diphosphate esters are biologically active for animals but not for lactic acid bacteria. The optical isomer L-pantothenic acid appears physiologically inert. Some organisms may utilize a portion of the molecule. Bacteria appeared to require only the dihydroxydimethylbutyric acid, and some yeasts utilize only g-alanine. Animals, however, need the entire pantothenic acid molecule or its reduced alcohol form.

Positive Functions

Pantothenic acid is part of acetyl coenzyme A which occurs in many enzymatic processes involving 2-carbon compounds. It has been shown to be required by all animal species studied and by many micro-organisms.

The acetyl coenzyme A system is involved in the acetylation of aromatic amines and choline; condensation reactions for synthesis of acetate, fatty acids, and citrate; the oxidation of pyruvate and acetaldehyde; and is essential for the development of the central nervous system. The 2-carbon fragment called 'active acetate', or acetyl coenzyme A, is an essential intermediate in metabolism. It is involved in acylation of acetate, succinate, benzoate, propionate and butyrate. Pantothenic acid is involved in adrenal function and for the production of cholesterol. Coenzyme A is also involved in many other steps of intermediate metabolism of carbohydrates, fats and proteins.

Deficiency Syndromes

Under standard test conditions with deficient diet fed in 10-15°C water systems, salmon and trout exhaust pantothenic acid stores within 8-12 weeks. Fish stop feeding and close examination of gill filament show proliferation of epithelial surface plus swelling and clubbing together of the filaments and lamellae. The opercules become distended and the surface of the gills is often covered with an exudate. Fish become prostrate or sluggish. Necrosis, scarring and cellular atrophy of the tender gill elements occur and anemia develops after prolonged deficiency. Dietary gill disease has been adequately described and correlated with pantothenic acid deficiency. The same type of symptom has been observed in salmon, trout, eel, carp and catfish. After replacement of pantothenic acid in the diet, recovery is rapid for those fish still feeding and gross deficiency symptoms disappear after about four weeks on the recovery diet although evidence of necrosis and scarring remains.

Sources and Protection

Good sources for pantothenic acid are cereal bran, yeast, liver, kidney, heart, spleen and lung. Fish flesh is a relatively rich source, although the content is only about 20 percent of pantothenic acid found in animal glandular tissue. Royal jelly probably contains the greatest amount as it contains over 500 μ g of pantothenol/g dry weight. The calcium or sodium salt of pantothenic acid is relatively stable and can be incorporated into either moist or dry fish diets. Some loss is incurred during autoclaving and excessive heat should therefore be minimized during diet preparations. Since the free acid is labile to heat and also to acid and alkali, some loss can be expected during moist diet preparation or during storage. Certain cereal brans may have pantothenic acid bound in a form unavailable to fish because of the low digestibility coefficient and should not be relied upon as the sole pantothenic acid source in the diet.

Antimetabolites and Inactivation

Since pantothenic acid affects the respiration of many types of cells, compounds like 6-mercaptopurine, 2, 6-diaminopurine, and 8-azaguanine, which inhibit growth of tumors, is antagonistic toward pantothenic acid. Pantoyltaurine is an antimetabolite of pantothenic acid and has been used to accelerate deficiency syndromes in experimental animals.

Methyl-w -pantothenic acid was reported to interfere with the formation of acetyl coenzyme A and accelerates deficiency syndromes in animals. This compound inhibits sulfanilamide acetylation in pigeon liver homogenates but did not prevent citric acid formation. Pantothenic acid can be used to overcome these inhibitory effects, including the reversal of mitosis blockage by 7-mecaptopurine in animals. High levels of calcium pantothenate in the diet also have a transient effect on the migratory urge of salmon.

Clinical Assessment

Assay of pantothenic acid content in the diet may be misleading unless care is exercised in proper hydrolysis of the raw materials being assayed since pantothenic acid is only slowly liberated by normal hydrolytic procedures. Complete hydrolysis with enzyme preparations will liberate all of pantothenic acid from biologically active material of glandular tissues, fish flesh, yeast, and bran.

Salmon feeding actively in the oceans showed liver pantothenic acid content of 18-20 m /g of fresh tissue. Young chinook and coho salmon fingerlings reared in fresh water at 12-15°C showed maximum liver storage at about 14-16 μ g of pantothenic acid/g of fresh liver tissue. Load tests and acetylation reactions of sulfanilamide have been used in man and other experimental animals but have not yet been extended for assessment of pantothenic acid status in fish.

Niacin

Nicotinic acid was synthesized in 1873 but was left on the shelf as an organic compound unrelated to the severe pellagra afflictions occurring throughout the world at that time.

Chemistry

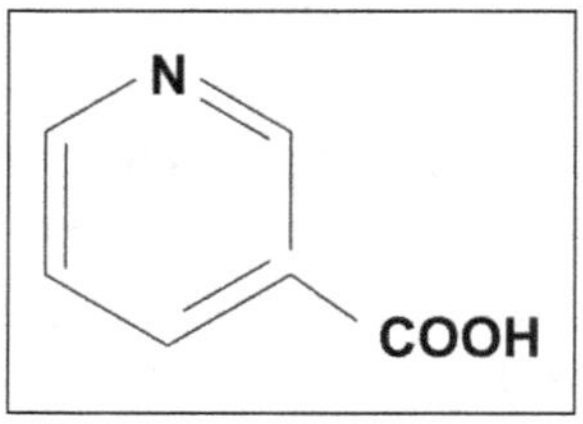

Figure: Nicotinic acid

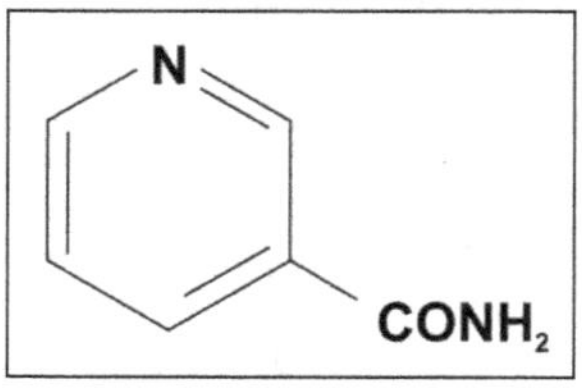

Figure: Niacinamide

Niacin is the preferred nomenclature. Nicotinic acid amide or niacinamide is the common form in which the vitamin is physiologically active. Niacin is a white, crystalline solid, soluble in water and alcohol. It is stable in the dry state and may be autoclaved for short periods without destruction. It is also stable to heat in mineral acids and alkali. Niacin is both a carboxylic acid and an amine and forms quaternary ammonium compounds because of its basic nature. Acidic characteristics include salt formation with alkali. Niacin can be esterified easily, and then converted to amides. Niacinamide is a crystalline powder soluble in water and ethanol and the dry material is stable up to about 60°C. In aqueous solutions it is stable for a short period when autoclaved. It is the form in which the vitamin is normally found in niacinamide adenine dinucleotide (NAD), and in niacinamide adenine dinucleotide phosphate (NADP).

Positive Functions

The major function of niacin in NAD and NADP is hydrogen transport in intermediary metabolism. Most of these enzyme systems function by alternating between the oxidized and reduced state of the coenzymes NAD-NADH and NADP-NADPH. Oxidation-reduction reactions may be anaerobic as when pyruvate acts as the hydrogen acceptor and lactate is formed, or the reactions may be coupled to electron transport systems with oxygen as the ultimate hydrogen acceptor; such aerobic reactions occur in respiration. Both NAD and NADP are involved in the synthesis of high energy phosphate bonds which furnish energy for certain steps in glycolysis, in pyruvate metabolism, amino acid and protein metabolism, and in photosynthesis. An interrelationship between thiamine and niacin exists since both vitamins are coenzymes in intermediary metabolism whereby food is oxidized to furnish energy for physiological functions, to maintain homeostasis, and for body temperature maintenance in homeotherms.

Deficiency Syndrome

Stores of niacin are more slowly exhausted under experimental conditions than are some of the other vitamins resulting in less defined and more slowly developing symptoms.

Niacin deficiencies in fish were experimentally induced in the late forties and early fifties by using basal diets which had low niacin content. Loss of appetite and poor food conversion were the first signs noted. Then the fish turned dark and went off feed, followed by the appearance of lesions in the colon, erratic motion, oedema of the stomach and colon and muscle spasms while fish were apparently resting. A predisposition to sunburn in fish confined in the open in shallow ponds or raceways was described. Common carp showed a congestion of the skin with subcutaneous hemorrhages. Common symptoms of niacin deficiency in most fish studied were muscular weakness and spasms, coupled with poor growth and poor food conversion.

Requirements

In homeotherms on a balanced test ration the niacin requirement is generally estimated to be about ten times that of the thiamine requirement. These rations generally contain considerable carbohydrate material to furnish energy to maintain body temperature. In fish the requirement appears to be twenty to thirty times that of the thiamine needs determined for the same test conditions and test rations. This difference may be due to low carbohydrate content of young fish diets and the higher protein content of these rations. Conversion of tryptophan to niacin occurs in the mammalian liver and possibly also in the liver of fish. This conversion may account for the slow development of the niacin-deficiency syndrome in fish. However, after 10-14 weeks on diets devoid of niacin, deficiency symptoms did occur in several species of fish. The symptoms were reduced by replacement of niacin in the ration even when high protein diets containing an excess of tryptophan were fed. Too much niacin inhibits growth.

Sources and Protection

Niacin is found in most animal and plant tissues. Rich sources are yeast, liver, kidney, heart, legumes, and green vegetables. Wheat contains more niacin than corn and the vitamin is also found in milk and egg products. The vitamin is very stable since it is generally found in coenzyme form in raw materials. Niacin added to the diet as a supplement remains relatively unaltered during diet manufacture, processing, and storage.

Antimetabolites and Inactivation

Pyridine-3-sulphonic acid and 3-acetylpyridine are compounds structurally related to niacin and are antimetabolites for this vitamin in animals and in micro-organisms. Additional niacin can overcome the anti-metabolic effect. Deficiency symptoms in rats may be induced by 6-amino niacinamide. The symptoms are reversed by addition of ten times more niacinamide than the antimetabolite. Thioacetamide has been reported to be a niacin antagonist in fish.

Clinical Assessment

Salmon feeding actively in the oceans showed liver niacin content of 70-80 μ g of niacin/g of fresh tissue. About half of this amount is present in fingerling salmon raised in fresh water at 12-15°C and fed test rations containing 40-50 percent protein and niacin supplements 500-750 mg/kg dry diet. Urinary metabolities of niacin have been measured in other animals on standard niacin load in test rations containing a standard tryptophan load. The technique is well developed to measure the N^1-methyl derivative in mammalian urine. These data have not been reported for fish but metabolism chambers are available for collecting branchial and urinary wastes from large fish intubated with different diet material.

Biotin

Certain foods, notably liver and kidney, were found to be protective against a form of dermatitis resulting from the consumption of egg white by rats, in the early thirties. It was soon learned that a specific component of egg albumin, avidin, rendered dietary biotin unavailable, hence producing the symptoms. Biotin was variously called coenzyme R and 'vitamin H'. It was isolated by Du Vigneaud in 1941 and synthesized by workers of Merck and Company in 1943. Biotin was once thought to be part of factor H for fish. Blue slime patch disease due to biotin deficiency was reported in trout.

Chemistry

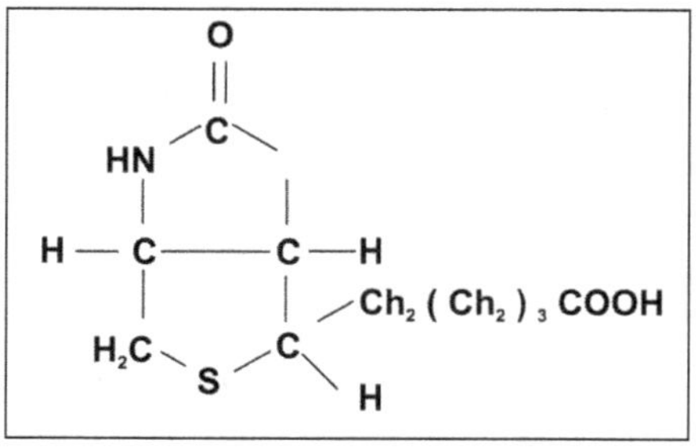

Biotin is a monocarboxylic acid slightly soluble in water and alcohol and insoluble in organic solvents. Salts of the acid are soluble in water. Aqueous solutions or the dry material are stable at 100 C and to light. The vitamin is destroyed by acids and alkalis and by oxidizing agents such as peroxides or permanganate. Biocytin is a bound form of biotin isolated from yeast, plant, and animal tissues. Other bound forms of the vitamin can generally be liberated by peptic digestion. Oxybiotin has partial vitamin activity but oxybiotin sulphonic acid and other analogues are antimetabolites inhibiting the growth of bacteria.

Avidin, a protein found in raw egg white, binds biotin and makes it unavailable to fish and other animals. Heating to denature the protein makes the bound biotin available again to the fish. Biocytin or e -biotinyl lysine (the epsilon amino group of lysine and the carboxyl of biotin being combined in a peptide bond) is hydrolyzed by the enzyme biotinase making the protein-bound biotin available.

Positive Functions

Biotin is required in several specific carboxylation and decarboxylation reactions, including the carboxylation of pyruvic acid to form oxaloacetic acid. It is part of the coenzyme of several carboxylating enzymes fixing CO_2 such as propionyl coenzyme A involved in the conversion of propionic acid to succinic acid in methylmalonyl coenzyme A. Biotin is also involved in the conversion of acetyl CO_2 to malonyl coenzyme A in the formation of long chain fatty acids. It has possible involvement in citrulline synthesis and may have effects on purine and pyrimidine synthesis. It is involved in the conversion of unsaturated fatty acids to the stable cis form in the synthesis of biologically active fatty acids.

Deficiency Syndrome

Some signs of biotin deficiency in salmonids are skin disorders, muscle atrophy, lesions in the colon, loss of appetite, and spastic convulsions. Haematology discloses fragmentation of erythrocytes. Poor growth is a common symptom and has been reported for salmonids, common carp, goldfish (Carassius auratus) and eel. Blue slime patch disease in brook trout deficient in biotin appears typical for this species. Fish reared in 10 -15 C water exhaust biotin stores in 8-12 weeks and the first signs are anorexia, poor food conversion, and general listlessness before the more acute deficiency symptoms become detectable.

Requirements

The biotin requirements for young salmon, trout, carp, goldfish and eel raised under experimental conditions appear to be about the same. Brown trout appear to require nearly twice as much biotin in the diet as do brook or rainbow trout.

Sources and Protection

Rich sources of biotin are liver, kidney, yeast, milk products, and egg yolks. Nut meats contain good supplies of biotin. The diet should be protected from strong oxidizing agents or conditions which promote oxidation of ingredients. Raw egg white should not be incorporated into moist fish diets. Cooking will inactivate the avidin.

Antimetabolites and Inactivation

Raw egg white has already been discussed which irreversibly binds biotin and makes it unavailable to young fish. Many biotin homologues with different side chain lengths inhibit the growth of bacteria. Oxybiotin, in which sulphur is replaced by oxygen, has about the same biological activity as the natural biotin. On the other hand, oxybiotin sulphonic acid inhibits biotin activity.

Clinical Assessment

Measurement or urinary excretion of biotin in animals does not prove a good clinical method since biotin is synthesized by several organisms in the gut. In fish, this technique needs to be explored and may well be valuable as a clinical tool since the gastrointestinal tract of many freshwater fish contains only small quantities of bacteria. Biotin is one of the most expensive vitamins to add to fish rations. Salmon feeding actively in the oceans had liver biotin concentrations of 10-12 mg of wet liver tissue. The concentrations in the liver of young salmon fingerlings in fresh water fed test diets containing an excess of biotin were between 6-8 mg of the vitamin/g of tissue. Fish with these levels of biotin in the liver should probably be in sound biotin nutritional status.

Folic Acid (Folacin)

A factor effective in curing metaloblastic anemia in monkeys was found in yeast and liver concentrates and was designated vitamin M in 1935. In 1939 an anti-anemic factor was found in liver and called vitamin B_C. These were later shown to be the same substance with folic acid as the active ingredient. Folic acid was synthesized in 1946 and was soon used in fish diets for preventing purified diet anemia.

Chemistry

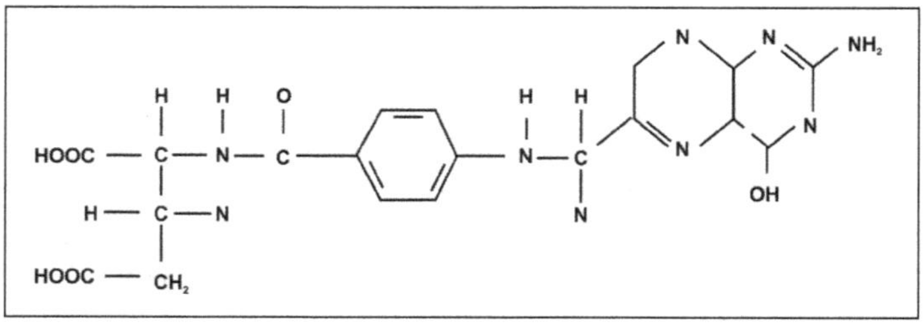

Folic acid crystallizes into yellow spear-shaped leaflets which are soluble in water and dilute alcohol. It can be precipitated with heavy metal salts. It is stable to heat in neutral or alkaline solution, but unstable in acid solution. It deteriorates when exposed to sunlight, or during prolonged storage. Several analogues have biological activity including pteroic acid, rhizopterin, folinic acid, xanthopterin and several formyltetrahydropteroyl-glutamic acid derivatives. These have closely allied ring structures and many have been isolated as derivatives in various animals or microbiological preparations. One simple form, xanthopterin, present in the pigments of insects, is shown below and is of special interest because of early work with this compound as the anti-anaemic factor H for fish.

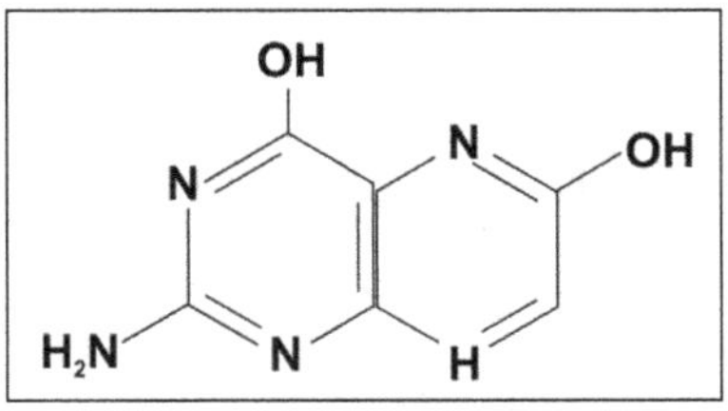

Figure: Xanthopterin

Positive Functions

Folic acid is required for normal blood cell formation and is involved as a coenzyme in one-carbon transfer mechanisms. In the presence of ascorbic acid, folic acid is transformed into the active (5-formyl-5, 6, 7, 8) tetrahydrofolic acid. Folic acid is involved in many one-carbon metabolism systems such as serine and glycine interconversion, methionine-homocysteine synthesis, histidine synthesis, and pyrimidine synthesis.

Several coenzyme forms of the active vitamin have been isolated. Folic acid is involved in the conversion of megaloblastic bone marrow to normoblastic type. It has a role in blood glucose regulation and improves cell membrane function and hatchability of eggs.

Deficiency Syndrome

Macrocytic normochromic anemia occurs in several experimental animals, including fish fed diets devoid of the folic acid. Increasing numbers of senile cells are observed as the deficiency progresses until only a few old and degenerating cells are found in the blood of deficient fish. Anterior kidney imprints disclose only adult cells and no preforms present. Other signs observed have been poor growth, anorexia, general anemia, lethargy, fragile fins, dark skin pigmentation, and infarction of spleen.

Requirements

The requirement seems to be about the same for trout and salmon. Marginal macrocytic anaemias occur in fish fed diets containing marginal amounts of folacin. Individual fish ingesting adequate amounts of the vitamin show little variation in total erythrocyte counts.

Sources and Protection

Yeast, green vegetables, liver, kidney, glandular tissue, fish tissue, and fish viscera are good sources of folic acid. Insects contain xanthopterin which has folic acid activity. At one time the yellow pigment of xanthopterin was identified as the fish anti-anemic factor H, but subsequent experiments showed only partial activity and that folic acid itself was a much more potent antimacrocytic anaemia factor. Insects may contribute significantly to the folic acid requirements of wild fish, but in scientific fish husbandry artificial diets are more reliable sources. Activity is lost during extended storage and when material is exposed to sunlight. Therefore, dry feeds should be carefully protected during manufacture and moist diet rations should be carefully preserved. Both types of fish diets should be fed soon after manufacture to assure minimal loss of folic acid activity.

Antimetabolites and Inactivation

One antagonist of folacin is 4-aminopteroylglutamic acid or aminopterin. This material, when incorporated in the diet of guinea pigs and rats, induces anaemia and leucopenia and has been used to treat leukemia in man. Amethopterin (4-amino-N^{10}-methylpteroylglutamic acid) can also be used to induce deficiency by inhibiting purine, pyrimidine, and nucleic acid protection; viz., inhibition of nucleic acid synthesis results in macroytic anaemia.

Clinical Assessment

Haematology is used as a simple clinical tool to assess haemopoiesis in fish. Anterior kidney imprints easily disclose normal distribution of immature cells and preforms undergoing reticulosis. Salmon actively feeding in the ocean and young salmon fingerlings raised in fresh water and fed diets rich in folacin show liver storage of 3-4 μg of folic acid/g of wet tissue. Microbiological assay is preferred for assessment of total folic acid in dietary raw materials because the total biological activity it measures includes all the various coenzyme forms and folic acid analogues. Assessment of the dietary intake of folic acid is important for intensive cold water fish husbandry. In pond culture, aquatic and terrestrial insects, algae, etc., may also be available and folic acid in the supplementary feed may not be as critical. Since folic acid is labile in storage, excess amounts are generally added to manufacture feed in anticipation of storage losses. However, prudent fish husbandry dictates rapid use of manufactured rations with minimum storage. Routine periodic haematology of fish assures proper nutritional status for maximum production and sound health.

Vitamin B_{12}

The antipernicious anaemia factor found to be contained in liver was isolated and crystallized in the mid-forties. This substance, named vitamin B_{12} by its discoverers, was later to be recognized as essential for growth of chicken fed diets entirely of plant origin and was designated animal protein factor (APF). When anaemic salmon were injected with crystalline B_{12} in combination with folic acid and xanthopterin positive haemopoiesis occurred within a few days, and the salmon showed rapid recovery from the anaemia.

Chemistry

Vitamin B_{12} or cynacobalamin has the following approximate chemical structure.

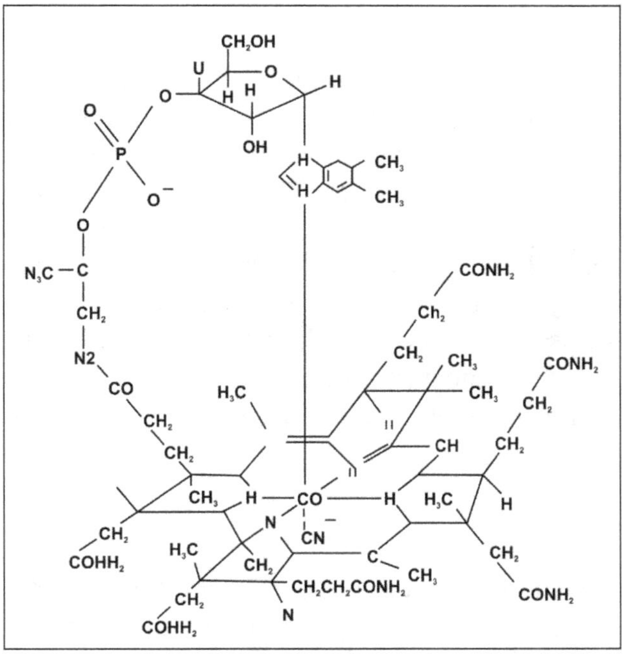

Figure: Cyanocobalamin

The molecule has a planar group and a nucleotide group lying nearly at right angles to one another. This cobalt-containing vitamin has a net charge of one at the central cobalt atom to which is attached a replaceable cyano group. Vitamin B_{12} is stable to mild heat in neutral solution, but is rapidly destroyed by heating in dilute acid or alkali. Crude concentrates are more unstable and rapidly lose activity. The compound is similar to the porphyrins in its spatial configuration with a central cobalt atom linked to four reduced pyrrole rings in the haeme series. Replacing the cyanide ion with a variety of anions, produce derivatives which have comparable biological activities; viz., hydroxocobalamin, nitritocobalamin, chlorocobalamin and sulphatocobalamin.

Positive Functions

Cyanocobalamin is involved with folic acid in haemopoiesis. It is required by many micro-organisms and is a growth factor for many animals. The animal protein factor present in fish and animal by-products was not recognized until crystalline vitamin B_{12} was injected into anaemic chinook salmon fingerlings in 1949 and positive haemopoiesis was observed. A coenzyme incorporating vitamin B_{12} is involved in the reversible isomerization of methyl-malonyl coenzyme A to succinyl coenzyme A and in the isomerization of methylaspartate to glutomate. Cyanocobalamin is involved in the coenzyme for the methylation of homocystine to form methionine. It is also involved in several other one-carbon reactions and in the synthesis of labile methyl compounds. One vitamin B_{12} containing coenzyme acts in methylation of the purine ring during thymine synthesis. Vitamin B_{12} is also involved in cholesterol metabolism, in purine and pyrimidine biosynthesis, and in the metabolism of glycols.

Deficiency Syndrome

Deficiency signs in young pigs, chicks, and rats show abnormal blood elements, poor growth, and pernicious anaemia. An intrinsic factor is necessary for good absorption of the vitamin from the gut. This factor is a low molecular weight mucoprotein which normally occurs in gastric juice, and especially in hog gut mucosa. Pernicious anaemia in chinook and coho salmon is characterized by fragmented, erythrocytes with many aberrant forms present. Haemoglobin levels are inconsistent and erythrocyte counts have a range extending from frank anaemia to a near normal blood pattern. Cyanocobalamin stores in fish tissues are slowly exhausted and only after 12-16 weeks on test do the symptoms appear in deficient salmon populations. Poor appetite, poor growth, poor food conversion, and some dark pigmentation can be observed before frank anaemia is detected.

Requirements

Requirement based on fish that showed normal haematology at the end of the 16-week feeding period, and maximum liver storage of the vitamin determined by Lactobaccilis leichmanii microbiological assay.

Sources and Protection

Rich sources of vitamin B_{12} are found in fish meal, fish viscera, liver, kidney, glandular tissues, and slaughter house wastes. Since vitamin B_{12} is labile on storage, and in mild acid solution is easily destroyed by heating, care must be exercised in diet preparation containing flesh or meat scraps.

Antimetabolites and Inactivation

The vitamin B_{12} coenzymes are very unstable under light, which rapidly decomposes the coenzymes. Photo-sensitivity is increased in dilute acid solutions.

Clinical assessment

Generalized anaemia with fragmentation of erythrocytes and extremely variable haemoglobin levels and erythrocyte counts indicate possible B_{12} deficiency. Prompt response in individual fish is obtained by injecting B_{12} alone or in combination with folic acid in the ratio of 1 part vitamin B_{12} to 100 parts folic acid. Careful interpretation of haemotological data will enable one to distinguish one form of anaemia from the other.

Ascorbic Acid

The isolation of ascorbic acid was due to Szent-Györgyi of Hungary and C.G. King of the U.S.A. Vitamin C synthesis was accomplished in 1933 after the chemical structure of ascorbic acid was established by British and Swiss workers.

McCay and Tunison reported scoliosis in brook trout fed formalin-preserved meat in 1934 and McLaren observe hemorrhages in trout fed rations low in ascorbic acid. It was not until the sixties that a critical need for L-ascorbic acid by trout and salmon was demonstrated.

Chemistry

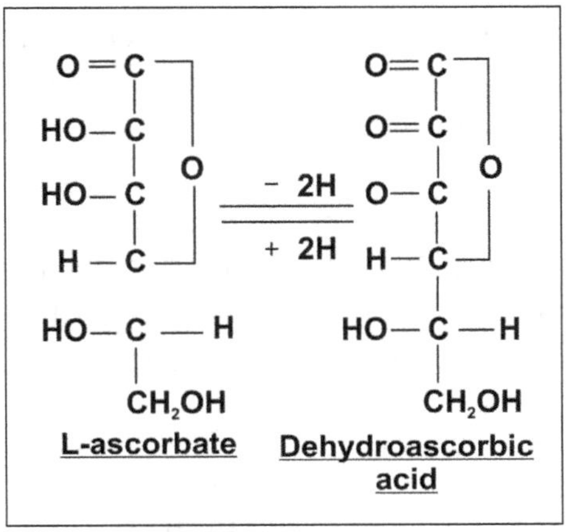

Figure: Cyanocobalamin

L-ascorbic acid is a white, odorless, crystalline compound, soluble in water but insoluble in fat solvents. It is readily oxidized to dehydroascorbic acid, the less biologically potent form. Ascorbic acid is very stable in acid solution because of the preservation of the lactone ring, but in alkaline solution hydrolysis occurs rapidly and vitamin activity is lost. It is very heat labile and prone to atmospheric oxidation, especially in the presence of copper, iron, or several other metallic catalysts. The reduced form is the most biologically active but several derivatives or salts are obtainable which have varying degrees of ascorbate activity.

Positive Functions

L-ascorbic acid acts as a biological reducing agent in hydrogen transport. It is involved in many enzyme systems for hydroxylation; i.e., hydroxylation of tryptophan, tyrosine, or proline. It is involved in the detoxification of aromatic drugs and also acts in the production of adrenal steroids.

Ascorbic acid is necessary for the formation of hydroxy proline which is a constituent of collagen, a component of intercellular material in bones and soft tissues. Ascorbic acid plays a synergistic role with vitamin E as intracellular antioxidants and free radical traps. The conversion of folic acid to folinic acid requires vitamin C. Ascorbic acid is involved in the formation of chondroitin sulphate and intercellular ground substance. Labelled ascorbic acid fed to fish previously deficient in the vitamin was shown to be rapidly mobilized and fixed in areas of rapid collagen synthesis and became concentrated in the thick collagen of the skin and in cartilagenous bones, as well as in the glands of the anterior kidney. Ascorbic acid is also involved in erythrocyte maturation.

Deficiency Syndrome

Scurvy with impaired collagen formation, perifollicular hemorrhages; loose teeth and poor bone formation, anaemia, and oedema have been reported in other animals. Deficiency signs in fish are generally related to impaired collagen formation. Fish soon show hyperplasia of jaw and snout. The same symptoms have been observed in trout, salmon, yellowtail, carp, guppies and char. Histologically, hypertrophy of the adrenal tissues and hemorrhage at the bases of fins have been observed in coho salmon. Deficiency signs cease to develop and new growth becomes normal upon replacement of ascorbic acid in the ration. Anaemia eventually develops in extremely deficient fish and scoliosis and lordosis do not repair but are walled off by new growth around the afflicted areas of the spine when ascorbic acid is once again added to the ration.

Requirements

In the rainbow trout, reasonable blood and anterior kidney storage levels were obtained with an intake of about 100 mg of vitamin C/kg of dry ration in 10°, 12°, or 15° C water systems. When wound repair experiments were initiated, however, or when fish were exposed to other stress then the requirements doubled or tripled. When severe abdominal or intramuscular wounds were inflicted, young fish needed at least 500 mg of active ascorbate for tissue repair comparable with control fish receiving 1 g or more of ascorbate in the diet/kg of dry diet. Coho salmon appear to need about half of these requirements for adequate tissue levels and for maximum severe wound repair rates. The requirement for ascorbic acid is related to stress, growth rate and size of the animal, as well as to the other nutrients present in the diet. A compromise value of about 200 mg of ascorbic acid/kg diet for trout and salmon raised in freshwater systems between 10-15°C would ensure reasonable tissue storage levels and furnish some excess for mild stress conditions and for ascorbic acid loss from the diet through oxidation. Large common carp can synthesize some ascorbate and the requirement for this species may be dependent on fish size and the environment in which they are reared.

Table: Growth and Tissue Ascorbate.

Vitamin C diet treatment	Trout			Salmon		
	Average weight at 24 weeks	Ascorbate concentrate 1/		Average weight at 24 weeks	Ascorbate concentrate 1/	
		blood	kidney		blood	kidney
mg/100 g	g	m g/g	m g/g	g	m g/g	m s/s
0	2.4	2/	2/	5.0	22.3±2.2	89
5	9.6	34.4±2.9	125	6.0	30.5±1.2	132

10	10.6	34.6±1.3	137	5.7	35.8±1.6	265
20	10.1	38.8±3.3	132	6.1	34.2±2.3	183
40	10.2	46.8±6.2	162	6.3	33.7±2.0	225
100	10.8	51.0±4.6	247	6.0	37.8±2.3	321

1/ Average of five samples for blood (± S.D.) and two for head kidney tissue.

2/ No fish available for assay.

Sources and Protection

Ascorbic acid is widely distributed in nature with citrus fruits, cabbage, liver, and kidney tissue good sources for the vitamin. Fresh insects and fish tissues contain reasonable amounts of the vitamin. Synthetic ascorbic acid is also readily available. Fish food should be protected from oxidizing agents and kept sealed or frozen until used to prevent loss of the vitamin.

Antimetabolites and Inactivation

D-ascorbic acid, the optical isomer of the active form, has no vitamin activity and competes for sites of several enzyme reactions mediated by L-ascorbic acid. 6-deoxy-L-ascorbic acid, dehydroascorbic acid and L-glucoascorbic acid have very little activity.

Clinical Assessment

Ascorbic acid status for experimental animals is normally attempted by tissue ascorbate analysis. Most of the assays previously used measure total ascorbate and not biologically active L-ascorbic acid. Consequently these are fraught with errors and misconception of true vitamin C status. In fish tissues, blood and liver do not adequately reflect the ascorbic acid intake and status, whereas assay of the anterior kidney which contains adrenal tissue provides a fairly representative picture of tissue storage of the vitamin. Stress rapidly reduces the ascorbic acid content of this tissue with concurrent production of adrenal steroids. Conversely, dietary repletion is reflected by up to four or five-fold storage levels from the deficient state. Examination of fragile support cartilage in the gill filaments under low magnification will detect early hypovitaminosis before clinically acute symptoms become noticeable. However, the best tissue for routine clinical analysis to assess vitamin C status in trout and salmon appears to be the anterior kidney with samples selected from the junction of the two forward wings. Tissues are blotted free of blood with filter paper, and then assayed for total ascorbate by one of the improved quick methods to determine total ascorbate.

Inositol

Muscle 'sugar' was discovered by Scherer in 1850 and was characterized as inositol in

1887. Inositol was shown to be an alopecia (a form of hairlessness) preventing factor for mice in 1940. Poor growth and poor food passage in inositol-deficient fish was observed in salmon and carp.

Chemistry

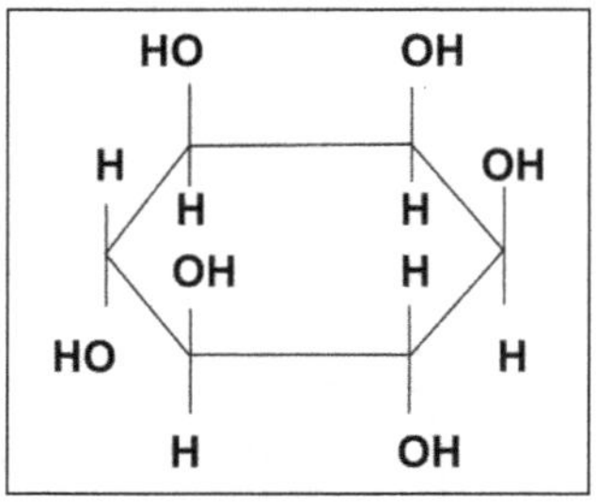

Seven optically inactive and two optically active isomers of hexahydroxycyclohexane can exist. One of the optically active forms, myo-inositol, is a white crystalline powder soluble in water and insoluble in alcohol and ether. The material can be synthesized, but is easily isolated from biological material in free or combined forms. The mixed calcium-magnesium salt of the hexophosphate is phytin. Isomers have little biological activity but will compete in chemical reactions. Inositol is a highly stable compound.

Positive Functions

Myo-inositol is a structural component in living tissues. It has lipotropic action by preventing accumulation of cholesterol in one type of fatty liver disease and is involved with choline in maintaining normal lipid/metabolism. It is a growth-promoting substance for micro-organisms and prevents alopecia in mice. It is a reserve carbohydrate in muscle as well as a major component of phosphoglycerides in animal tissues.

Deficiency Syndrome

Poor growth, increased gastric emptying time, oedema, dark colour, and distended stomachs are symptoms observed in salmon, trout, carp and catfish held for long periods on inositol-deficient test rations.

The major deficiency sign is inefficiency in digestion and food utilization and concomitant poor growth leading to a population of fish with distended abdomens.

Requirements

Inositol needs have been measured in only two species of salmon and carp and the requirement is high for maximum growth and for maximum liver storage. Whether liver storage is accurate criteria to determine requirements is debatable since inositol intake was compared with maximum growth rate and diet conversion to develop a tentative requirement for young fish for this 'muscle' sugar.

Sources and Protection

Myo-inositol occurs ubiquitously in large amounts wherever biological tissue is found. Wheat germ, dried peas, and beans are rich sources. Brain, heart, and glandular tissues are very good sources of biologically active inositol. Citrus fruit pulp and dried yeast also contain inositol. The compound is stable.

Antimetabolites and Inactivation

Seven optically inactive and one optically active but biologically inactive stereo isomers occur. Since inositol is synthesized in the biologically active form by many microorganisms in the gut, only large quantities of chemically synthesized inactive isomers added to diets would interfere with the metabolism of inositol for growth and normal physiological function. Biologically inactive stereoisomers of myo-inositol do not compete for critical sites in metabolism. Methyl derivatives and mono-, di-, and triphosphoric acid esters occur naturally. Salts of the hexaphosphate or phytin make the bound inositol practically unavailable to the animal.

Clinical Assessment

Assessment in fish has been based on lack of deficiency signs coupled with the most efficient food conversion. Salmon feeding actively in oceans show 1-1.5 mg of inositol/g of fresh liver tissue and young fingerlings raised in freshwater at 10-15°C had 600-700 m g/g of liver tissue. An alternate, better assessment may be based on a standard muscle section or whole carcass analysis for free or for bound inositol. Projection of inositol intake from normal fish diet ingredients should indicate an excess of this particular vitamin.

Choline

Methylation as a basic metabolic process was postulated by Hoffmeister. Methyl transfer was shown in vivo by Thompson and the interrelationships between choline, methionine, and homo-cystine were shown by du Vigneaud in 1939-42. Trout fed low choline rations developed haemorrhagic kidneys and salmon showed an aversion to food in choline-deficient diet.

Chemistry

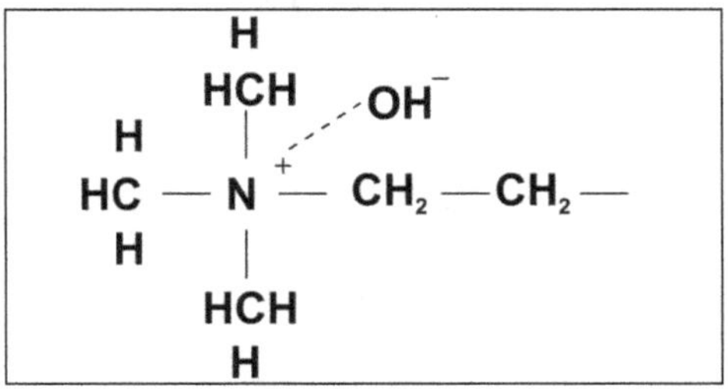

Choline is a very strong organic base and forms many derivatives widely distributed in animal and vegetable tissue. One derivative, acetylcholine, is involved in the transmission of nerve impulses across synapses. Choline is very hygroscopic, very soluble in water, and is stable to heat in acid, but decomposes in alkaline solutions.

Positive Functions

Choline acts as a methyl donor in trans-methylation reactions. It is a lipotropic and antihaemorrhagic factor preventing the development of fatty livers. It is involved in the synthesis of phospholipids and in fat transport. Acetylcholine transmits the excitory state across the ganglionic synapses and neuromuscular junctions. Choline is essential for growth and good food conversion in fish.

Deficiency Syndrome

Deficiency signs include poor growth and poor food conversion accompanied by impaired fat metabolism. Haemorrhagic kidneys and intestines have been reported in trout and increased gastric emptying time has been observed in salmon.

Sources and Protection

Rich sources of choline are wheat germ, beans, brain, and heart tissue. Choline hydrochloride, the commercially available form, may inactivate a -tocopherol and vitamin K when in direct contact with these vitamins and care should be exercised in selecting properly protected (gelatin coated) fat soluble vitamins in fish diet preparation.

Clinical Assessment

Choline status of fish can be estimated from the assay of choline content of the dietary ingredients with the absence of deficiency signs. Maximum liver storage may not be the best criteria to determine choline nutritional status but has been used to assess the tentative requirement listed for the two species of salmon.

p-Aminobenzoic Acid

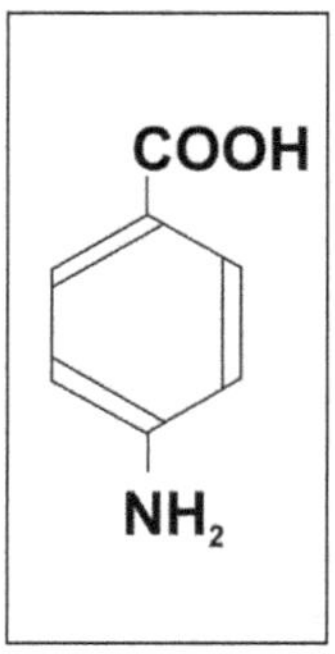

p-Aminobenzoic Acid acid is a white crystalline powder which is water soluble and heat and light stable in aqueous and mild alkaline solution. It is a growth promoting vitamin for micro-organisms which require the vitamin for folic acid synthesis. Large intake has been shown to counteract the antimetabolite effect of sulphonamides in bacterial culture. No positive function or deficiency signs have been observed in fish.

Lipoic Acid

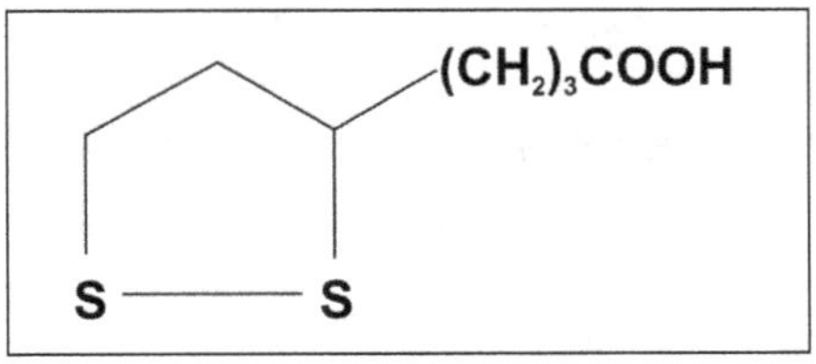

Lipoic acid is both fat soluble and water soluble. Its active form is the amide derivative known as lipoamide. Lipoic acid functions as a coenzyme in a a -ketoacid decarboxylation. It was discovered independently in several laboratories during the period 1945-50 and shown to be an essential component of multienzyme, the pyruvate dehydrogenase complex. Pyruvate is converted to 'active acetaldehyde' which in turn is picked up by lipoamide. Subsequent oxidation of the aldehyde results in the reduction of lipoamide to a disulphydryl form. The multi-enzyme unit also includes thiamine pyrophosphate, coenzyme A, and flavin adenine dinucleotide. Glandular tissues are good sources of lipoic acid. No requirements have been determined for fish.

Fat-Soluble Vitamins

Fat-soluble vitamins A, D, E, and K differ from the water-soluble vitamins in their accumulative action. Little evidence has been recorded for hypervitaminosis with the water-soluble vitamins since these compounds are rapidly metabolized and excreted when intake exceeds liver or tissue storage capacity, but hypervitaminosis is a common occurrence in fish and other animals when large quantities of any one of the fat-soluble vitamins are ingested. Toxicity symptoms involving vitamins A and D are indistinguishable from deficiency symptoms for the same vitamins. On the other hand, symptoms of excess vitamins E and K intake are more discrete. Fish rations may often be enriched with fish oils to increase caloric density of the ration resulting in excessive intake of the fat-soluble vitamins.

Vitamin A

A fat-soluble factor that promoted growth in rats was described by Hopkins and by Osborne and Mendel at the beginning of this century. McCollum and Simmonds cured xerophthalmia, a disease of the eye, with this material. The chemical structure of vitamin A and its relationship to b -carotene was shown by Von Euler in 1928. Active vitamin A was synthesized in the mid-thirties.

Chemistry

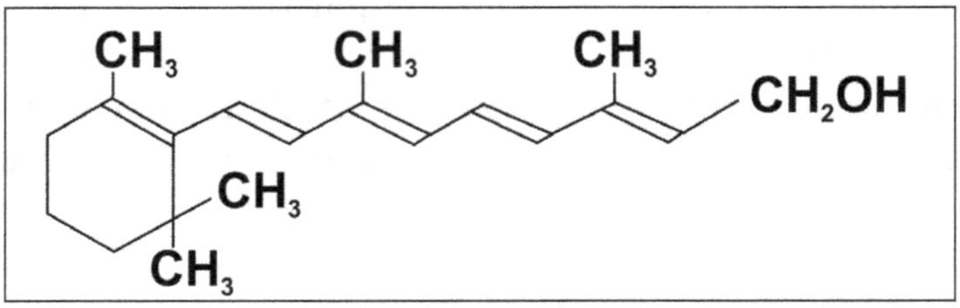

Figure: Vitamin A alcohol

The relationship of the vitamin A alcohols to naturally occurring b -carotene is as follows:

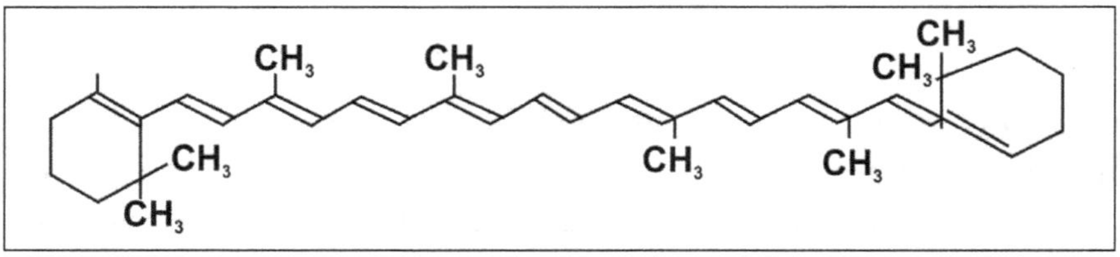

Figure: Beta-carotene.

Retinene, the aldehyde form of vitamin A, has been isolated from the retina of dark adapted eyes and is involved in vision in dim light. Retinoic acid, which is the oxidized form of vitamin A alcohol, has been shown to have some vitamin A activity. Vitamin A_1 is found in saltwater fish, whereas vitamin A is more abundant in freshwater fish. Interconversion of the two forms in living fish tissue has been demonstrated. Fish oils contain vitamin A as free alcohols or esters. Vitamin A alcohol occurs as light colored viscous oil which is heat labile and subject to air oxidation. Beta-carotene occurs as an orange, crystalline compound which is more stable to heat and oxidation. Vitamin A is water insoluble but is soluble in fat and organic solvent.

Positive Functions

Vitamin A is essential in maintaining epithelial cells, preventing atrophy and keratinization of epithelial tissues. It is combined with a protein in visual purple and is important in night vision. Vitamin A also prevents xerophthalmia in rats and young children. Vitamin A promotes growth of new cells and aids in maintaining resistance to infection. The interrelationships of cis- and trans-vitamin A in the rhodopsin cycle in mammalian vision are shown below.

The Syndrome of Deficiency or Excess

Hypovitaminosis A is characterized by poor growth, poor vision, keratinization of epithelial tissue, xerophthalmia, night blindness, hemorrhage in the anterior chamber of the eye, hemorrhage of the base of the fins, and abnormal bone formation. Nerve degeneration has been reported in pigs, chickens, rats, rabbits, and ducks, but only occasionally observed in fish after long periods of deficiency. Hypervitaminosis A has been described in fish and in other animals and involved enlargement of liver and spleen, abnormal growth, skin lesions, epithelial keratinization, hyperplasia. of head cartilage, and abnormal bone formation resulting in ankylosis and fusion of vertebrae. Hypervitaminosis A is reflected in very high liver oil vitamin A content and elevated serum alkaline phosphatase. Removal of excess vitamin A from the diet promotes rapid recovery.

Requirements

Fish apparently require vitamin A for growth in light, but not in darkness. Therefore, the requirement for maximum growth and reproduction is related to exposure to light and reflects observations in other animals that near normal growth will occur at very low vitamin A intake in protected environments where fish are not exposed to stress, infection, and ultraviolet radiation.

Sources and Protection

Cod liver oil is the best known source of vitamin A although black sea bass, swordfish, or ling cod oils contain much more of the vitamin. Whale liver oil contains kitol which has little or no biological activity until heated above 200° C when one molecule of biologically active vitamin A is generated per molecule of whale kitol. This biologically inactive kitol may be deposited in the whale to avoid hypervitaminosis A during excessive vitamin A intake. The possibility of hypervitaminosis A occurs when tuna, shark, or ling cod viscera are used in preparation of moist fish diets. Synthetic vitamin A preparations, such as vitamin A palmitate, are available and are often used to supplement rations low in fish meal, fish viscera, or carotenes. Some fish species seem able to utilize b-carotene as a vitamin A source, whereas others are unable to split the g-carotene molecule and vitamin A must be added to the diet.

Clinical Assessment

Vitamin A status can best be assessed by the absence of deficiency signs and by assay of liver oil for vitamin A content. Assay for the vitamin in blood or plasma has not been found to be useful.

Vitamin D_2

Rickets was induced with test diets by Hopkins, and Mellanby cured the disease in dogs by adding cod liver oil to the ration. Ultraviolet light exposure was shown to have an anti-rachitic effect, and provitamin D activity had been ascribed to ergosterol. Crystalline vitamin D was isolated by Angus and activated 7-dehydrocholesterol was isolated by Windaus.

Chemistry

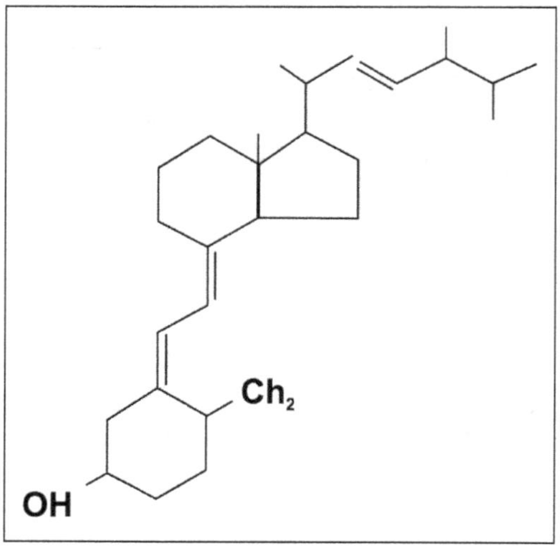

Figure: Vitamin D_2.

Vitamin D_2 or ergocalciferol is one of several biologically active forms of vitamin D. Vitamin D_3 or activated 7-dehydrocholesterol has the chemical formula $C_{27}H_{44}O$ and contains a more simplified, unsaturated 8-carbon side chain. Vitamin D_3, also known as cholecalciferol, is formed in most animal tissue by the rupture of one of the ring bonds of 7-dehydrocholesterol by ultraviolet radiation. Cholecalciferol is a white, crystalline compound soluble in fat and organic solvents and is stable to heat and oxidation in mild alkali or acid solution. The conversion of ergosterol to vitamin D_2 and several side compounds is shown.

Positive Functions

Vitamin D is essential for maintaining calcium and inorganic phosphate homeostasis. It is involved in alkaline phosphatase activity, promotes intestinal absorption of calcium, and influences the action of parathyroid hormone on bone. Fish may sequester calcium from water through the gill membrane; thus the major function of vitamin D for other animals may not be necessary to satisfy calcium requirements for fish.

Syndrome of Deficiency or Excess

Hypovitaminosis D for fish has not been described. Rickets and abnormal bone formation described in detail for animals has not been observed in fish fed low vitamin D diets. However little work has been done under carefully controlled conditions with young growing fish and only alteration in alkaline phosphatase activity has been reported on different vitamin D diet intake. Hypervitaminosis D, however, has been reported. Brook trout fed large doses of vitamin D showed impaired growth, lethargy, and dark coloration. High intake of vitamin D mobilizes phosphorus and calcium from the bone and tissues and may result in fragile bones, poor growth, and poor appetite related to the nausea described in man afflicted with hyper-vitaminosis D. Arterial and kidney lesions due to excessive intake of vitamin D reported for rats and dogs have not been described histologically for fish nor has hypercalcaemia been described. This area needs to be explored because of the potential for hypervitaminosis D in fish fed diets containing various fish viscera which might contain large amounts of the vitamin D. Tuna liver oil may contain, for example, 100 to 1 000 times as much active vitamin D as cod liver oil.

Requirements

No requirements of fish for vitamin D have been described to date, but little work has been done in this area using highly purified diets and controlled experiments with young growing fish. Likewise, no demonstration of synthesis of the vitamin in fish reared on diets devoid of vitamin D or vitamin D precursors has been reported. Therefore, actual requirement of vitamin D for maintenance of calcium-phosphorus homeostasis in the young growing animal has not been adequately investigated and the true requirements of vitamin D in young fish have not been defined.

Sources and Protection

Vitamin D requirements of many animals can be met by ultraviolet irradiation of the skin where cholesterol derivatives are converted to calciferol. Since the vitamin is fat soluble and accumulates in lipid stores, fish liver oil is a rich source of the material. Content varies tremendously in liver oil, however, with values of about 25 I.U. /g present in shark liver oil and over 200 000 I.U. /g in albacore tuna liver oil. Cod liver oil contains from 100-500 I.U./g and animal liver contains some vitamin D. One international unit (I.U.) is equal to 0.025 mg of crystalline vitamin D.

Clinical Assessment

Absorption maxima in the ultraviolet region can be used to detect provitamins D in the non-saponifiable fraction of oils. Concentrated preparations of vitamin D can be assayed by the Carr-Price antimony trichloride reaction when assay is necessary to determine biologically active materials in liver oil of fish on different treatments. The chick assay may not apply to fish liver storage levels because the biologically active form for fish has not been determined. Therefore, clinical assessment for hypervitaminosis A must rely on crude methods for determination of vitamin D in liver oil samples by the Carr-Price reaction or by measuring absorption in the UV spectrum.

Vitamin E

The existence of an antisterility vitamin was postulated by Evans and Bishop. This factor was named 'vitamin E' by Sure. The active tocopherol was isolated, characterized, and synthesized by Karrer.

Chemistry

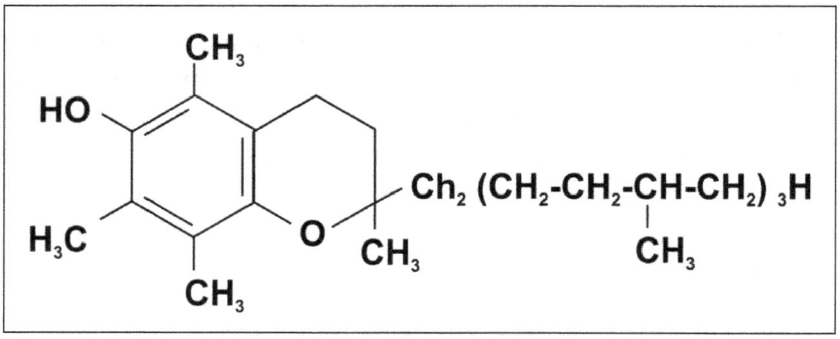

Figure: Alpha-tocopherol.

Vitamin E is composed of a class of compounds known as tocopherols. One of the most important tocopherols is a -tocopherol. Eight naturally occurring tocopherol derivatives have been isolated and all belong to the D series. Synthetic a -tocopherol is a racemic DL-a -tocoperhol mixture. The derivatives of tocol or of tocotrienol are named, alpha, beta, gamma, delta, epsilon, eta, $zeta_1$ and $zeta_2$-tocopherol. The pure tocopherols are fat-soluble oils which are capable of esterification to form crystalline compounds. The tocopherols are stable to heat and acids in the absence of oxygen, but are rapidly oxidized in the presence of nascent oxygen, peroxides, or other oxidizing agents. The tocopherols are sensitive to ultraviolet light and are excellent antioxidants in the free form. The esters are more stable and are commonly used as dietary supplements-anticipating hydrolysis in the gut and absorption of the free alcohol to act as an active intra- and intercellular antioxidant. Ethyl derivatives on the aromatic ring are also active. Oxidation products of a-tocopherol can be reduced with hydrosulphite to a -tocopherylhydroquinone or, in the presence of ascorbic acid, to a -tocopherol.

Table: The Tocopherols.

a -Tocopherol (alpha)	5,7,8-Trimethyltocol
b -Tocopherol (beta)	5,8-Dimethyltocol
g -Tocopherol (gamma)	7,8-Dimethyltocol
z_2-Tocopherol ($zeta_2$)	5,7-Dimethyltocol
h -Tocopherol (eta)	7-Methyltocol
d -Tocopherol (delta)	8-Methyltocol
e -Tocopherol (epsilon)	5,8-Dimethyltocotrienol
z_1-Tocopherol ($zeta_1$)	5,7,8-Trimethyltocotrienol

Positive Functions

The tocopherols act as extra and intracellular antioxidants to maintain homeostasis of labile metabolites in the cell and tissue plasma. As physiological antioxidants, these usually protect oxidizable vitamins and labile unsaturated fatty acids. Vitamin E prevents encephalomalacia in chicks, erythrocyte haemolysis in several animals and steatitis in mink, pigs, and farm animals. The tocopherols also prevent exudative diathesis in chicks, white muscle disease in lambs and calves, and dietary liver necrosis in rats. They act with selenium and with vitamin C for normal reproductive activity and are involved in prevention of nutritional muscular dystrophy in the chick, the yellowtail and carp. The tocopherols act as free radical traps to stop the chain reaction during peroxide formation and stabilize unsaturated carbon bonds of polyunsaturated fatty acids and other long-chain labile compounds.

Vitamin E is involved in the maintenance of normal blood capillary permeability and the integrity of heart muscle. It was first shown to be involved in prevention of sterility and foetal resorption in rats. It may likewise affect embryo membrane permeability and hatch-ability of fish eggs.

Syndrome of Deficiency or Excess

Deficiency signs in fish are listed in table. One of the first signs is erythrocyte fragility closely followed by anaemia, ascites, xerophthalmia, poor growth, poor food conversion, epicarditis, and ceroid deposits in spleen and liver. Muscle dystrophy and xerophthalmia have been described in yellowtail and carp. Non-specific forms of degenerative conditions have been described in several species of fish fed large quantities of polyunsaturated fatty acids with inadequate tocopherol in the ration. Hypervitaminosis E results in poor growth, toxic liver reaction, and death.

Requirements

The exact requirement of the fish for a -tocopherol may depend upon the amount and type of polyunsaturated fatty acids content of the ration. Polyunsaturated labile fish oils may invoke an increased requirement for intracellular antioxidants.

In addition, the amount of tocopherol needed as a supplement to the ration will depend upon the form of the vitamin used, the method of diet preparation, and the storage conditions before feeding.

Sources and Protection

Vegetable oils are rich sources of tocopherols. Synthetic a -tocopherol in esterfied acetate or phosphate form is commonly used as a diet supplement. These esters are much more stable than the free form which is rapidly lost by air oxidation or in the presence of labile compounds like the polyunsaturated fish oils. Addition of antioxidants such as BHT (butylated hydroxyanisole) and BHT (butylated hydroxytoluene) protects fats and other labile compounds in the ration from oxidation, but these antioxidants have no vitamin E activity.

Clinical Assessment

The erythrocyte fragility test indicates the physiological state of fish. Absence of histologically detectable ceroid in liver and spleen from representative samples in the population is a good clue on the presence of adequate amounts of physiological antioxidants in the fish. A barbituric acid test for oxidation of components has not been applied to fish tissues as a clinical tool for assessment of nutrition state except when liver oils become saturated with very labile polyunsaturated fatty acids such as when feeding squid or saury oils. These assays are good indicators of the state of oxidation of the finished ration, but the absence of deficiency signs and normal erythrocyte fragility are better clinical tests. Analysis for tocopherol is difficult and time-consuming and only applicable under critical research experiment situation.

Vitamin K

The name vitamin K (for 'koagulation') was proposed by Dam. Dam isolated the vitamin from alfalfa and from fish meal in 1939. It was synthesized later that year.

Chemistry

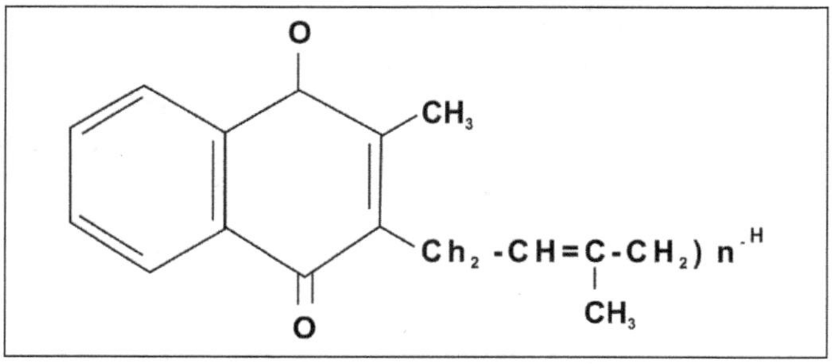

Figure: Vitamin K2 series; n may equal 6, 7 or 9 isoprene units.

The K vitamins K_2 contain 6, 7, or 9 isoprene units in the side chain which varies from 30-45 carbon atoms. Many isosteres of vitamin K have been identified in animal tissues, plant tissues, and micro-organisms. The structure of phthiocol and menadione (K_3) are shown below:

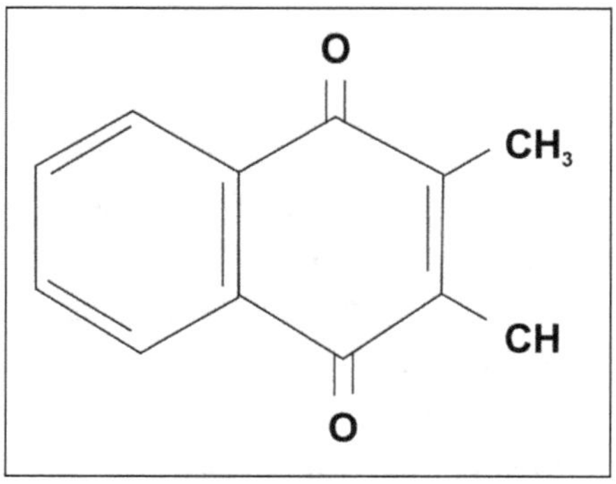

Figure: Pthiocol

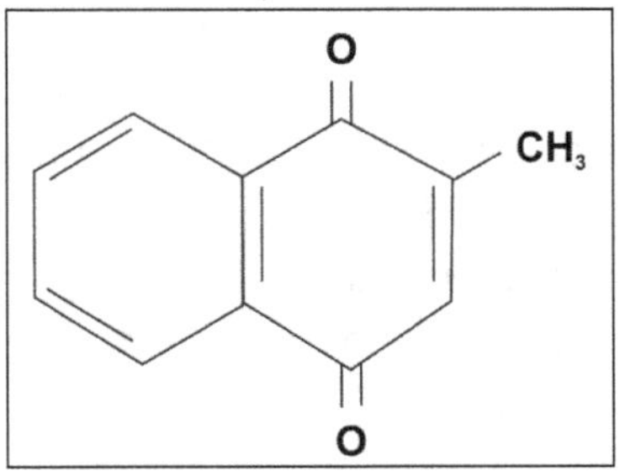

Figure: Menadione

Although fairly stable compounds, they are destroyed upon oxidation and exposure to ultraviolet radiation. Menadione is very reactive and is subject in aqueous media to chemical interaction.

Positive Functions

Vitamin K is involved in the hepatic synthesis of blood clotting proteins - prothrombin and proconvertin. A simplified scheme of blood coagulation is shown Substituted forms of vitamin K are strongly bacteriostatic and may serve as an alternate defence mechanism for bacterial infections. Vitamin K is structurally related to flavo compounds which function as electron carriers in the electron transport system. The primary role of vitamin K is to maintain a fast normal blood clotting rate which is so important to fish living in a water environment.

Syndrome of Deficiency or Excess

Prothrombin time in salmon fed diets devoid of vitamin K was increased three to five times and, during prolonged deficiency states, anaemia and hemorrhagic areas appeared in the gills, eyes, and vascular tissues. Increased blood clotting time has also been reported for other fish reared on diets with low vitamin K content. Interrelationships with other vitamins have not been documented in fish where the primary deficiency signs are slow blood clotting and haemorrhage, severe anaemia, or death in wounded fish. Haemorrhagic areas often appear in fragile tissues such as the gills.

Requirements

Nutritional deficiency signs in fish occur within 10-14 weeks. Quantitative requirement studies have not been completed are needed in order to define the vitamin K-requirement of rapidly growing young fish, especially those held in high population density under intensive fish husbandry conditions.

Sources and Protection

Vitamin K sources are green, leafy vegetables. Alfalfa leaves are among the best sources of vitamin K. Low levels are found in soybeans and animal liver. Synthetic menadione is also available. Although vitamin K in ground alfalfa is fairly stable, synthetic material should be protected from exposure to ultraviolet light and to excessive oxidizing or reducing conditions. The use of rapidly cured dehydrated alfalfa is essential to minimize formation of the physiological antagonist, dicumarol. The diet should be kept dry, prepared with minimum exposure to air oxidation, and fed as soon as practicable after manufacture to minimize vitamin K loss.

Antimetabolites and Inactivation

Two vitamin K antagonists, dicumarol and warfarin are shown below:

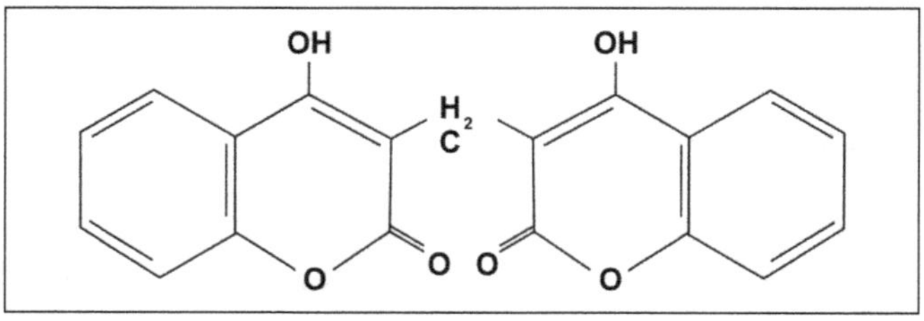

Figure: Dicumarol

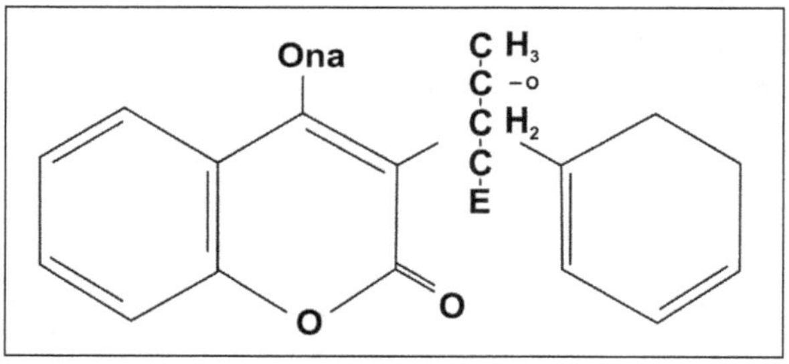

Figure: Warfarin

Dicumarol was isolated from spoiled sweet clover hay and shown to prevent the normal function of vitamin K in maintenance of normal blood clotting times. Early work was with cattle and hogs but was soon extended to rats, other experimental animals, and man. Dicumarol is an anticoagulant and has been used to prevent thrombosis in animals and man. It is not an antimetabolite competing for vitamin K sites but plays another role in preventing normal blood clotting. Vitamin K counteracts the dicumarol effect quantitatively. Another anticoagulant, warfarin, is a common rat poison which has five to ten times the anticoagulant activity of dicumarol. The effects of warfarin can also be reversed by administration of vitamin K.

Clinical Assessment

Vitamin K status of fish is determined by measuring blood clotting time. Chemical methods for determining menadione content of active metabolite after storage are available but have not been applied to measure vitamin K activity in the liver or tissues of young, growing fish.

Absorption of Vitamins

Vitamins are organic molecules necessary for normal metabolism in animals, but either is not synthesized in the body or is synthesized in inadequate quantities and must be obtained from the diet. Essentially all vitamin absorption occurs in the small intestine.

Absorption of vitamins in the intestine is critical in avoiding deficiency states, and impairment of intestinal vitamin absorption can results from a number of factors, including intestinal disease, genetic disorders in transport molecules, excessive alcohol consumption and interactions with drugs.

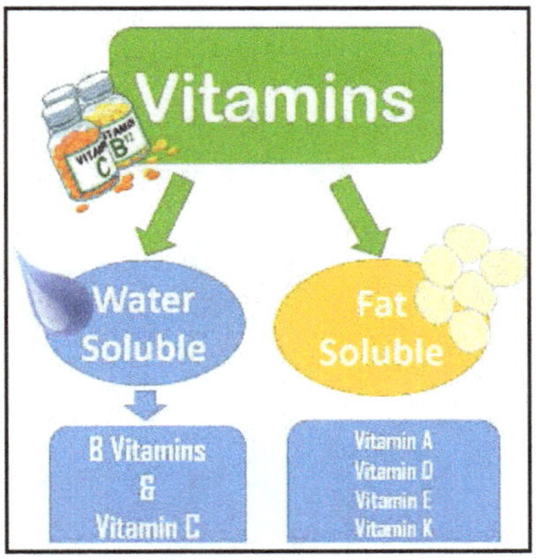

Absorption of Water-Soluble Vitamins

Most water soluble vitamins are available for intestinal absorption from two sources:

- The diet.
- Synthesis by microbes in the large intestine or, in the case of ruminants, the rumen.

These dual-origin vitamins include biotin, folic acid, pantothenic acid, riboflavin and thiamin. Ascorbic acid can be synthesized by many animals, but not by primates or guinea pigs, in which it is a true vitamin and must be obtained from dietary sources. Niacin is also a bit different - it can be synthesized within the body from tryptophan but is also absorbed in the intestine from dietary sources.

Water soluble vitamins of dietary origin are absorbed predominantly in the small intestine, whereas those synthesized by microbes in the large intestine are absorbed there. For most of these vitamins, specific carrier-mediated transport systems have been identified that allow uptake from the intestinal lumen into the enterocyte and for export from the basolateral surface of the enterocyte. Some of these transporters are sodium-dependent, while others are not.

Absorption of Fat-Soluble Vitamins

The fat soluble vitamins A, D, E and K are absorbed from the intestinal lumen using the same mechanisms used for absorption of other lipids. In short, they are incorporated into mixed micelles with other lipids and bile acids in the lumen of the small intestine and enter the enterocyte largely by diffusion. Within the enterocytge, they are incorporated into chylomicrons and exported via exocytosis into lymph.

5

Minerals

Minerals are chemical elements required in small amounts as essential nutrients by organisms to perform normal metabolism. Minerals are of two types; macrominerals and trace elements. Minerals and other related topics are discussed at lenght in this chapter.

Mineral

Minerals are important for your body to stay healthy. Your body uses minerals for many different jobs, including keeping your bones, muscles, heart, and brain working properly. Minerals are also important for making enzymes and hormones.

There are two kinds of minerals: macrominerals and trace minerals. You need larger amounts of macrominerals. They include calcium, phosphorus, magnesium, sodium, potassium, chloride and sulfur. You only need small amounts of trace minerals. They include iron, manganese, copper, iodine, zinc, cobalt, fluoride and selenium.

Most people get the amount of minerals they need by eating a wide variety of foods. In some cases, your doctor may recommend a mineral supplement. People who have certain health problems or take some medicines may need to get less of one of the minerals. For example, people with chronic kidney disease need to limit foods that are high in potassium.

List of Mineral Nutrients

Boron (B)

Boron can be found in many fruits, vegetables and nuts.

Boron is needed by the body in tiny quantities. Boron helps the body to use both calcium and magnesium effectively. Boron is thought to be useful in bone development and maintenance, muscle development and strength and can help alleviate problems associated with Vitamin D deficiency. Boron may also help to prevent arthritis.

Calcium (Ca)

Calcium is found in milk and other dairy products including cheese and yoghurt, lower fat dairy products contain more calcium as less of their volume is taken up with fat. Nuts, seeds, oily fish and dark green vegetables can also be rich sources of calcium.

Calcium is required for the production and upkeep of bones and teeth. Calcium also plays key roles in nerve signalling, muscle contraction, as well as controlling levels of some hormones. Too much calcium is dangerous and can lead to serious problems like stroke and heart attack whereas too little can cause muscle cramps, numbness in the extremities and abnormal heartbeats.

Chromium (Cr)

Chromium helps the body breakdown fat, carbohydrates and some hormones like insulin. Chromium is also fundamental in the body's production of some fatty acids and cholesterol – essential for brain function. Needed in small quantities and common in many foods, we get most of our chromium through meat, fish, whole grains, fruit and vegetables.

Cobalt (Co)

Cobalt is one of the elements found in vitamin B12. Helping with the production of red blood cells cobalt is needed in small quantities in our diet. (More about Vitamins).

Copper (Cu)

Copper is needed by the body to make healthy haemoglobin (red blood cells) and bones. Copper is also necessary for effective healing of wounds as it helps the blood to clot, for the colouring or pigmentation of hair and fertility. There is a correlation between copper and levels of certain fat in the blood, especially cholesterol, the more copper the less cholesterol and vice-versa. However you should only increase your copper intake if you are told by a health-care professional that you have a deficiency.

Copper is stored in tiny amounts in the body and therefore does not need to be replenished every day. As well as from natural sources such as lamb, liver, oysters, nuts, cherries, whole grains, seeds, and many fruit and vegetables traces of copper may be found in water supplies using copper pipes or transferred to the body via copper cooking implements and pans.

Fluorine (F)

Fluorine is good for the teeth, helping to prevent and even reverse tooth decay and is found in many toothpastes and mouthwash products.

Fluorine is also added, sometimes controversially, to the water supply mainly in USA, Canada, Brazil, Australia, New Zealand, Philippines and parts of Europe including the UK, Ireland and Spain. Fluorine can also be naturally present in water supplies in varying levels - sometimes water is treated to remove excess fluorine. People have speculated that adding fluorine to water would cause health problems, cancer being a particular concern, however, apart from a discolouring of the teeth at high levels, there is no evidence that fluorine is toxic. As fluorine is found naturally or added to fresh water it is also present in many foods.

Iodine (I)

Iodine helps in the production of thyroid hormones. These hormones help your body to keep a healthy metabolism, digesting food thoroughly and at the right speed. Iodine may also help prevent certain cancers. Good sources of Iodine include sea fish other seafood, cereals and grains depending on the amount of naturally occurring iodine in the soil where they were grown.

Iron (Fe)

Iron an important nutrient helping to make red blood cells, which carry oxygen around the body. A lack of iron can lead to iron deficiency anaemia, a potentially serious condition, which may include some of the following symptoms: tiredness, feeling faint and being easily made breathless, heart palpitations, fragile nails, hair loss and in extreme cases heart failure. Iron deficiency anaemia occurs most commonly in women during heavy menstruation and in pregnancy and can usually be easily corrected with iron supplements.

Manganese (Mn)

Manganese is an essential element useful in the formation of bone and performing functions in the pituitary gland, liver, pancreas, kidney. Manganese also aids the breaking down of carbohydrates, cholesterol and amino acids in the body. Manganese is found in whole grains, many fruits and vegetables and tea.

Molybdenum (Mo)

Pronounced mol-ib-de-num, molybdenum is found in many foods, including liver, eggs, green beans, sunflower seeds, lentils, cucumbers and whole grains – the amount of molybdenum found in foods is dependent upon the area in which they were grown. Molybdenum plays some key roles in the body, including enabling enzymes to function. Enzymes are large molecules that increase the speed of chemical reactions within the body without being changed themselves in the process.

Molybdenum can help protect against certain cancers, but in high doses can also interfere with the body's ability to process copper.

Nickel (Ni)

Nickel is needed in very small quantities in the body and its exact purpose is unclear. However having too much or too little nickel can cause problems. A deficiency can lead to depression, hypotension, liver disease and anaemia. People with nickel deficiency can also have high blood sugar. Too much nickel on the other hand can mean low blood sugar levels and increased risk of chest pains (angina) and asthma. Nickel is found in nuts, seeds, whole grains, cocoa powder and dark chocolate as well as many other foods.

Selenium (Se)

Selenium is needed, in very small amounts, as part of our daily diet. Selenium protects your body's cells from damage caused by oxidisation it helps to strengthen the immune system and supports thyroid function for a healthy metabolism. Selenium can also help keep your hair and nails looking good.

Selenium occurs naturally in many foods – selenium levels in foods are dependent on the naturally occurring selenium levels in soil and therefore vary by geographic location. Brazil Nuts are particularly high in Selenium but the element can also be found in some cereals, meat, fish – especially shrimp, tuna and salmon, mushrooms, and eggs. Eating one Brazil nut a day as part of a healthy balanced diet will keep your selenium levels topped up.

Silicon (Si)

Although rarely written about as an essential mineral, silicon plays some important roles in the body. Silicon helps to make bone, blood vessels, cartilage, tendons and strong nails. Silicon also helps the skin to remain flexible and avoid premature ageing.

Being the most abundant element in the soil, silicon is present in many foods especially whole grains, sugar, fresh herbs, salad greens and cucumbers. Areas of hard drinking water may also be a good source.

Sodium (Na)

Most modern diets provide sodium in levels far higher than needed by the body due to the amount of sodium chloride (salt) contained in processed and manufactured foods. Salt is made up of approximately 40% sodium and 60% chloride. According to the U.S. Department of Health and Human Services the average daily American diet contains around 3,400 mg of sodium. The body needs only around 1,500 mg of sodium (less than a teaspoon of salt) a day. The sodium helps regulate the amount of water in cells, control the overall fluid balances in the body and help keep nerves and muscles working correctly.

Sodium chloride or salt intake has an effect of blood pressure; high salt diets increase blood pressure whereas reduced sodium intake can help lower blood pressure. High blood pressure can result in serious health problems including heart and kidney disease.

Vanadium (V)

Vanadium is needed in only tiny amounts in the body. Most people get enough vanadium from the food they eat and vanadium deficiency is very rare. Vanadium supplements are usually not recommended as high levels can be toxic. Vanadium is essential for proper growth and development of bones.

With the help of 'Popeye the Sailor Man' many people believe that spinach is a good source of iron – it is, however spinach also contains iron absorption-inhibiting substances that render most of the iron in spinach unusable by the human body. Tea and coffee also contain substances that can make it harder for the body to absorb iron. Good sources of iron include: liver (and liver pâté), fortified breakfast cereals, kale, nuts, beans and whole grains.

Zinc (Zn)

Zinc is an essential mineral and of paramount importance to health. Zinc deficiency is a huge problem in developing nations and it is estimated that zinc deficiency affects around two billion people. In children, lack of zinc can hinder natural growth and sexual maturity, increase the likelihood of developing infections and can cause diarrhoea. In adults, Zinc deficiency is usually due to inadequate diet. There are many symptoms of zinc deficiency, these can include: depressed growth, diarrhoea, impotence, hair loss, eye and skin lesions, reduced appetite, reduced concentration and other brain functions and a weaker immune system.

Zinc is present in many foods, including meat – especially red meats, seeds and nuts, seafood, cocoa powder and dark chocolate. Zinc supplements are widely available and are sometimes recommended for people on vegetarian and vegan diets.

Dietary Nutrition

Dietitians may recommend that minerals are best supplied by ingesting specific foods rich with the chemical element(s) of interest. The elements may be naturally present in the food (e.g., calcium in dairy milk) or added to the food (e.g., orange juice fortified with calcium; iodized salt fortified with iodine). Dietary supplements can be formulated to contain several different chemical elements (as compounds), a combination of vitamins and/or other chemical compounds, or a single element (as a compound or mixture of compounds), such as calcium (as calcium carbonate, calcium citrate, etc.) or magnesium (as magnesium oxide, etc.), or iron (as ferrous sulfate, iron bis-glycinate, etc.).

The dietary focus on chemical elements derives from an interest in supporting the biochemical reactions of metabolism with the required elemental components. Appropriate intake levels of certain chemical elements have been demonstrated to be required to maintain optimal health. Diet can meet all the body's chemical element requirements, although supplements can be used when some requirements (e.g., calcium, which is found mainly in dairy products) are not adequately met by the diet, or when chronic or acute deficiencies arise from pathology, injury, etc. Research has supported that altering inorganic mineral compounds (carbonates, oxides, etc.) by reacting them with organic ligands (amino acids, organic acids, etc.) improves the bioavailability of the supplemented mineral.

Macrominerals

Macrominerals are inorganic nutrients that the human body requires in large quantities because they carry out several critical bodily functions. The most important macrominerals include potassium, calcium, magnesium, sodium, chloride, sulfur and phosphorus. The recommended daily allowance of each of these in the human diet varies widely, from 320 mg each day for magnesium to 4,700 mg each day for potassium. If a person has a balanced diet, he typically consumes the macrominerals required each day.

Most people know that calcium is important for bone strength and density as well as for dental health, but it also plays a role in the dilation and contraction of the blood vessels, the communication of nerve signals, the movement of muscles and hormonal secretion.

Phosphorus is also important for strong teeth and bones, but it also helps the renal system filter toxins out of the blood. In addition, phosphorus is a basic building block of genetic material and helps the body store energy until it is needed.

Potassium has the important job of regulating the electrical currents that manage the heartbeat while helping with the building of proteins and muscles. Potassium helps the body break carbohydrates down so that the body converts them into energy sources. If potassium levels are off, heart rhythm suffers as well.

Calcium

Calcium is crucial in growing new bone and maintaining bone strength. Calcium supplements are standard for treating and preventing osteoporosis -- weak and easily broken bones -- and its precursor, osteopenia.

Calcium is used for many other conditions. It's an ingredient in many antacids. Doctors also use calcium to control high levels of magnesium, phosphorus, and potassium in the blood. There's good evidence that calcium can help prevent or control high blood pressure. It also may reduce PMS symptoms as well as play a role in preventing certain cancers. Calcium with vitamin D, for instance, may help protect against breast cancer in premenopausal women.

The data, though, are still inconclusive as to whether it might do the same for postmenopausal women. Calcium also has been looked at for other uses, for example, aiding weight loss. But so far, these studies have been inconclusive.

The people at highest risk of a calcium deficiency are postmenopausal women. Since dairy products are one of the most common sources of calcium, people who are lactose intolerant or vegan are also at increased risk of calcium deficiency.

How much Calcium should you Take?

The Institute of Medicine has set Dietary Reference Intakes (DRI) and Recommended Daily Allowances (RDA) for calcium. Getting this amount from diet, with or without supplements, may be enough to keep your bones healthy. Doctors may recommend higher doses.

Category	Calcium: (DRI)
0-6 months	Adequate Intake: 200 mg/day
7-12 months	AI: 260 mg/day
1-3 years	700 mg/day
4-8 years	1,000 mg/day
9-18 years	1,300 mg/day
19-50 years	1,000 mg/day
51- 70 years	1,200 mg/day (women) 1,000 mg/day (men)
70+ years	1,200 mg/day

Women who are pregnant or breastfeeding do not need extra calcium beyond the recommendations above.

The tolerable upper intake levels (UL) of a supplement are the highest amount that most people can take safely. For calcium, it's 1000 mg/day for infants 0-6 months, 1500 mg/day for infants 7-12 months, 2,500 mg/day for children 1-8 years, 3000 mg/day for children/teens 9-18 years, 2500 mg/day for adults 19-50 years, and 2000 mg/day for adults over the age of 51 years.

In general, it's best to take calcium supplements with food. For better absorption, don't take more than 500 milligrams at one time. Split up larger doses over the course of the day. For the body to make use of calcium properly, you also need to get enough vitamin D and magnesium.

Can you Get Calcium Naturally from Foods?

Good sources of calcium include:

- Milk.
- Cheese.
- Yogurt.
- Broccoli, kale, and Chinese cabbage.

- Fortified cereals, juices, soy products, and other foods.
- Tofu.

Experts say that most adults in the U.S. don't get enough calcium. While improving one's diet will help, many people do need to take calcium supplements as well.

What are the Risks of Taking Calcium?

- Side effects. At normal doses, calcium supplements may cause bloating, gas, and constipation. Very high doses of calcium can cause kidney stones. Research has found an increased risk of heart attacksand strokes in some people taking calcium supplements in addition to a diet high in calcium, though the true accuracy of these findings is being actively debated by experts.
- Interactions. If you take any prescription or over-the-counter medicines regularly, ask your doctor if it's safe to use calcium supplements. Calcium can interact with drugs for heart disease, diabetes, epilepsy, and other conditions. Excessive doses of vitamin D can result in dangerously high levels of calcium. High doses of calcium can also interfere with the absorption of other minerals, like iron and zinc. In general, take calcium one to two hours apart from other supplements or medications. When taken at the same time, calcium can bind those products and pass them unabsorbed from the body.
- Risks. People with kidney disease, heart problems, sarcoidosis, or bone tumors should not take calcium supplements unless their doctors suggest it.
- Overdose. Excessive levels of calcium in the blood can cause nausea, dry mouth, abdominal pain, irregular heartbeat, confusion, and even death.

There is no need to use products identified as "coral calcium." Claims made that coral calcium is superior to regular calcium are unsubstantiated. Also, coral calcium products may contain dangerous amounts of lead.

Phosphorus

Phosphorus is an essential mineral primarily used for growth and repair of body cells and tissues. According to the University of Maryland Medical Center, all body cells contain phosphorus, with 85 percent found in bones and teeth. There, together with calcium, phosphorus provides structure and strength. Phosphorus is also required for a variety of biochemical processes including energy production and pH regulation.

Energy Production

Phosphorus is commonly found in the body as phosphate. Phosphates play an important role in energy production as components of ATP, or adenosine triphosphate. ATP is readily used to fuel your body's many functions. Structurally, ATP consists of adenosine, an organic compound, and three phosphate molecules. When bonding between one phosphate and adenosine is severed, energy is released which then fires cellular activity. According to the authors of "Nutrition," energy released from ATP is used quickly, so your body contains only a small amount at any one time.

Protein Synthesis

Phosphorus is a component of deoxyribonucleic acid, or DNA, and ribonucleic acid, or RNA, long molecules which carry genetic information used to make proteins. Synthesis begins in the cell nucleus, where a portion of DNA serves as a template for RNA manufacture. RNA then carries specific coding instructions for building needed body proteins to the ribosomes, where proteins are assembled from amino acids. Without sufficient phosphorus, body protein manufacture is impaired, which eventually affects overall health.

Secondary Functions

Phosphorus also acts as a buffer, neutralizing acids to maintain normal pH in the blood. Many enzymes and hormones also contain phosphorus as a structural component. Hemoglobin, the important oxygen-carrying protein in the bloodstream, also depends upon phosphorus contained in its structure for proper function.

Food Sources and Requirements

Good food sources of phosphorus include protein foods, such as meat, fish, eggs, milk, nuts and legumes, and also cereals and grains. Carbonated beverages supply significant amounts of phosphorus in the diet, too. Gordon Wardlaw and Anne Smith, in their book "Contemporary Nutrition," report that between 20 and 30 percent of dietary phosphorus comes from food additives contained in processed foods. The Institute of Medicine's Recommended Dietary Allowance for adults is 700 milligrams of phosphorus per day. The Tolerable Upper Intake Limit, or UL, also set by the Institute of Medicine, is 4 grams per day. Intakes above this are considered unsafe.

Precautions

Because phosphorus is found in a wide variety of foods, deficiencies are rare, except in diseases that affect absorption, such as diabetes or Crohn's disease. In children, phosphorus deficiency affects normal bone and teeth development. According to the University of Maryland Medical Center, many individuals consume over twice as much phosphorus as they do calcium. Equal amounts of both minerals are necessary to avoid calcium depletion from bones. As your intake of phosphorus increases, so should your intake of calcium in order to prevent bone abnormalities.

Potassium

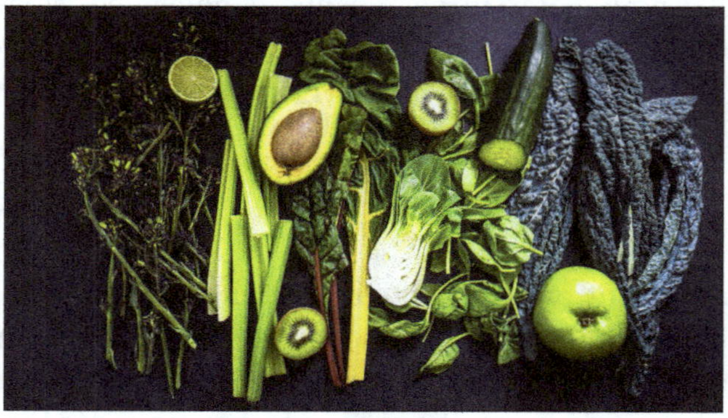

Potassium is the third most abundant mineral in the body.

It helps the body regulate fluid, send nerve signals and regulate muscle contractions.

Roughly 98% of the potassium in your body is found in your cells. Of this, 80% is found in your muscle cells, while the other 20% can be found in your bones, liver and red blood cells.

Once inside your body, it functions as an electrolyte.

When in water, an electrolyte dissolves into positive or negative ions that have the ability to conduct electricity. Potassium ions carry a positive charge.

Your body uses this electricity to manage a variety of processes, including fluid balance, nerve signals and muscle contractions.

Therefore, a low or high amount of electrolytes in the body can affect many crucial functions.

Potassium is a mineral that, among other things, helps muscles contract, helps regulate fluids and mineral balance in and out of body cells, and helps maintain normal blood pressure by blunting the effect of sodium. Potassium also may reduce the risk of recurrent kidney stones and bone loss as we age.

Potassium is found in a wide range of foods, especially fruits and vegetables such as leafy greens, tomatoes, cucumbers, zucchini, eggplant, pumpkins, potatoes, carrots and beans. It's also found in dairy foods, meat, poultry, fish and nuts.

Sources of Potassium

Our bodies cannot store potassium, that's why it's so important for us to have a diet rich enough in this valuable nutrient. In the absence of a healthy diet, we could be deficient in potassium without even knowing it. If we don't get enough potassium, we may suffer from heart disease, high blood pressure, or digestive and muscle disorders, among other conditions. Here is a table that shows how much potassium people of different age groups' should have per day.

Ages	Adequate Intake Per Day
0-6 months	400 mg
7-12 months	700 mg
1-3 years	3,000 mg
4-8 years	3,800 mg
9-13 years	4,500 mg
14 years and up	4,700 mg
Pregnant women	4,700 mg
Breastfeeding women	5,100 mg

Daily potassium recommendations.

Do you love green leafy vegetables? What do you think about beans? If you do, the good news is, these are key sources of potassium that can help you meet your daily intake of this essential element. Here are some excellent potassium-rich sources, shown in milligrams per serving size.

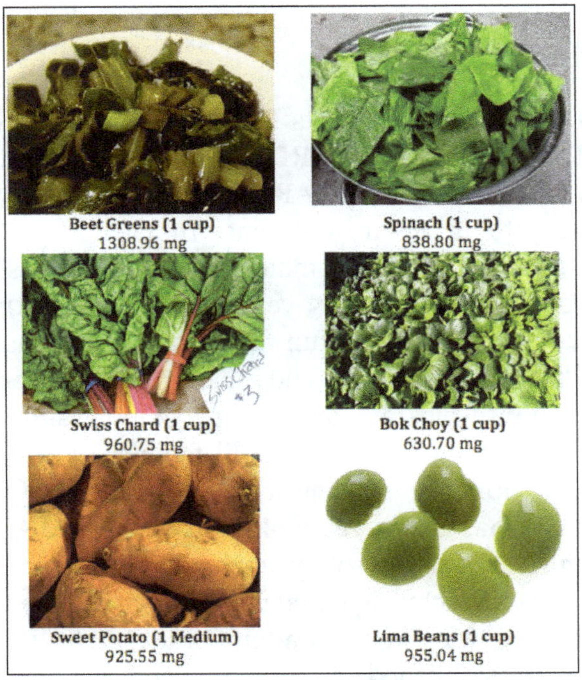
Beet Greens (1 cup)
1308.96 mg
Spinach (1 cup)
838.80 mg
Swiss Chard (1 cup)
960.75 mg
Bok Choy (1 cup)
630.70 mg
Sweet Potato (1 Medium)
925.55 mg
Lima Beans (1 cup)
955.04 mg

Sources rich in potassium.

If you are not too fond of the previously mentioned food sources, there are others that also have a high potassium content. Here are some fruits and other vegetables that are also great sources of potassium.

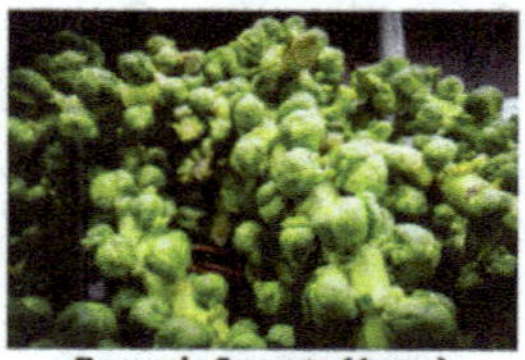

Brussels Sprouts (1 cup)
494.52 mg

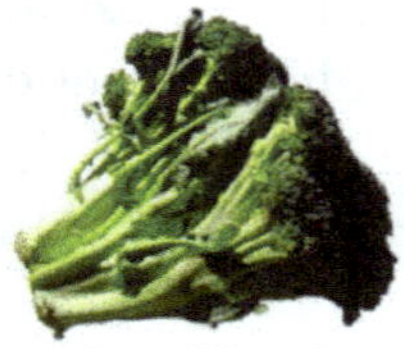

Broccoli (1 cup)
457.08 mg

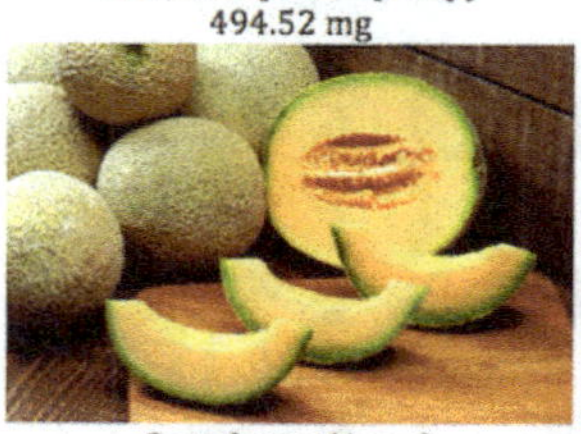

Cantaloupe (1 cup)
427.20 mg

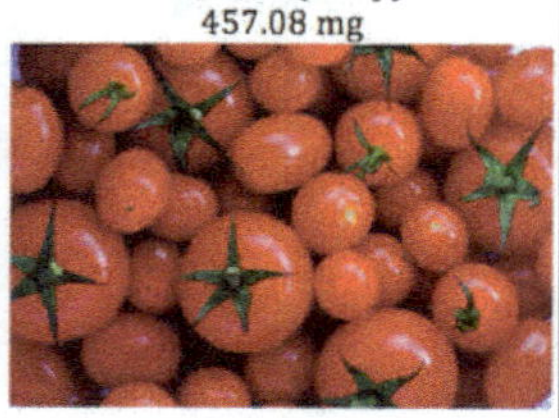

Tomatoes (1 cup)
426.60 mg

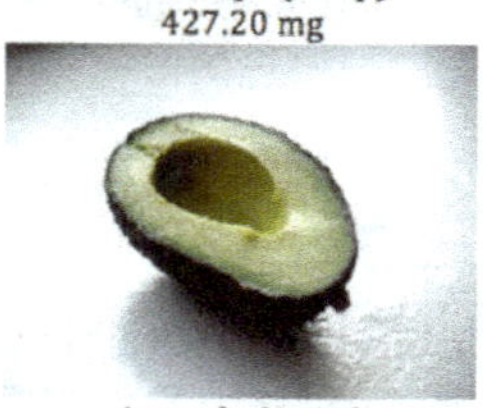

Avocado (1 cup)
727.50 mg

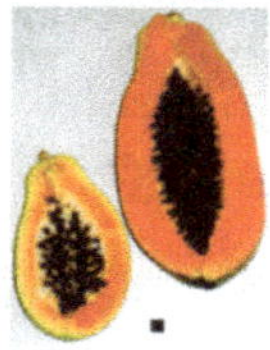

Papaya (1 medium)
502.32 mg

Nutrition

Dietary Recommendations

The U.S. Institute of Medicine (IOM) sets Estimated Average Requirements (EARs) and Recommended Dietary Allowances (RDAs), or Adequate Intakes (AIs) for when there is not sufficient information to set EARs and RDAs. Collectively the EARs, RDAs, AIs and ULs are referred to as Dietary Reference Intakes. The AIs for potassium are: 400mg of potassium for 0-6-month-old males, 700mg of potassium for 7-12-month-old males, 3,000mg of potassium for 1-3-year-old males, 3,800mg of potassium for 4-8-year-old males, 4,500mg of potassium for 9-13-year-old males, and 4,700mg of potassium for males that are 14 years old and older. The AIs for potassium are: 400mg of potassium for 0-6-month-old females, 700mg of potassium for 7-12-month-old females, 3,000mg of potassium for 1-3-year-old females, 3,800mg of potassium for 4-8-year-old females, 4,500mg of potassium for 9-13-year-old females, and 4,700mg of potassium for females that are 14 years old and older. The AIs for potassium are: 4,700mg of potassium for 14-50-year-old pregnant females; furthermore, 5,100mg of potassium for 14-50-year-old lactating females. As for safety, the IOM also sets Tolerable upper intake levels (ULs) for vitamins and minerals, but for potassium the evidence was insufficient, so no UL established.

Most Americans consume only half that amount per day.

Likewise, in the European Union, in particular in Germany and Italy, insufficient potassium intake is somewhat common. However, the British National Health Service recommends a lower intake, saying that adults need 3,500 mg per day and that excess amounts may cause health problems such as stomach pain and diarrhoea.

Food Sources

Potassium is present in all fruits, vegetables, meat and fish. Foods with high potassium concentrations include yam, parsley, dried apricots, milk, chocolate, all nuts (especially almonds and pistachios), potatoes, bamboo shoots, bananas, avocados, coconut water, soybeans, and bran.

The USDA lists tomato paste, orange juice, beet greens, white beans, potatoes, plantains, bananas, apricots, and many other dietary sources of potassium, ranked in descending order according to potassium content. A day's worth of potassium is in 5 plantains or 11 bananas.

Deficient Intake

Diets low in potassium can lead to hypertension and hypokalemia.

Supplementation

Supplements of potassium are most widely used in conjunction with diuretics that block reabsorption of sodium and water upstream from the distal tubule (thiazides and loop diuretics), because this promotes increased distal tubular potassium secretion, with resultant increased potassium excretion. A variety of prescription and over-the counter supplements are available. Potassium chloride may be dissolved in water, but the salty/bitter taste make liquid supplements unpalatable. Typical doses range from 10 mmol (400 mg), to 20 mmol (800 mg). Potassium is also available in tablets or capsules, which are formulated to allow potassium to leach slowly out of a matrix, since very high concentrations of potassium ion that occur adjacent to a solid tablet can injure the gastric or intestinal mucosa. For this reason, non-prescription potassium pills are limited by law in the US to a maximum of 99 mg of potassium.

Since the kidneys are the site of potassium excretion, individuals with impaired kidney function are at risk for hyperkalemia if dietary potassium and supplements are not restricted. The more severe the impairment, the more severe is the restriction necessary to avoid hyperkalemia.

A meta-analysis concluded that a 1640 mg increase in the daily intake of potassium was associated with a 21% lower risk of stroke. Potassium chloride and potassium bicarbonate may be useful to control mild hypertension.

Detection by Taste Buds

Potassium can be detected by taste because it triggers three of the five types of taste sensations, according to concentration. Dilute solutions of potassium ions taste sweet, allowing moderate concentrations in milk and juices, while higher concentrations become increasingly bitter/alkaline, and finally also salty to the taste. The combined bitterness and saltiness of high-potassium solutions makes high-dose potassium supplementation by liquid drinks a palatability challenge.

It Helps Regulate Fluid Balance

The body is made of approximately 60% water.

40% of this water is found inside your cells in a substance called intracellular fluid (ICF).

The remainder is found outside your cells in areas such as your blood, spinal fluid and between cells. This fluid is called extracellular fluid (ECF).

Interestingly, the amount of water in the ICF and ECF is affected by their concentration of electrolytes, especially potassium and sodium.

Potassium is the main electrolyte in the ICF, and it determines the amount of water inside the cells. Conversely, sodium is the main electrolyte in the ECF, and it determines the amount of water outside the cells.

The number of electrolytes relative to the amount of fluid is called osmolality. Under normal conditions, the osmolality is the same inside and outside your cells.

Simply put, there's an equal balance of electrolytes outside and inside your cells.

However, when osmolality is unequal, water from the side with fewer electrolytes will move into the side with more electrolytes to equalize electrolyte concentrations.

This may cause cells to shrink as water moves out of them, or swell up and burst as water moves into them.

That's why it's important to make sure you consume the right electrolytes, including potassium.

Maintaining good fluid balance is important for optimal health. Poor fluid balance can lead to dehydration, which in turn affects the heart and kidneys.

Eating a potassium-rich diet and staying hydrated can help maintain good fluid balance.

Potassium Is Important for the Nervous System

The nervous system relays messages between your brain and body.

These messages are delivered in the form of nerve impulses and help regulate your muscle contractions, heartbeat, reflexes and many other body functions.

Interestingly, nerve impulses are generated by sodium ions moving into cells and potassium ions moving out of cells.

The movement of ions changes the voltage of the cell, which activates a nerve impulse.

Unfortunately, a drop in blood levels of potassium can affect the body's ability to generate a nerve impulse.

Getting enough potassium from your diet can help you maintain healthy nerve function.

Potassium Helps Regulate Muscle and Heart Contractions

The nervous system helps regulate muscle contractions.

However, altered blood potassium levels can affect nerve signals in the nervous system, weakening muscle contractions.

Both low and high blood levels can affect nerve impulses by altering the voltage of nerve cells.

The mineral is also important for a healthy heart, as its movement in and out of cells helps maintain a regular heartbeat.

When blood levels of the mineral are too high, the heart may become dilated and flaccid. This can weaken its contractions and produce an abnormal heartbeat.

Likewise, low levels in the blood can also alter the heartbeat.

When the heart does not beat properly, it cannot effectively pump blood to the brain, organs and muscles.

In some cases, heart arrhythmia, or an irregular heartbeat, can be fatal and lead to sudden death.

Sodium

Sodium is a mineral that's essential for life. It's regulated in the body by your kidneys, and it helps control your body's fluid balance. It also helps send nerve impulses and affects muscle function.

What are the Common Sources of Sodium?

More than 70% of the sodium we consume comes from packaged, prepared and restaurant foods. The rest of the sodium in our diets occurs naturally in food (about 15 percent) or is added by us when we're cooking food or sitting down to eat.

The latter only makes up only about 11 percent of our total sodium intake, so even if you never use the salt shaker, you're probably getting too much sodium.

Role of Sodium

As much as sodium has been demonized in the American diet—mostly because we consume far too much—it actually plays as vital a role in the functioning of our bodies.

Sodium (like calcium, magnesium, phosphate, and potassium) is an electrolyte, meaning that it creates an electrically charged ion when dissolved in fluids like blood. Our bodies need electrolytes are they facilitate nerve impulses and regulate body functions such as heart rate, digestion, respiration, brain activity, and blood pressure.

For its part, sodium helps maintain the fluid balance in and around cells (including the volume of fluid in the blood) and helps regulate nerve and muscle function.

An excess amount of sodium—above 145 milliequivalents per liter (mEq/L)—can affect the fluid balance and contribute to high blood pressure. By contrast, the excessive loss of sodium (below 135 mEq/L) will not only decrease blood pressure but interfere with the activity of nerve cells and the muscles of the heart and digestive tract.

In humans, sodium is an essential mineral that regulates blood volume, blood pressure, osmotic equilibrium and pH; the minimum physiological requirement for sodium is 500 milligrams per day. Sodium chloride is the principal source of sodium in the diet, and is used as seasoning and preservative in such commodities as pickled preserves and jerky; for Americans, most sodium chloride comes from processed foods. Other sources of sodium are its natural occurrence in food and such food additives as monosodium glutamate (MSG), sodium nitrite, sodium saccharin, baking soda (sodium bicarbonate), and sodium benzoate. The US Institute of Medicine set its Tolerable Upper Intake Level for sodium at 2.3 grams per day, but the average person in the United States consumes 3.4 grams per day. Studies have found that lowering sodium intake by 2 g per day tends to lower systolic blood pressure by about two to four mm Hg. It has been estimated that such a decrease in sodium intake would lead to between 9 and 17% fewer cases of hypertension.

Hypertension causes 7.6 million premature deaths worldwide each year. (Note that salt contains about 39.3% sodium—the rest being chlorine and trace chemicals; thus, 2.3 g sodium is about 5.9 g, or 2.7 ml of salt—about one US teaspoon.) The American Heart Association recommends no more than 1.5 g of sodium per day.

One study found that people with or without hypertension who excreted less than 3 grams of sodium per day in their urine (and therefore were taking in less than 3 g/d) had a *higher* risk of death, stroke, or heart attack than those excreting 4 to 5 grams per day. Levels of 7 g per day or more in people with hypertension were associated with higher mortality and cardiovascular events, but this was not found to be true for people without hypertension. The US FDA states that adults with hypertension and prehypertension should reduce daily intake to 1.5 g.

The renin–angiotensin system regulates the amount of fluid and sodium concentration in the body. Reduction of blood pressure and sodium concentration in the kidney result in the production of renin, which in turn produces aldosterone and angiotensin, retaining sodium in the urine. When the concentration of sodium increases, the production of renin decreases, and the sodium concentration returns to normal. The sodium ion (Na^+) is an important electrolyte in neuron function, and in osmoregulation between cells and the extracellular fluid. This is accomplished in all animals by Na^+/K^+-ATPase, an active transporter pumping ions against the gradient, and sodium/potassium channels. Sodium is the most prevalent metallic ion in extracellular fluid.

Unusually low or high sodium levels in humans are recognized in medicine as hyponatremia and hypernatremia. These conditions may be caused by genetic factors, ageing, or prolonged vomiting or diarrhea.

In C4 plants, sodium is a micronutrient that aids metabolism, specifically in regeneration of phosphoenolpyruvate and synthesis of chlorophyll. In others, it substitutes for potassium in several roles, such as maintaining turgor pressure and aiding in the opening and closing of stomata. Excess sodium in the soil can limit the uptake of water by decreasing the water potential, which may result in plant wilting; excess concentrations in the cytoplasm can lead to enzyme inhibition, which in turn causes necrosis and chlorosis. In response, some plants have developed mechanisms to limit sodium uptake in the roots, to store it in cell vacuoles, and restrict salt transport from roots to leaves; excess sodium may also be stored in old plant tissue, limiting the damage to new growth. Halophytes have adapted to be able to flourish in sodium rich environments.

Causes of Sodium Deficiency

While you lose a little sodium every day when you sweat or urinate, it is generally not enough to cause a sodium deficiency unless you are severely malnourished. By and large, the foods we eat provide us with more than enough sodium to replace whatever we lost.

With that being said, it is possible to be sodium-deficient if you overexert yourself and lose excessive amounts of sodium in sweat. On the flip side, you can drive your sodium levels down by drinking too much water and diluting its concentration.

Both of these things can lead to a potentially dangerous condition known as hyponatremia. With hyponatremia, the extreme loss of sodium can trigger symptoms ranging from muscle cramps, nausea, vomiting, and dizziness to shock, coma, and death.

This is why athletes are routinely advised to consume electrolyte-rich sports drinks during strenuous activities to compensate for the loss of sodium and other essential minerals.

In term of the excessive consumption of water, it generally doesn't happen in daily life as you would need to drink no less than six gallons of water for many days or weeks before it becomes an issue. However, if you drink too much during an endurance event, such as a marathon, you can quickly develop hyponatremia even if it's a sports drink.

This is because our kidneys can eliminate between five and eight gallons of water a day but can't get rid of more than 27 to 33 ounces per hour. As a result, endurance athletes are today advised to drink when thirsty rather than forcing extra fluids.

There are other conditions that can cause hyponatremia by either depleting fluid level or causing the excessive retention of fluids. This is especially true among older adults who take medications or have medical conditions that place them at risk.

The risk factor includes:

- Chronic kidney disease.
- Cirrhosis.
- Congestive heart failure.
- Diuretics ("water pills") used to treat high blood pressure and edema(fluid overload).
- Hypothyroidism (low thyroid function).
- Remeron (mirtazapine), a tetracyclic antidepressant.
- Tegretol (carbamazepine), an anticonvulsant.
- Tricyclic antidepressants.
- Lung cancer and secondary adrenal gland tumors.

Recommended Sodium Intake

According to the Office of Disease Prevention and Health Promotion (ODPHP), you need around 1,500 milligrams (mg) of sodium per day to replace whatever you lose in urine and sweat. In most cases, we consume enough in our regular diet and then some.

Consider how quickly the sodium levels add up if you eat just four ounces of beef (60 mg), a cup of milk (140 mg), one cup of greens (100 mg), two eggs (350 mg), an ounce of blue cheese (375 mg), and one slice of refined white bread (175 mg), and a cup of plain yogurt (150 mg). Even without a grain of added salt, you're already more than halfway to your 1,500-milligram target.

Unfortunately, Americans tend to eat far more than this. In fact, according to ODPHP, the average American consumes around 3,400 milligrams of sodium day due in large part to the packaged and processed foods we grab at the grocery store.

To this end, the ODPHP recommends that American adults consume less than 2,300 milligrams of sodium per day as part of a healthy dietary routine. Furthermore, African Americans, people with high blood pressure, and those over 50 are advised to limit their intake to 1,500 milligrams per day due to the increased risk of cardiovascular disease.

Magnesium

Magnesium, an abundant mineral in the body, is naturally present in many foods, added to other food products, available as a dietary supplement, and present in some medicines (such as antacids and laxatives). Magnesium is a cofactor in more than 300 enzyme systems that regulate diverse biochemical reactions in the body, including protein synthesis, muscle and nerve function, blood glucose control, and blood pressure regulation [1-3]. Magnesium is required for energy production, oxidative phosphorylation, and glycolysis. It contributes to the structural development of bone and is required for the synthesis of DNA, RNA, and the antioxidant glutathione. Magnesium also plays a role in the active transport of calcium and potassium ions across cell membranes, a process that is important to nerve impulse conduction, muscle contraction, and normal heart rhythm.

An adult body contains approximately 25 g magnesium, with 50% to 60% present in the bones and most of the rest in soft tissues. Less than 1% of total magnesium is in blood serum, and these levels are kept under tight control. Normal serum magnesium concentrations range between 0.75 and 0.95 millimoles (mmol)/L [1,5]. Hypomagnesemia is defined as a serum magnesium level less than 0.75 mmol/L. Magnesium homeostasis is largely controlled by the kidney, which typically excretes about 120 mg magnesium into the urine each day. Urinary excretion is reduced when magnesium status is low.

Assessing magnesium status is difficult because most magnesium is inside cells or in bone. The most commonly used and readily available method for assessing magnesium status is measurement of serum magnesium concentration, even though serum levels have little correlation with total body magnesium levels or concentrations in specific tissues. Other methods for assessing magnesium status include measuring magnesium concentrations in erythrocytes, saliva, and urine; measuring ionized magnesium concentrations in blood, plasma, or serum; and conducting a magnesium-loading (or "tolerance") test. No single method is considered satisfactory. Some experts but not others consider the tolerance test (in which urinary magnesium is measured after parenteral infusion of a dose of magnesium) to be the best method to assess magnesium status in adults. To comprehensively evaluate magnesium status, both laboratory tests and a clinical assessment might be required.

Recommended Intakes

Intake recommendations for magnesium and other nutrients are provided in the Dietary Reference Intakes (DRIs) developed by the Food and Nutrition Board (FNB) at the Institute of Medicine of the National Academies (formerly National Academy of Sciences). DRI is the general term for a set of reference values used to plan and assess nutrient intakes of healthy people. These values, which vary by age and sex, include:

- Recommended Dietary Allowance (RDA): Average daily level of intake sufficient to meet the nutrient requirements of nearly all (97%–98%) healthy individuals; often used to plan nutritionally adequate diets for individuals.
- Adequate Intake (AI): Intake at this level is assumed to ensure nutritional adequacy; established when evidence is insufficient to develop an RDA.
- Estimated Average Requirement (EAR): Average daily level of intake estimated to meet the requirements of 50% of healthy individuals; usually used to assess the nutrient intakes of groups of people and to plan nutritionally adequate diets for them; can also be used to assess the nutrient intakes of individuals.
- Tolerable Upper Intake Level (UL): Maximum daily intake unlikely to cause adverse health effects.

Table lists the current RDAs for magnesium. For infants from birth to 12 months, the FNB established an AI for magnesium that is equivalent to the mean intake of magnesium in healthy, breastfed infants, with added solid foods for ages 7–12 months.

Table: Recommended Dietary Allowances (RDAs) for Magnesium

Age	Male	Female	Pregnancy	Lactation
Birth to 6 months	30 mg*	30 mg*		
7–12 months	75 mg*	75 mg*		
1–3 years	80 mg	80 mg		
4–8 years	130 mg	130 mg		
9–13 years	240 mg	240 mg		
14–18 years	410 mg	360 mg	400 mg	360 mg
19–30 years	400 mg	310 mg	350 mg	310 mg
31–50 years	420 mg	320 mg	360 mg	320 mg
51+ years	420 mg	320 mg		

*Adequate Intake (AI)

Sources of Magnesium

Food

Magnesium is widely distributed in plant and animal foods and in beverages. Green leafy vegetables, such as spinach, legumes, nuts, seeds, and whole grains, are good sources. In general, foods containing dietary fiber provide magnesium. Magnesium is also added to some breakfast cereals and other fortified foods. Some types of food processing, such as refining grains in ways that remove the nutrient-rich germ and bran, lower magnesium content substantially. Selected food sources of magnesium are listed in Table.

Tap, mineral, and bottled waters can also be sources of magnesium, but the amount of magnesium in water varies by source and brand (ranging from 1 mg/L to more than 120 mg/L).

Approximately 30% to 40% of the dietary magnesium consumed is typically absorbed by the body [2,9].

Table: Selected Food Sources of Magnesium.

Food	Milligrams (mg) per Percent	
Serving DV*		
Almonds, dry roasted, 1 ounce	80	20
Spinach, boiled, ½ cup	78	20
Cashews, dry roasted, 1 ounce	74	19
Peanuts, oil roasted, ¼ cup	63	16
Cereal, shredded wheat, 2 large biscuits	61	15
Soymilk, plain or vanilla, 1 cup	61	15
Black beans, cooked, ½ cup	60	15
Edamame, shelled, cooked, ½ cup	50	13
Peanut butter, smooth, 2 tablespoons	49	12
Bread, whole wheat, 2 slices	46	12
Avocado, cubed, 1 cup	44	11
Potato, baked with skin, 3.5 ounces	43	11
Rice, brown, cooked, ½ cup	42	11
Yogurt, plain, low fat, 8 ounces	42	11
Breakfast cereals, fortified with 10% of the DV for magnesium	40	10
Oatmeal, instant, 1 packet	36	9
Kidney beans, canned, ½ cup	35	9
Banana, 1 medium	32	8
Salmon, Atlantic, farmed, cooked, 3 ounces	26	7
Milk, 1 cup	24–27	6–7
Halibut, cooked, 3 ounces	24	6
Raisins, ½ cup	23	6
Chicken breast, roasted, 3 ounces	22	6
Beef, ground, 90% lean, pan broiled, 3 ounces	20	5
Broccoli, chopped and cooked, ½ cup	12	3
Rice, white, cooked, ½ cup	10	3
Apple, 1 medium	9	2
Carrot, raw, 1 medium	7	2

*DV = Daily Value. DVs were developed by the U.S. Food and Drug Administration (FDA) to help consumers compare the nutrient contents of products within the context of a total diet. The DV for magnesium is 400 mg for adults and children aged 4 and older. However, the FDA does not require food labels to list magnesium content unless a food has been fortified with this nutrient. Foods providing 20% or more of the DV are considered to be high sources of a nutrient.

The U.S. Department of Agriculture's (USDA's) Nutrient Databaseexternal link disclaimer Web site lists the nutrient content of many foods and provides comprehensive list of foods containing magnesium arranged by nutrient content and by food name.

Dietary Supplements

Magnesium supplements are available in a variety of forms, including magnesium oxide, citrate, and chloride. The Supplement Facts panel on a dietary supplement label declares the amount of elemental magnesium in the product, not the weight of the entire magnesium-containing compound.

Absorption of magnesium from different kinds of magnesium supplements varies. Forms of magnesium that dissolve well in liquid are more completely absorbed in the gut than less soluble forms [2,11]. Small studies have found that magnesium in the aspartate, citrate, lactate, and chloride forms is absorbed more completely and is more bioavailable than magnesium oxide and magnesium sulfate [11-15]. One study found that very high doses of zinc from supplements (142 mg/day) can interfere with magnesium absorption and disrupt the magnesium balance in the body.

Medicines

Magnesium is a primary ingredient in some laxatives. Phillips' Milk of Magnesia®, for example, provides 500 mg elemental magnesium (as magnesium hydroxide) per tablespoon; the directions advise taking up to 4 tablespoons/day for adolescents and adults. (Although such a dose of magnesium is well above the safe upper level, some of the magnesium is not absorbed because of the medication's laxative effect.) Magnesium is also included in some remedies for heartburn and upset stomach due to acid indigestion. Extra-strength Rolaids®, for example, provides 55 mg elemental magnesium (as magnesium hydroxide) per tablet , although Tums® is magnesium free.

Magnesium Intakes and Status

Dietary surveys of people in the United States consistently show that intakes of magnesium are lower than recommended amounts. An analysis of data from the National Health and Nutrition Examination Survey (NHANES) of 2005–2006 found that a majority of Americans of all ages ingest less magnesium from food than their respective EARs; adult men aged 71 years and older and adolescent females are most likely to have low intakes. In a study using data from NHANES 2003–2006 to assess mineral intakes among adults, average intakes of magnesium from food alone were higher among users of dietary supplements (350 mg for men and 267 mg for women, equal to or slightly exceeding their respective EARs) than among nonusers (268 mg for men and 234 for women). When supplements were included, average total intakes of magnesium were 449 mg for men and 387 mg for women, well above EAR levels.

No current data on magnesium status in the United States are available. Determining dietary intake of magnesium is the usual proxy for assessing magnesium status. NHANES has not determined serum magnesium levels in its participants since 1974 , and magnesium is not evaluated in routine electrolyte testing in hospitals and clinics.

Magnesium Deficiency

Symptomatic magnesium deficiency due to low dietary intake in otherwise-healthy people is uncommon because the kidneys limit urinary excretion of this mineral. However, habitually low intakes or excessive losses of magnesium due to certain health conditions, chronic alcoholism, and/or the use of certain medications can lead to magnesium deficiency.

Early signs of magnesium deficiency include loss of appetite, nausea, vomiting, fatigue, and weakness. As magnesium deficiency worsens, numbness, tingling, muscle contractions and cramps, seizures, personality changes, abnormal heart rhythms, and coronary spasms can occur. Severe magnesium deficiency can result in hypocalcemia or hypokalemia (low serum calcium or potassium levels, respectively) because mineral homeostasis is disrupted.

Groups at Risk of Magnesium Inadequacy

Magnesium inadequacy can occur when intakes fall below the RDA but are above the amount required to prevent overt deficiency. The following groups are more likely than others to be at risk of magnesium inadequacy because they typically consume insufficient amounts or they have medical conditions (or take medications) that reduce magnesium absorption from the gut or increase losses from the body.

People with Gastrointestinal Diseases

The chronic diarrhea and fat malabsorption resulting from Crohn's disease, gluten-sensitive enteropathy (celiac disease), and regional enteritis can lead to magnesium depletion over time. Resection or bypass of the small intestine, especially the ileum, typically leads to malabsorption and magnesium loss.

People with Type 2 Diabetes

Magnesium deficits and increased urinary magnesium excretion can occur in people with insulin resistance and/or type 2 diabetes. The magnesium loss appears to be secondary to higher concentrations of glucose in the kidney that increase urine output.

People with Alcohol Dependence

Magnesium deficiency is common in people with chronic alcoholism. In these individuals, poor dietary intake and nutritional status; gastrointestinal problems, including vomiting, diarrhea, and steatorrhea (fatty stools) resulting from pancreatitis; renal dysfunction with excess excretion of magnesium into the urine; phosphate depletion; vitamin D deficiency; acute alcoholic ketoacidosis; and hyperaldosteronism secondary to liver disease can all contribute to decreased magnesium status.

Older Adults

Older adults have lower dietary intakes of magnesium than younger adults. In addition, magnesium absorption from the gut decreases and renal magnesium excretion increases with age. Older adults are also more likely to have chronic diseases or take medications that alter magnesium status, which can increase their risk of magnesium depletion.

Magnesium and Health

Habitually low intakes of magnesium induce changes in biochemical pathways that can increase the risk of illness over time. This section focuses on four diseases and disorders in which magnesium might be involved: hypertension and cardiovascular disease, type 2 diabetes, osteoporosis, and migraine headaches.

Hypertension and Cardiovascular Disease

Hypertension is a major risk factor for heart disease and stroke. Studies to date, however, have found that magnesium supplementation lowers blood pressure, at best, to only a small extent. A meta-analysis of 12 clinical trials found that magnesium supplementation for 8–26 weeks in 545 hypertensive participants resulted in only a small reduction (2.2 mmHg) in diastolic blood pressure. The dose of magnesium ranged from approximately 243 to 973 mg/day. The authors of another meta-analysis of 22 studies with 1,173 normotensive and hypertensive adults concluded that magnesium supplementation for 3–24 weeks decreased systolic blood pressure by 3–4 mmHg and diastolic blood pressure by 2–3 mmHg. The effects were somewhat larger when supplemental magnesium intakes of the participants in the nine crossover-design trials exceeded 370 mg/day. A diet containing more magnesium because of added fruits and vegetables, more low-fat or non-fat dairy products, and less fat overall was shown to lower systolic and diastolic blood pressure by an average of 5.5 and 3.0 mmHg, respectively. However, this Dietary Approaches to Stop Hypertension (DASH) diet also increases intakes of other nutrients, such as potassium and calcium, that are associated with reductions in blood pressure, so any independent contribution of magnesium cannot be determined.

Several prospective studies have examined associations between magnesium intakes and heart disease. The Atherosclerosis Risk in Communities study assessed heart disease risk factors and levels of serum magnesium in a cohort of 14,232 white and African-American men and women aged 45 to 64 years at baseline. Over an average of 12 years of follow-up, individuals in the highest quartile of the normal physiologic range of serum magnesium (at least 0.88 mmol/L) had a 38% reduced risk of sudden cardiac death compared with individuals in the lowest quartile (0.75 mmol/L or less). However, dietary magnesium intakes had no association with risk of sudden cardiac death. Another prospective study tracked 88,375 female nurses in the United States to determine whether serum magnesium levels measured early in the study and magnesium intakes from food and supplements assessed every 2 to 4 years were associated with sudden cardiac death over 26 years of follow-up. Women in the highest compared with the lowest quartile of ingested and plasma magnesium concentrations had a 34% and 77% lower risk of sudden cardiac death, respectively. Another prospective population study of 7,664 adults aged 20 to 75 years in the Netherlands who did not have cardiovascular disease found that low urinary magnesium excretion levels (a marker for low dietary magnesium intake) were associated with a higher risk of ischemic heart disease over a median follow-up period of 10.5 years. Plasma magnesium concentrations were not associated with risk of ischemic heart disease. A systematic review and meta-analysis of prospective studies found that higher serum levels of magnesium were significantly associated with a lower risk of cardiovascular disease, and higher dietary magnesium intakes (up to approximately 250 mg/day) were associated with a significantly lower risk of ischemic heart disease caused by a reduced blood supply to the heart muscle.

Higher magnesium intakes might reduce the risk of stroke. In a meta-analysis of 7 prospective trials with a total of 241,378 participants, an additional 100 mg/day magnesium in the diet was associated with an 8% decreased risk of total stroke, especially ischemic rather than hemorrhagic stroke. One limitation of such observational studies, however, is the possibility of confounding with other nutrients or dietary components that could also affect the risk of stroke.

A large, well-designed clinical trial is needed to better understand the contributions of magnesium from food and dietary supplements to heart health and the primary prevention of cardiovascular disease.

Type 2 Diabetes

Diets with higher amounts of magnesium are associated with a significantly lower risk of diabetes, possibly because of the important role of magnesium in glucose metabolism [39,40]. Hypomagnesemia might worsen insulin resistance, a condition that often precedes diabetes, or it might be a consequence of insulin resistance. Diabetes leads to increased urinary losses of magnesium, and the subsequent magnesium inadequacy might impair insulin secretion and action, thereby worsening diabetes control.

Most investigations of magnesium intake and risk of type 2 diabetes have been prospective cohort studies. A meta-analysis of 7 of these studies, which included 286,668 patients and 10,912 cases of diabetes over 6 to 17 years of follow-up, found that a 100 mg/day increase in total magnesium intake decreased the risk of diabetes by a statistically significant 15%. Another meta-analysis of 8 prospective cohort studies that followed 271,869 men and women over 4 to 18 years found a significant inverse association between magnesium intake from food and risk of type 2 diabetes; the relative risk reduction was 23% when the highest to lowest intakes were compared.

A 2011 meta-analysis of prospective cohort studies of the association between magnesium intake and risk of type 2 diabetes included 13 studies with a total of 536,318 participants and 24,516 cases of diabetes. The mean length of follow-up ranged from 4 to 20 years. Investigators found an inverse association between magnesium intake and risk of type 2 diabetes in a dose-responsive fashion, but this association achieved statistical significance only in overweight (body mass index [BMI] 25 or higher) but not normal-weight individuals (BMI less than 25). Again, a limitation of these observational studies is the possibility of confounding with other dietary components or lifestyle or environmental variables that are correlated with magnesium intake.

Only a few small, short-term clinical trials have examined the potential effects of supplemental magnesium on control of type 2 diabetes and the results are conflicting [40,44]. For example, 128 patients with poorly controlled diabetes in a Brazilian clinical trial received a placebo or a supplement containing either 500 mg/day or 1,000 mg/day magnesium oxide (providing 300 or 600 mg elemental magnesium, respectively). After 30 days of supplementation, plasma, cellular, and urine magnesium levels increased in participants receiving the larger dose of the supplement, and their glycemic control improved. In another small trial in Mexico, participants with type 2 diabetes and hypomagnesemia who received a liquid supplement of magnesium chloride (providing 300 mg/day elemental magnesium) for 16 weeks showed significant reductions in fasting glucose and glycosylated hemoglobin concentrations compared with participants receiving a placebo, and their serum magnesium levels became normal. In contrast, neither a supplement of magnesium aspartate (providing 369 mg/day elemental magnesium) nor a placebo taken for 3 months had any effect on glycemic control in 50 patients with type 2 diabetes who were taking insulin.

The American Diabetes Association states that there is insufficient evidence to support the routine use of magnesium to improve glycemic control in people with diabetes.

Osteoporosis

Magnesium is involved in bone formation and influences the activities of osteoblasts and osteoclasts. Magnesium also affects the concentrations of both parathyroid hormone and the active form of vitamin D, which are major regulators of bone homeostasis. Several population-based studies have found positive associations between magnesium intake and bone mineral density in both men and women. Other research has found that women with osteoporosis have lower serum magnesium levels than women with osteopenia and those who do not have osteoporosis or osteopenia. These and other findings indicate that magnesium deficiency might be a risk factor for osteoporosis.

Although limited in number, studies suggest that increasing magnesium intakes from food or supplements might increase bone mineral density in postmenopausal and elderly women. For example, one short-term study found that 290 mg/day elemental magnesium (as magnesium citrate) for 30 days in 20 postmenopausal women with osteoporosis suppressed bone turnover compared with placebo, suggesting that bone loss decreased.

Diets that provide recommended levels of magnesium enhance bone health, but further research is needed to elucidate the role of magnesium in the prevention and management of osteoporosis.

Migraine Headaches

Magnesium deficiency is related to factors that promote headaches, including neurotransmitter release and vasoconstriction. People who experience migraine headaches have lower levels of serum and tissue magnesium than those who do not.

However, research on the use of magnesium supplements to prevent or reduce symptoms of migraine headaches is limited. Three of four small, short-term, placebo-controlled trials found modest reductions in the frequency of migraines in patients given up to 600 mg/day magnesium. The authors of a review on migraine prophylaxis suggested that taking 300 mg magnesium twice a day, either alone or in combination with medication, can prevent migraines.

In their evidence-based guideline update, the American Academy of Neurology and the American Headache Society concluded that magnesium therapy is "probably effective" for migraine prevention. Because the typical dose of magnesium used for migraine prevention exceeds the UL, this treatment should be used only under the direction and supervision of a healthcare provider.

Health Risks from Excessive Magnesium

Too much magnesium from food does not pose a health risk in healthy individuals because the kidneys eliminate excess amounts in the urine. However, high doses of magnesium from dietary supplements or medications often result in diarrhea that can be accompanied by nausea and abdominal cramping. Forms of magnesium most commonly reported to cause diarrhea include magnesium carbonate, chloride, gluconate, and oxide. The diarrhea and laxative effects of magnesium salts are due to the osmotic activity of unabsorbed salts in the intestine and colon and the stimulation of gastric motility.

Very large doses of magnesium-containing laxatives and antacids (typically providing more than 5,000 mg/day magnesium) have been associated with magnesium toxicity , including fatal hypermagnesemia in a 28-month-old boy and an elderly man. Symptoms of magnesium toxicity, which usually develop after serum concentrations exceed 1.74–2.61 mmol/L, can include hypotension, nausea, vomiting, facial flushing, retention of urine, ileus, depression, and lethargy before progressing to muscle weakness, difficulty breathing, extreme hypotension, irregular heartbeat, and cardiac arrest. The risk of magnesium toxicity increases with impaired renal function or kidney failure because the ability to remove excess magnesium is reduced or lost.

The FNB has established ULs for magnesium that apply only to supplemental magnesium for healthy infants, children, and adults (Table below).

Table: Tolerable Upper Intake Levels (ULs) for Supplemental Magnesium.

Age	Male	Female	Pregnant	Lactating
Birth to 12 months	None established	None established		
1–3 years	65 mg	65 mg		
4–8 years	110 mg	110 mg		
9–18 years	350 mg	350 mg	350 mg	350 mg
19+ years	350 mg	350 mg	350 mg	350 mg

Interactions with Medications

Several types of medications have the potential to interact with magnesium supplements or affect magnesium status. A few examples are provided below. People taking these and other medications on a regular basis should discuss their magnesium intakes with their healthcare providers.

Bisphosphonates

Magnesium-rich supplements or medications can decrease the absorption of oral bisphosphonates, such as alendronate (Fosamax®), used to treat osteoporosis. Use of magnesium-rich supplements or medications and oral bisphosphonates should be separated by at least 2 hours.

Antibiotics

Magnesium can form insoluble complexes with tetracyclines, such as demeclocycline (Declomycin®) and doxycycline (Vibramycin®), as well as quinolone antibiotics, such as ciprofloxacin (Cipro®) and levofloxacin (Levaquin®). These antibiotics should be taken at least 2 hours before or 4–6 hours after a magnesium-containing supplement.

Diuretics

Chronic treatment with loop diuretics, such as furosemide (Lasix®) and bumetanide (Bumex®), and thiazide diuretics, such as hydrochlorothiazide (Aquazide H®) and ethacrynic acid (Edecrin®), can increase the loss of magnesium in urine and lead to magnesium depletion. In contrast, potassium-sparing diuretics, such as amiloride (Midamor®) and spironolactone (Aldactone®), reduce magnesium excretion.

Proton Pump Inhibitors

Prescription proton pump inhibitor (PPI) drugs, such as esomeprazole magnesium (Nexium®) and lansoprazole (Prevacid®), when taken for prolonged periods (typically more than a year) can cause hypomagnesemia. In cases that FDA reviewed, magnesium supplements often raised the low serum magnesium levels caused by PPIs. However, in 25% of the cases, supplements did not raise magnesium levels and the patients had to discontinue the PPI. FDA advises healthcare professionals to consider measuring patients' serum magnesium levels prior to initiating long-term PPI treatment and to check magnesium levels in these patients periodically.

Trace Element

Trace Element is usually defined as mineral elements that occur in living systems in micrograms per gram of body weight or less. A majority of elements of the periodic table probably could be considered trace elements. However, the presence of most of these elements in higher animals quite likely is just a manifestation of our geochemical origin or the result of environmental exposure. Only eight trace elements are generally accepted as being essential for health and wellbeing in higher animals through the consumption of food and beverages; these are cobalt, copper, iodine, iron, manganese, molybdenum, selenium, and zinc. Persuasive evidence has recently appeared that indicates two other trace elements, boron and chromium, may also be essential; however, general acceptance of their essentiality is still lacking. Based on findings with experimental animals and lower life forms, numerous other trace elements have been suggested as being essential for higher animals including aluminum, arsenic, fluorine, lithium, nickel, silicon, and vanadium. However, conclusive evidence for essentiality, such as a defined biochemical function, is lacking for these elements. Thus, their nutritional importance remains to be determined. Of the elements mentioned, assuring the consumption of foods providing adequate amounts of iodine, iron, and zinc is of greatest practical concern for human health. Evidence is emerging, however, suggesting that the amount of cobalt (as vitamin B12), copper, selenium, boron, and chromium provided through foods should be considered a practical nutritional concern in assuring or promoting health and well-being.

Copper

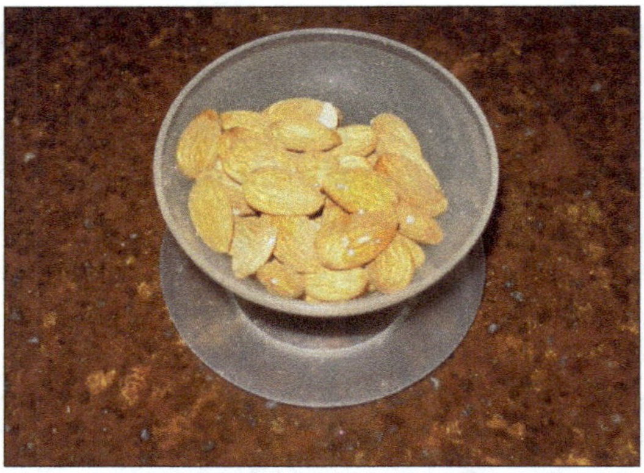

Almonds and other nuts are a source of copper.

Copper is a metal element and an essential dietary trace mineral required for several important metabolic reactions in your body. Chemically, copper is considered an inorganic element and is represented by the symbol Cu, but exists in several forms such as Cu^{2+} and Cu^{1+}.

In its inorganic form copper has a variety of uses as a conductor of heat and electricity, a constituent of metal alloys, and as a building and sculpting material.

As an essential dietary nutrient found in a variety of foods, copper is found in organic forms in living organisms most often bound to individual amino acids within proteins. Your body contains about 100 mg of copper in various tissues and cells as a component of several biologically important enzymes.

Copper, in its organic form may also be used in bacteriostatic and fungal preparations, as well as wood preservatives.

Within your body, copper containing metalloenzymes are generally involved in oxygen consuming reactions or reactions which involve oxygen radicals.

Copper Sources

Copper is derived from two sources: exogenous or dietary sources, and endogenous or from within your body.

Exogenous dietary sources of copper include legumes, whole grains, nuts, seeds, organ meats, shell fish, and potatoes. The copper content of food depends on the copper content of soil and water where the food originated and how the food has been processed and prepared for use.

Water is also a source of copper, but the copper content depends on the type of plumbing materials, and also the hardness of the water which is dependent on the minerals in the soil and rock through which the water passes.

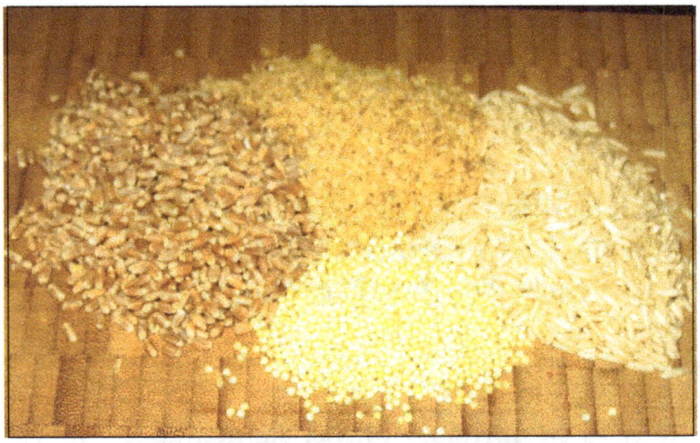

Adding grains to your diet will add copper.

Endogenous sources of copper refer to available copper within your body. As part of your metabolic processes copper is secreted into your gastrointestinal tract in your digestive juices. Your saliva may contain up to 400 mcg, gastric juices up to 1000 mcg, pancreatic juice 1300 mcg and your duodenal juices 2200 mcg. Copper secretion occurs daily.

However, low intakes of copper overtime will reduce the amount of copper that is in these various body secretions.

Functions

Copper containing enzymes have a variety of functions:

Oxidation of minerals

Copper is a co-factor for the enzyme ceruloplasmin which is found in your blood and bound to cell membranes. As an oxidative enzyme, ceruloplasmin catalyses the binding of iron to transferrin which transports iron to various tissues including bone marrow, and is involved in hemoglobin synthesis.

Ceruloplasmin is also involved in manganese oxidation. As an antioxidant ceruloplasmin protects cells by scavenging free radicals.

Iodine

Iodine is a trace mineral found naturally in some foods and added to others. It is essential for metabolism and normal thyroid function in the human body. Lack of iodine in foods is often the result of deficient soil in which foods are grown. Iodine deficiency can lead to goiter, a disease featured by an abnormally enlarged thyroid gland. Though virtually eliminated in the United States and other Western nations with the iodination of salt in the 1920's, this condition still affects about 187 million people in other parts of the world.

How is Iodine Used in the Human Body?

Iodine is an essential component of the thyroid hormones thyroxine (T4) and triiodothyronine (T3). Both T4 and T3 can function as hormones and trigger signal transduction cascades via membrane receptors. They can also function as nuclear receptors and turn genes on or off by directly binding to the promoter region of the DNA. When regulating gene expression, T4 and T3 directly control the metabolic rate of the human body and also brain development during times of rapid growth.

Forms of Iodine

Iodine occurs naturally in two primary forms, elemental and ionic. Elemental iodine refers to the atom itself, which is found primarily in the ocean. Single iodine atoms don't float around by themselves in nature. Atomic iodine refers to two iodine atoms bonded together. In this form, it's usually highly corrosive.

Potassium Iodide

More commonly, iodine is found in combination with other substances, such as potassium, where it's known as potassium iodide, and is the type that's usually added to processed salt.

SSKI is a concentrated solution of potassium iodide. It does have uses, such as topical applications to alleviate some skin disorders, but should not be used as a dietary supplement.

Colloidal Iodine

However, a form of iodine that provides both iodide's safety and the purity of atomic iodine has been developed. It's known by different terms: nascent, atomic, and colloidal iodine. Atomic iodine makes iodine highly available to the body's metabolism and is safe to use both internally and externally.

6 Reasons to Eat More Iodine-Rich Foods

1. Supports Thyroid Health

The thyroid must have high enough levels of iodine present in order to make key hormones, including thyroxine. Thyroid hormones regulate many important biochemical reactions every day — some of the most significant include the synthesis of amino acids from proteins, digestive enzyme activity, and proper skeletal and central nervous system development.

Healthy, normal thyroid function is primarily regulated by thyroid-stimulating hormones (TSH), also known as thyrotropin. This hormone is secreted by the pituitary gland and works to control thyroid hormone production and secretion throughout the body — it's what allows our bodies to protect us from hypothyroidism and hyperthyroidism (too much or too little thyroid hormones production). TSH secretion increases uptake of iodine in the thyroid and stimulates the synthesis and release of hormones T3 and T4, so in the absence of iodine, TSH levels remains dangerously elevated.

When thyroid disorders occur because of a diet low in iodine-rich foods, symptoms can range from a sluggish metabolism, heart complications, changes in appetite and body temperature, changes in thirst and perspiration, weight fluctuations, and mood changes.

2. Helps Prevent Cancer

Iodine improves immunity and helps induce apoptosis — the self-destruction of dangerous, cancerous cells. While iodine can help destroy mutated cancer cells, it doesn't destroy healthy cells in the process. For example, evidence shows the ability of iodine-rich seaweed to inhibit breast tumor development. This is supported by the relatively low rate of breast cancer in parts of the world like Japan, where women consume a diet high in iodine-rich seaweed.

3. Prevents Impaired Growth and Development in Children

Research shows that an iodine deficiency during pregnancy and infancy can disturb healthy growth and brain development. Infants with iodine deficiency are more susceptible to mortality and at a higher risk for neuro-degenerative problems like a form of mental disability known as cretinism, low growth rate, motor-function problems and learning disabilities.

Although doctors commonly test women during pregnancy for iodine deficiency, it's difficult to get an accurate reading of iodine levels. Thus, many health experts now encourage women to increase their intake of iodine-rich foods and supplement with iodine considering how common deficiencies are.

4. Maintains Healthy Brain Function

Iodine plays a big role in healthy brain development and ongoing cognitive abilities, therefore iodine deficiency is believed to be one of the most common preventable causes of mental disorders in the world.

5. Preserves Skin Health

A common sign of iodine deficiency is dry, rough and irritated skin that becomes flaky and inflamed. Iodine also helps regulate perspiration, so people might experience changes in how much they sweat if their iodine levels become imbalanced.

6. Helps Control Sweating and Body Temperature

Sweating is an important detoxification method that the body uses to discard toxins and even excess calories. Iodine deficiency can disturb the natural way we flush waste from the body through our pores and control our body temperature. Similar to an ability to produce enough sweat, a lack of iodine also can cause dry mouth due to an abnormally low production of saliva. This makes it difficult to enjoy eating and can impair digestion to some degree.

Iron

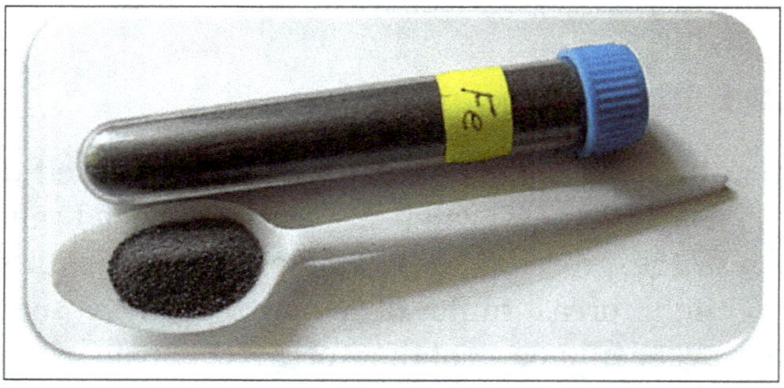

Elemental iron.

Iron is an essential nutrient: a mineral which is required in small amounts by your body. Although iron is found in a wide range of foods many people do not obtain sufficient amounts of this mineral from their diet.

These people may experience symptoms associated with iron deficiency which is the most common nutrient deficiency.

Almost 50% of pre-school children and pregnant women in developing countries experience iron-deficiency anaemia. In North America up to 10% of young children, adolescent girls and pre-menopausal women suffer from iron-deficiency anaemia.

Conversely some people absorb too much iron which is also associated with adverse healtheffects. As with most nutrients, both essential and non-essential, too little or too much iron poses potential health risks.

Iron has many functions within your body and is used by cells and tissues throughout your body for essential metabolic activities and maintaining an adequate supply of iron is essential to good health.

Although your body does not readily excrete iron small amounts of iron are lost from your body on a daily basis. Women experience greater iron loses due to menstruation, pregnancy and child birth. Iron losses need to be replaced on a daily basis.

Just as there are many sources of iron there are many factors which influence iron absorption and iron excretion.

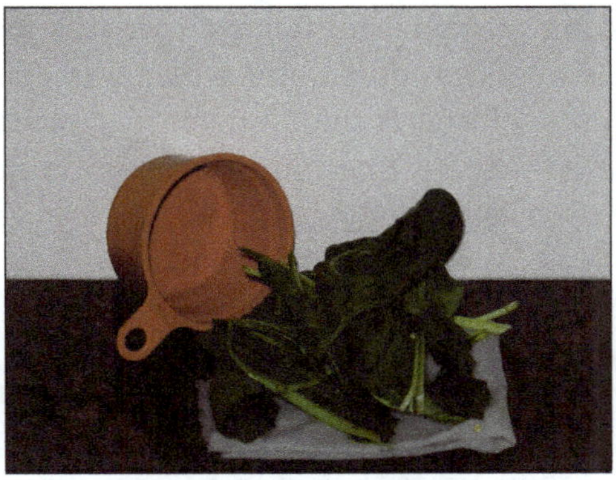

Spinach is a good source of iron.

Knowing which foods are good sources of iron, and understanding the factors which influence iron absorption and excretion can help you obtain the iron that your body needs for optimum function.

Functions

The primary function of iron, and probably the most well known function, is as a component of hemoglobin and myoglobin: two proteins involved in transporting oxygen in your body.

Hemoglobin transports approximately 98% of total body oxygen in the blood. Myoglobin is found in muscles where it functions as a temporary oxygen store which provides oxygen for muscle contractions and other metabolic activities.

Iron is also involved in energy metabolism pathways as part of cytochromes and enzymes in the electron transport chain in the mitochondria of your cells.

Iron is required for life. The iron–sulfur clusters are pervasive and include nitrogenase, the enzymes responsible for biological nitrogen fixation. Iron-containing proteins participate in transport, storage and used of oxygen. Iron proteins are involved in electron transfer.

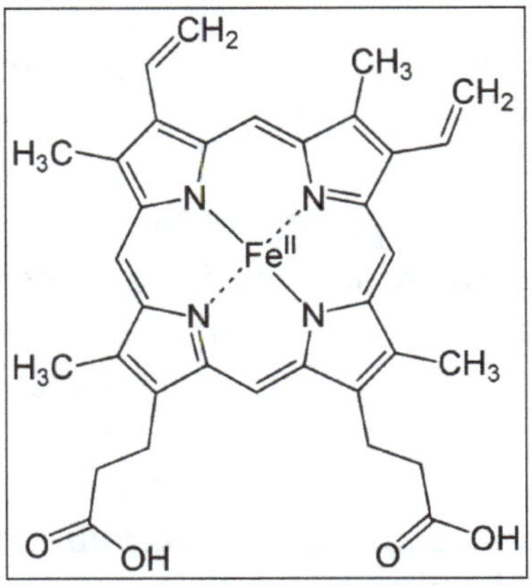

Structure of Heme b; in the protein additional ligand(s) would be attached to Fe.

Examples of iron-containing proteins in higher organisms include hemoglobin, cytochrome, and catalase. The average adult human contains about 0.005% body weight of iron, or about four grams, of which three quarters is in hemoglobin – a level that remains constant despite only about one milligram of iron being absorbed each day, because the human body recycles its hemoglobin for the iron content.

Biochemistry

Iron acquisition poses a problem for aerobic organisms because ferric iron is poorly soluble near neutral pH. Thus, these organisms have developed means to absorb iron as complexes, sometimes taking up ferrous iron before oxidising it back to ferric iron. In particular, bacteria have evolved very high-affinity sequestering agents called siderophores.

After uptake in human cells, iron storage is precisely regulated. A major component of this regulation is the protein transferrin, which binds iron ions absorbed from the duodenum and carries it in the blood to cells. Transferrin contains Fe^{3+} in the middle of a distorted octahedron, bonded to one nitrogen, three oxygens and a chelating carbonate anion that traps the Fe^{3+} ion: it has such a high stability constant that it is very effective at taking up Fe^{3+} ions even from the most stable complexes. At the bone marrow, transferrin is reduced from Fe^{3+} and Fe^{2+} and stored as ferritin to be incorporated into hemoglobin.

The most commonly known and studied bioinorganic iron compounds (biological iron molecules) are the heme proteins: examples are hemoglobin, myoglobin, and cytochrome P450. These compounds participate in transporting gases, building enzymes, and transferring electrons. Metalloproteins are a group of proteins with metal ion cofactors. Some examples of iron metalloproteins are ferritin and rubredoxin. Many enzymes vital to life contain iron, such as catalase, lipoxygenases, and IRE-BP.

Hemoglobin is an oxygen carrier that occurs in red blood cells and contributes their color, transporting oxygen in the arteries from the lungs to the muscles where it is transferred to myoglobin, which stores it until it is needed for the metabolic oxidation of glucose, generating energy. Here the hemoglobin binds to carbon dioxide, produced when glucose is oxidized, which is transported through the veins by hemoglobin (predominantly as bicarbonate anions) back to the lungs where it is exhaled. In hemoglobin, the iron is in one of four heme groups and has six possible coordination sites; four are occupied by nitrogen atoms in a porphyrin ring, the fifth by an imidazole nitrogen in a histidine residue of one of the protein chains attached to the heme group, and the sixth is reserved for the oxygen molecule it can reversibly bind to. When hemoglobin is not attached to oxygen (and is then called deoxyhemoglobin), the Fe^{2+} ion at the center of the heme group (in the hydrophobic protein interior) is in a high-spin configuration. It is thus too large to fit inside the porphyrin ring, which bends instead into a dome with the Fe^{2+} ion about 55 picometers above it. In this configuration, the sixth coordination site reserved for the oxygen is blocked by another histidine residue.

When deoxyhemoglobin picks up an oxygen molecule, this histidine residue moves away and returns once the oxygen is securely attached to form a hydrogen bond with it. This results in the Fe^{2+} ion switching to a low-spin configuration, resulting in a 20% decrease in ionic radius so that now it can fit into the porphyrin ring, which becomes planar. (Additionally, this hydrogen bonding results in the tilting of the oxygen molecule, resulting in a Fe–O–O bond angle of around 120° that avoids the formation of Fe–O–Fe or Fe–O_2–Fe bridges that would lead to electron transfer, the oxidation of Fe^{2+} to Fe^{3+}, and the destruction of hemoglobin.) This results in a movement of all the protein chains that leads to the other subunits of hemoglobin changing shape to a form with larger oxygen affinity. Thus, when deoxyhemoglobin takes up oxygen, its affinity for more oxygen increases, and vice versa. Myoglobin, on the other hand, contains only one heme group and hence this cooperative effect cannot occur. Thus, while hemoglobin is almost saturated with oxygen in the high partial pressures of oxygen found in the lungs, its affinity for oxygen is much lower than that of myoglobin, which oxygenates even at low partial pressures of oxygen found in muscle tissue. As described by the Bohr effect (named after Christian Bohr, the father of Niels Bohr), the oxygen affinity of hemoglobin diminishes in the presence of carbon dioxide.

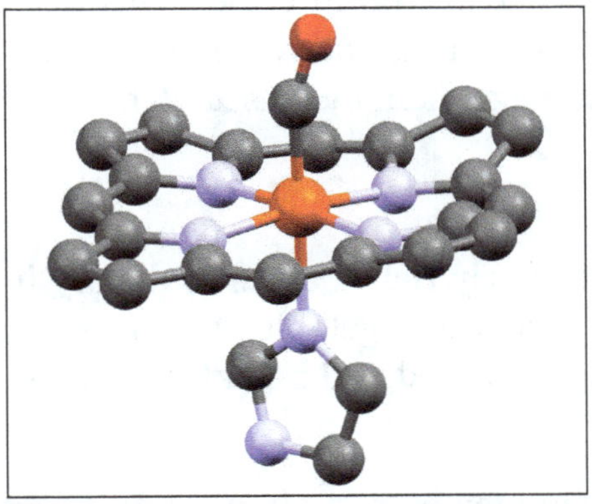

A heme unit of human carboxyhemoglobin, showing the carbonyl ligand at the apical position, *trans* to the histidine residue.

Carbon monoxide and phosphorus trifluoride are poisonous to humans because they bind to hemoglobin similarly to oxygen, but with much more strength, so that oxygen can no longer be transported throughout the body. Hemoglobin bound to carbon monoxide is known as carboxyhemoglobin. This effect also plays a minor role in the toxicity of cyanide, but there the major effect is by far its interference with the proper functioning of the electron transport protein cytochrome a. The cytochrome proteins also involve heme groups and are involved in the metabolic oxidation of glucose by oxygen. The sixth coordination site is then occupied by either another imidazole nitrogen or a methionine sulfur, so that these proteins are largely inert to oxygen – with the exception of cytochrome a, which bonds directly to oxygen and thus is very easily poisoned by cyanide. Here, the electron transfer takes place as the iron remains in low spin but changes between the +2 and +3 oxidation states. Since the reduction potential of each step is slightly greater than the previous one, the energy is released step-by-step and can thus be stored in adenosine triphosphate. Cytochrome a is slightly distinct, as it occurs at the mitochondrial membrane, binds directly to oxygen, and transports protons as well as electrons, as follows:

$$4\ Cytc^{2+} + O_2 + 8H^+_{inside} \rightarrow 4\ Cytc^{3+} + 2\ H_2O\ +\ 4H^+_{outside}$$

Although the heme proteins are the most important class of iron-containing proteins, the iron-sulfur proteins are also very important, being involved in electron transfer, which is possible since iron can exist stably in either the +2 or +3 oxidation states. These have one, two, four, or eight iron atoms that are each approximately tetrahedrally coordinated to four sulfur atoms; because of this tetrahedral coordination, they always have high-spin iron. The simplest of such compounds is rubredoxin, which has only one iron atom coordinated to four sulfur atoms from cysteine residues in the surrounding peptide chains. Another important class of iron-sulfur proteins is the ferredoxins, which have multiple iron atoms. Transferrin does not belong to either of these classes.

The ability of sea mussels to maintain their grip on rocks in the ocean is facilitated by their use of organometallic iron-based bonds in their protein-rich cuticles. Based on synthetic replicas, the presence of iron in these structures increased elastic modulus 770 times, tensile strength 58 times, and toughness 92 times. The amount of stress required to permanently damage them increased 76 times.

Health and Diet

Iron is pervasive, but particularly rich sources of dietary iron include red meat, oysters, lentils, beans, poultry, fish, leaf vegetables, watercress, tofu, chickpeas, black-eyed peas, and blackstrap molasses. Bread and breakfast cereals are sometimes specifically fortified with iron.

Iron provided by dietary supplements is often found as iron(II) fumarate, although iron(II) sulfate is cheaper and is absorbed equally well. Elemental iron, or reduced iron, despite being absorbed at only one-third to two-thirds the efficiency (relative to iron sulfate), is often added to foods such as breakfast cereals or enriched wheat flour. Iron is most available to the body when chelated to amino acids and is also available for use as a common iron supplement. Glycine, the cheapest and most common amino acid is most often used to produce iron glycinate supplements.

Dietary Recommendations

The U.S. Institute of Medicine (IOM) updated Estimated Average Requirements (EARs) and Recommended Dietary Allowances (RDAs) for iron in 2001. The current EAR for iron for women ages 14–18 is 7.9 mg/day, 8.1 for ages 19–50 and 5.0 thereafter (post menopause). For men the EAR is 6.0 mg/day for ages 19 and up. The RDA is 15.0 mg/day for women ages 15–18, 18.0 for 19–50 and 8.0 thereafter. For men, 8.0 mg/day for ages 19 and up. RDAs are higher than EARs so as to identify amounts that will cover people with higher than average requirements. RDA for pregnancy is 27 mg/day and, for lactation, 9 mg/day. For children ages 1–3 years 7 mg/day, 10 for ages 4–8 and 8 for ages 9–13. As for safety, the IOM also sets Tolerable upper intake levels (ULs) for vitamins and minerals when evidence is sufficient. In the case of iron the UL is set at 45 mg/day. Collectively the EARs, RDAs and ULs are referred to as Dietary Reference Intakes.

The European Food Safety Authority (EFSA) refers to the collective set of information as Dietary Reference Values, with Population Reference Intake (PRI) instead of RDA, and Average Requirement instead of EAR. AI and UL defined the same as in United States. For women the PRI is 13 mg/day ages 15–17 years, 16 mg/day for women ages 18 and up who are premenopausal and 11 mg/day postmenopausal. For pregnancy and lactation, 16 mg/day. For men the PRI is 11 mg/day ages 15 and older. For children ages 1 to 14 the PRI increases from 7 to 11 mg/day. The PRIs are higher than the U.S. RDAs, with the exception of pregnancy. The EFSA reviewed the same safety question did not establish a UL.

Infants may require iron supplements if they are bottle-fed cow's milk. Frequent blood donors are at risk of low iron levels and are often advised to supplement their iron intake.

For U.S. food and dietary supplement labeling purposes the amount in a serving is expressed as a percent of Daily Value (%DV). For iron labeling purposes 100% of the Daily Value was 18 mg, and as of May 27, 2016 remained unchanged at 18 mg. A table of all of the old and new adult Daily Values is provided at Reference Daily Intake. The original deadline to be in compliance was July 28, 2018, but on September 29, 2017 the U.S. Food and Drug Administration released a proposed rule that extended the deadline to January 1, 2020 for large companies and January 1, 2021 for small companies.

Deficiency

Iron deficiency is the most common nutritional deficiency in the world. When loss of iron is not adequately compensated by adequate dietary iron intake, a state of latent iron deficiency occurs, which over time leads to iron-deficiency anemia if left untreated, which is characterised by an insufficient number of red blood cells and an insufficient amount of hemoglobin. Children, pre-menopausal women (women of child-bearing age), and people with poor diet are most susceptible to the disease. Most cases of iron-deficiency anemia are mild, but if not treated can cause problems like fast or irregular heartbeat, complications during pregnancy, and delayed growth in infants and children.

Excess

Iron uptake is tightly regulated by the human body, which has no regulated physiological means of excreting iron. Only small amounts of iron are lost daily due to mucosal and skin epithelial cell sloughing, so control of iron levels is primarily accomplished by regulating uptake. Regulation of iron uptake is impaired in some people as a result of a genetic defect that maps to the HLA-H gene region on chromosome 6 and leads to abnormally low levels of hepcidin, a key regulator of the entry of iron into the circulatory system in mammals. In these people, excessive iron intake can result in iron overload disorders, known medically as hemochromatosis. Many people have an undiagnosed genetic susceptibility to iron overload, and are not aware of a family history of the problem. For this reason, people should not take iron supplements unless they suffer from iron deficiency and have consulted a doctor. Hemochromatosis is estimated to be the cause of 0.3 to 0.8% of all metabolic diseases of Caucasians.

NFPA 704 fire diamond

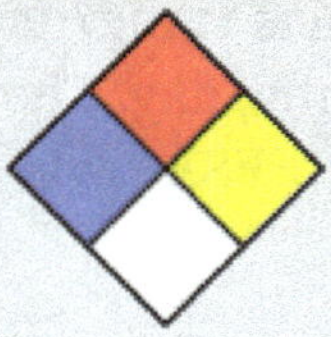

1

1

0

Fire diamond hazard sign for metallic iron

Overdoses of ingested iron can cause excessive levels of free iron in the blood. High blood levels of free ferrous iron react with peroxides to produce highly reactive free radicals that can damage DNA, proteins, lipids, and other cellular components. Iron toxicity occurs when the cell contains free iron, which generally occurs when iron levels exceed the availability of transferrin to bind the iron. Damage to the cells of the gastrointestinal tract can also prevent them from regulating iron absorption, leading to further increases in blood levels. Iron typically damages cells in the heart, liver and elsewhere, causing adverse effects that include coma, metabolic acidosis, shock, liver failure, coagulopathy, adult respiratory distress syndrome, long-term organ damage, and even death. Humans experience iron toxicity when the iron exceeds 20 milligrams for every kilogram of body mass; 60 milligrams per kilogram is considered a lethal dose. Overconsumption of iron, often the result of children eating large quantities of ferrous sulfate tablets intended for adult consumption, is one of the most common toxicological causes of death in children under six. The Dietary Reference Intake (DRI) sets the Tolerable Upper Intake Level (UL) for adults at 45 mg/day. For children under fourteen years old the UL is 40 mg/day.

The medical management of iron toxicity is complicated, and can include use of a specific chelating agent called deferoxamine to bind and expel excess iron from the body.

Zinc

Zinc is a metal. It is called an "essential trace element" because very small amounts of zinc are necessary for human health.

Zinc is used for treatment and prevention of zinc deficiency and its consequences, including stunted growth and acute diarrhea in children, and slow wound healing.

It is also used for boosting the immune system, treating the common cold and recurrent ear infections, and preventing lower respiratory infections. It is also used for malaria and other diseases caused by parasites.

Some people use zinc for an eye disease called macular degeneration, for night blindness, and for cataracts. It is also used for asthma; diabetes; high blood pressure; acquired immunodeficiency syndrome (AIDS); and skin conditions such as psoriasis, eczema, and acne.

Other uses include treating attention deficit-hyperactivity disorder (ADHD), blunted sense of taste (hypogeusia), ringing in the ears (tinnitus), severe head injuries, Crohn's disease, Alzheimer's disease, Down syndrome, Hansen's disease, ulcerative colitis, peptic ulcers and promoting weight gain in people with eating disorders such as anorexia nervosa.

Some people use zinc for benign prostatic hyperplasia (BPH), male infertility, erectile dysfunction (ED), weak bones (osteoporosis), rheumatoid arthritis, and muscle cramps associated with liver disease. It is also used for sickle cell disease and inherited disorders such as acrodermatitis enteropathica, thalassemia, and Wilson's disease.

Some athletes use zinc for improving athletic performance and strength.

Zinc is also applied to the skin for treating acne, aging skin, herpes simplex infections, and to speed wound healing.

There is a zinc preparation that can be sprayed in the nostrils for treating the common cold.

Zinc sulfate is used in products for eye irritation.

Zinc citrate is used in toothpaste and mouthwash to prevent dental plaque formation and gingivitis.

Note that many zinc products also contain another metal called cadmium. This is because zinc and cadmium are chemically similar and often occur together in nature. Exposure to high levels of cadmium over a long time can lead to kidney failure. The concentration of cadmium in zinc-containing supplements can vary as much as 37-fold. Look for zinc-gluconate products. Zinc gluconate consistently contains the lowest cadmium levels.

How does it Work?

Zinc is needed for the proper growth and maintenance of the human body. It is found in several systems and biological reactions, and it is needed for immune function, wound healing, blood clotting, thyroid function, and much more. Meats, seafood, dairy products, nuts, legumes, and whole grains offer relatively high levels of zinc.

Zinc deficiency is not uncommon worldwide, but is rare in the US. Symptoms include slowed growth, low insulin levels, loss of appetite, irritability, generalized hair loss, rough and dry skin, slow wound healing, poor sense of taste and smell, diarrhea, and nausea. Moderate zinc deficiency is associated with disorders of the intestine which interfere with food absorption (malabsorption syndromes), alcoholism, chronic kidney failure, and chronic debilitating diseases.

Zinc plays a key role in maintaining vision, and it is present in high concentrations in the eye. Zinc deficiency can alter vision, and severe deficiency can cause changes in the retina (the back of the eye where an image is focused).

Zinc might also have effects against viruses. It appears to lessen symptoms of the rhinovirus (common cold), but researchers can't yet explain exactly how this works. In addition, there is some evidence that zinc has some antiviral activity against the herpes virus.

Low zinc levels can be associated with male infertility, sickle cell disease, HIV, major depression, and type 2 diabetes, and can be fought by taking a zinc supplement.

Distribution of Zinc

Zinc is a widely distributed element in foodstuffs (shellfish, liver, milk, and wheat bran). In the human body, zinc is widely distributed in many tissues, blood cells, bone, and teeth.5,6 However, zinc at these sites is firmly bound to protein, and during deficiency and refeeding the concentrations of zinc in tissues (with the exception of blood, milk, hair, and liver) do not change significantly.7 Endogenous stores of zinc are mobilized in the fasting state, but do not meet metabolic needs during anabolism, because the net movement of zinc is into tissues and circulating zinc is reduced.

Although 86% is in skeletal muscle, there are certain areas where zinc concentration is especially high and may represent functional importance. They are the prostate, hippocampus, pancreas, and kidney cortex. Zinc has been identified as a part of about 120 enzymes.8 Among them are carbonic anhydrase, carboxypeptidase, alkaline phosphatase, oxidoreductases, transferases, ligases, hydrolases, lyases, and isomerases. Although the syndrome of zinc deficiency cannot be identified with the dearth of any 1 enzyme, zinc deficiency does have a pronounced effect on nucleic acid metabolism, thus influencing protein and amino acid metabolism.

References

- "Radiation and Radioactive Decay. Radioactive Human Body". Harvard Natural Sciences Lecture Demonstrations. Retrieved July 2, 2016
- "Phosphorus in diet". MedlinePlus, National Library of Medicine, US National Institutes of Health. 2 December 2016. Retrieved 24 December 2016
- Haynes, William M., ed. (2011). CRC Handbook of Chemistry and Physics (92nd ed.). Boca Raton, FL: CRC Press. p. 4.122. ISBN 1439855110

- Mitsuo Kakei, Toshiro Sakae and Masayoshi Yoshikawa (2012). “Aspects Regarding Fluoride Treatment for Reinforcement and Remineralization of Apatite Crystals”. Journal of Hard Tissue Biology. 21 (3): 475–6. Retrieved 2017-06-01
- Karger, S. (2004). “Energy and nutrient intake in the European Union”. Annals of Nutrition and Metabolism. 48 (2 (suppl)): 1–16. doi:10.1159/000083041

6

Role of Nutrition in Diet

The sum of usual food consumed by a person or other organism is known as diet. This chapter explains diet, dietary supplements, nootropics and raw foodism in an easy-to-understand manner. It closely examines the key concepts of nutrition and diet to provide an extensive understanding of the subject.

Diet

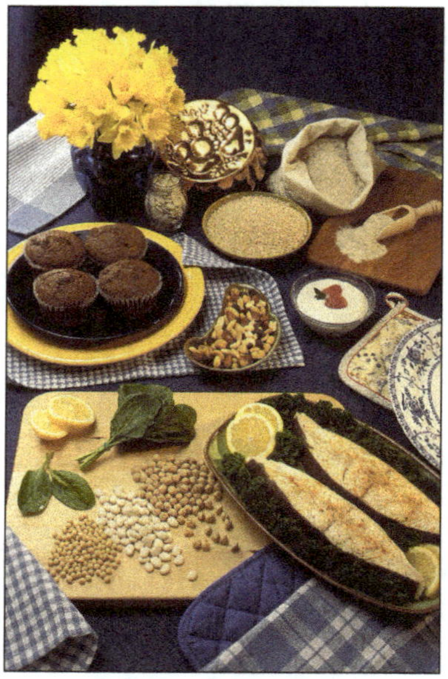

A selection of food consumed by humans. However, the human diet can vary widely.

In nutrition, diet is the sum of food consumed by a person or other organism. The word diet often implies the use of specific intake of nutrition for health or weight-management reasons (with the two often being related). Although humans are omnivores, each culture and each person holds some food preferences or some food taboos. This may be due to personal tastes or ethical reasons. Individual dietary choices may be more or less healthy.

Complete nutrition requires ingestion and absorption of vitamins, minerals, and food energy in the form of carbohydrates, proteins, and fats. Dietary habits and choices play a significant role in the quality of life, health and longevity.

Religious and Cultural Dietary Choices

Some cultures and religions have restrictions concerning what foods are acceptable in their diet. For example, only Kosher foods are permitted by Judaism, and Halal foods by Islam. Although Buddhists are generally vegetarians, the practice varies and meat-eating may be permitted depending on the sects. In Hinduism, vegetarianism is the ideal. Jains are strictly vegetarian and consumption of roots is not permitted.

Dietary Choices

Many people choose to forgo food from animal sources to varying degrees (e.g. flexitarianism, vegetarianism, veganism, fruitarianism) for health reasons, issues surrounding morality, or to reduce their personal impact on the environment, although some of the public assumptions about which diets have lower impacts are known to be incorrect. Raw foodism is another contemporary trend. These diets may require tuning or supplementation such as vitamins to meet ordinary nutritional needs.

Weight Management

A particular diet may be chosen to seek weight loss or weight gain. Changing a subject's dietary intake, or "going on a diet", can change the energy balance and increase or decrease the amount of fat stored by the body. Some foods are specifically recommended, or even altered, for conformity to the requirements of a particular diet. These diets are often recommended in conjunction with exercise. Specific weight loss programs can be harmful to health, while others may be beneficial and can thus be coined as healthy diets. The terms "healthy diet" and "diet for weight management" are often related, as the two promote healthy weight management. Having a healthy diet is a way to prevent health problems, and will provide the body with the right balance of vitamins, minerals, and other nutrients.

Eating Disorders

An eating disorder is a mental disorder that interferes with normal food consumption. It is defined by abnormal eating habits that may involve either insufficient or excessive diet.

Health

A healthy diet may improve or maintain optimal health. In developed countries, affluence enables unconstrained caloric intake and possibly inappropriate food choices.

Health agencies recommend that people maintain a normal weight by limiting consumption of energy-dense foods and sugary drinks, eating plant-based food, limiting consumption of red and processed meat, and limiting alcohol intake.

Dietary Supplement

A dietary supplement is intended to provide nutrients that may otherwise not be consumed in sufficient quantities.

Supplements as generally understood include vitamins, minerals, fiber, fatty acids, or amino acids, among other substances. U.S. authorities define dietary supplements as foods, while elsewhere they may be classified as drugs or other products.

There are more than 50,000 dietary supplements available. More than half of the U.S. adult population (53% – 55%) consume dietary supplements with most common ones being multivitamins.

These products are not intended to prevent or treat any disease and in some circumstances are dangerous, according to the U.S. National Institutes of Health. For those who fail to consume a balanced diet, the agency says that certain supplements "may have value."

Most supplements should be avoided, and usually people should not eat micronutrients except people with clearly shown deficiency. Those people should first consult a doctor. An exception is vitamin D, which is recommended in Nordic countries due to weak sunlight.

Definition

According to the United States Food and Drug Administration (FDA), dietary supplements are products which are not pharmaceutical drugs, food additives like spices or preservatives, or conventional food, and which also meet any of these criteria:

1. The product is intended to supplement a person's diet, despite it not being usable as a meal replacement.
2. The product is or contains a vitamin, dietary element, herb used for herbalism or botanical used as a medicinal plant, amino acid, any substance which contributes to other food eaten, or any concentrate, metabolite, ingredient, extract, or combination of these things.
3. The product is labeled as a dietary supplement.

In the United States, the FDA has different monitoring procedures for substances depending on whether they are presented as drugs, food additives, food, or dietary supplements. Dietary supplements are eaten or taken by mouth, and are regulated in United States law as a type of food rather than a type of drug. Like food and unlike drugs, no government approval is required to make or sell dietary supplements; the manufacturer checks the safety of dietary supplements but the government does not;

and rather than requiring risk–benefit analysis to prove that the product can be sold like a drug, risk–benefit analysis is only used to petition that food or a dietary supplement is unsafe and should be removed from market.

Medical Uses

The intended use of dietary supplements is to ensure that a person gets enough essential nutrients.

Dietary supplements should not be used to treat any disease or as preventive healthcare. An exception to this recommendation is the appropriate use of vitamins.

Supplements may create harm in several ways, including over-consumption, particularly of minerals and fat-soluble vitamins which can build up in the body. The products may also cause harm related to their rapid absorption in a short period of time, quality issues such as contamination, or by adverse interactions with other foods and medications.

Types

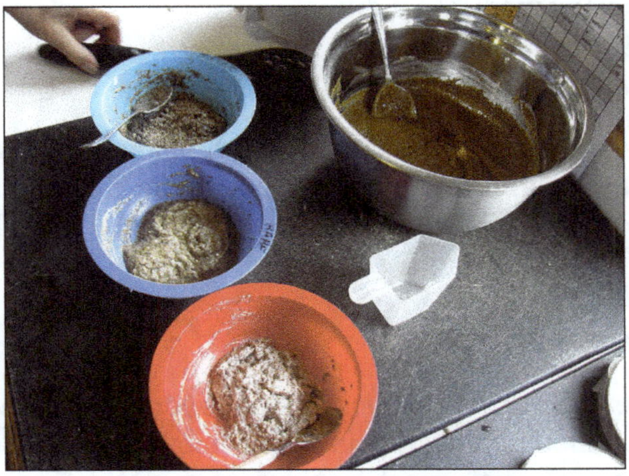

Dietary supplements being mixed into food for pigs.

There are many types of dietary supplements.

Vitamins

Vitamin is an organic compound required by an organism as a vital nutrient in limited amounts. An organic chemical compound (or related set of compounds) is called a vitamin when it cannot be synthesized in sufficient quantities by an organism, and must be obtained from the diet. Thus, the term is conditional both on the circumstances and on the particular organism. For example, ascorbic acid (vitamin C) is a vitamin for humans, but not for most other animals. Supplementation is important for the treatment of certain health problems but there is little evidence of benefit when used by those who are otherwise healthy.

Dietary Mineral

Dietary elements, commonly called "dietary minerals" or "minerals", are the chemical elements required by living organisms, other than the four elements carbon, hydrogen, nitrogen, and oxygen present in common organic molecules.

Amino Acids and Proteins

Amino acids are biologically important organic compounds composed of amine ($-NH_2$) and carboxylic acid (-COOH) functional groups, along with a side-chain specific to each amino acid. The key elements of an amino acid are carbon, hydrogen, oxygen, and nitrogen, though other elements are found in the side-chains of certain amino acids.

Amino acids can be divided into three categories: essential amino acids, non-essential amino acids, and conditional amino acids. Essential amino acids cannot be made by the body, and must be supplied by food. Non-essential amino acids are made by the body from essential amino acids or in the normal breakdown of proteins. Conditional amino acids are usually not essential, except in times of illness, stress, or for someone challenged with a lifelong medical condition.

Essential Fatty Acids

Essential fatty acids, or EFAs, are fatty acids that humans and other animals must ingest because the body requires them for good health but cannot synthesize them. The term "essential fatty acid" refers to fatty acids required for biological processes but does not include the fats that only act as fuel.

Bodybuilding Supplements

Bodybuilding supplements are dietary supplements commonly used by those involved in bodybuilding and athletics. Bodybuilding supplements may be used to replace meals, enhance weight gain, promote weight loss or improve athletic performance. Among the most widely used are vitamin supplements, protein drinks, branched-chain amino acids (BCAA), glutamine, essential fatty acids, meal replacement products, creatine, weight loss products and testosterone boosters. Supplements are sold either as single ingredient preparations or in the form of "stacks" – proprietary blends of various supplements marketed as offering synergistic advantages. While many bodybuilding supplements are also consumed by the general public their salience and frequency of use may differ when used specifically by bodybuilders.

Industry

In 2013, the global market of vitamins, minerals, and nutritional and herbal supplements (VMHS) was valued at $82 billion, with roughly 28 percent of that in the U.S., where sales increased by approximately $6 billion between 2007 and 2012.

The vitamins and dietary supplements sector in the U.S. grew 4% in 2015, to reach US$27.2 billion. The U.S. market was highly competitive in 2015, as no single company accounted for more than a 5% share of value sales.

Controversy

According to University of Helsinki food safety professor Marina Heinonen, more than 90% of dietary supplement health claims are incorrect. In addition, ingredients listed have been found to be different from the contents. For example, Consumer Reports reported unsafe levels of arsenic, cadmium, lead and mercury in several of the protein powders that were tested. Also, the CBC found that protein spiking (the addition of amino acid filler to manipulate analysis) was not uncommon, however many of the companies involved challenged their claim.

Adverse Effects

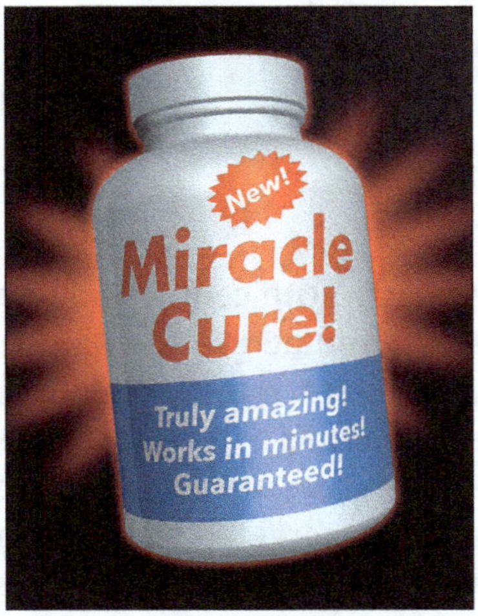

Some products make extraordinary claims and contain active ingredients which may not have been proven effective.

Among general reasons for harmful effects of dietary supplements are: a) absorption in a short time; b) quality and contamination; and c) enhancing both positive and negative effects at the same time. The number of incidents of liver damage from dietary supplements has tripled in a decade. Most of the products causing that effect were bodybuilding supplements. Some of the victims required liver transplants and some died. A third of the supplements involved contained unlisted steroids. Mild to severe toxicity has occurred on many occasions due to dietary supplements, even when the active ingredients were essential nutrients such as vitamins, minerals or amino acids. This has been a result of adulteration of the product, excessive usage on the part of the consumer, or use by persons at risk for the development of adverse effects. In addition, a number of supplements contain psychoactive drugs, whether of natural or synthetic origin.

Physical and Chemical Properties

Adulteration in North America

BMC Medicine published a study on herbal supplements in 2013. Most of the supplements studied were of low quality, one third did not contain the active ingredient(s) claimed, and one third contained unlisted substances.

An investigation by the New York Attorney General's office reported in 2015 analyzed 78 bottles of herbal supplements from Walmart, Target, Walgreens and GNC stores in New York State using DNA barcoding, a method used to detect labeling fraud in the seafood industry. Only about 20% contained the ingredient on the label.

Some supplements were contamined by rodent feces and urine.

Only 0.3% of the 55,000 U.S. market dietary supplements have been studied regarding their common side effects.

Society and Culture

Public Health

Work done by scientists in the early 20th century on identifying individual nutrients in food and developing ways to manufacture them raised hopes that optimal health could be achieved and diseases prevented by adding them to food and providing people with dietary supplements; while there were successes in preventing vitamin deficiencies, and preventing conditions like neural tube defects by supplementation and food fortification with folic acid, no targeted supplementation or fortification strategies to prevent major diseases like cancer or cardiovascular diseases have proved successful.

For example, while increased consumption of fruits and vegetables are related to decreases in mortality, cardiovascular diseases and cancers, supplementation with key factors found in fruits and vegetable, like antioxidants, vitamins, or minerals, do not help and some have been found to be harmful in some cases. In general as of 2016, robust clinical data is lacking, that shows that any kind of dietary supplementation does more good than harm for people who are healthy and eating a reasonable diet but there is clear data showing that dietary pattern and lifestyle choices are associated with health outcomes.

As a result of the lack of good data for supplementation and the strong data for dietary pattern, public health recommendations for healthy eating urge people to eat a plant-based diet of whole foods, minimizing processed food, salt and sugar and to get exercise daily, and to abandon Western pattern diets and a sedentary lifestyle.

Legal Regulation

United States

The regulation of food and dietary supplements by the U.S. Food and Drug Administration is governed by various statutes enacted by the United States Congress and interpreted by the U.S. Food and Drug Administration ("FDA"). Pursuant to the Federal Food, Drug, and Cosmetic Act ("the Act") and accompanying legislation, the FDA has authority to oversee the quality of substances sold as food in the United States, and to monitor claims made in the labeling about both the composition and the health benefits of foods.

Substances which the FDA regulates as food are subdivided into various categories, including foods, food additives, added substances (man-made substances which are not intentionally introduced into food, but nevertheless end up in it), and dietary supplements. The specific standards which the FDA exercises differ from one category to the next. Furthermore, the FDA has been granted a variety of means by which it can address violations of the standards for a given category of substances.

Regulation in European Union

The European Union's Food Supplements Directive of 2002 requires that supplements be demonstrated to be safe, both in dosages and in purity. Only those supplements that have been proven to be safe may be sold in the bloc without prescription. As a category of food, food supplements cannot be labeled with drug claims but can bear health claims and nutrition claims.

The dietary supplements industry in the United Kingdom (UK), one of the 28 countries in the bloc, strongly opposed the Directive. In addition, a large number of consumers throughout Europe, including over one million in the UK, and various doctors and scientists, had signed petitions by 2005 against what are viewed by the petitioners as unjustified restrictions of consumer choice.

In 2004, along with two British trade associations, the Alliance for Natural Health (ANH) had a legal challenge to the Food Supplements Directive referred to the European Court of Justice by the High Court in London.

Although the European Court of Justice's Advocate General subsequently said that the bloc's plan to tighten rules on the sale of vitamins and food supplements should be scrapped, he was eventually overruled by the European Court, which decided that the measures in question were necessary and appropriate for the purpose of protecting public health. ANH, however, interpreted the ban as applying only to synthetically produced supplements, and not to vitamins and minerals normally found in or consumed as part of the diet.

Nevertheless, the European judges acknowledged the Advocate General's concerns, stating that there must be clear procedures to allow substances to be added to the permitted list based on scientific evidence. They also said that any refusal to add the product to the list must be open to challenge in the courts.

Research

Effects of most dietary supplements have not been determined in randomized clinical trials and manufacturing is lightly regulated; randomized clinical trials of certain vitamins and antioxidants have found increased mortality rates.

Nootropic

Nootropics—also called smart drugs or cognitive enhancers—are drugs, supplements, or other substances that improve cognitive function, particularly executive functions, memory, creativity, or motivation, in healthy individuals. The use of cognition-enhancing drugs by healthy individuals in the absence of a medical indication is one of the most debated topics among neuroscientists, psychiatrists, and physicians which spans a number of issues, including the ethics and fairness of their use, concerns over adverse effects, and the diversion of prescription drugs for nonmedical uses, among others. Nonetheless, the international sales of cognition-enhancing supplements exceeded US$1 billion in 2015 and the global demand for these compounds is still growing rapidly.

The word *nootropic* was coined in 1972 by a Romanian psychologist and chemist, Corneliu E. Giurgea, from the Greek words (*nous*), or "mind", and (*trepein*), meaning to bend or turn.

Availability and Prevalence

There are only a few drugs that are known to improve some aspect of cognition. Many more are in different stages of development. The most commonly used class of drug is stimulants, such as caffeine.

These drugs are purportedly used primarily to treat cognitive or motor function difficulties attributable to disorders such as Alzheimer's disease, Parkinson's disease, Huntington's disease, and ADHD. Some researchers, however, report more widespread use despite concern for further research. Nevertheless, intense marketing may not correlate with efficacy. While scientific studies support the beneficial effects of some compounds, manufacturer's marketing claims for dietary supplements are usually not formally tested and verified by independent entities.

Use by Students

Among students, nootropics have been used to increase productivity, despite their long-term effects lacking conclusive research in healthy individuals. The use of prescription stimulants is especially prevalent among students attending academically competitive colleges. Surveys suggest that 0.7–4.5% of German students have used cognitive enhancers in their lifetime. Stimulants such as dimethylamylamine and methylphenidate are used on college campuses and by younger groups. Based upon studies of self-reported illicit stimulant use, 5–35% of college students use diverted ADHD stimulants, which are primarily used for performance enhancement rather than as recreational drugs.

Several factors positively and negatively influence the use of drugs to increase cognitive performance. Among them are personal characteristics, drug characteristics, and characteristics of the social context.

Side Effects

The main concern with pharmaceutical drugs is adverse effects, and these concerns apply to cognitive-enhancing drugs as well. Long-term safety data is typically unavailable for some types of nootropics (e.g., many non-pharmaceutical cognitive enhancers, newly developed pharmaceuticals and pharmaceuticals with short-term therapeutic use). Racetams—piracetam and other compounds that are structurally related to piracetam—have few serious adverse effects and low toxicity, but there is little evidence that they enhance cognition in individuals without cognitive impairments. While addiction to stimulants is sometimes identified as a cause for concern, a very large body of research on the therapeutic use of the "more addictive" psychostimulants indicate that addiction is fairly rare in therapeutic doses. On their safety profile, a systematic review from June 2015 asserted, "evidence indicates that at low, clinically relevant doses, psychostimulants are devoid of the behavioral and neurochemical actions that define this class of drugs and instead act largely as cognitive enhancers."

In the United States dietary supplements may be marketed if the manufacturer can show that it can manufacture the supplement safely, that the supplement is indeed generally recognized as safe, and if the manufacturer does not make any claims about the supplement's use to treat or prevent any disease or condition; supplements that contain drugs or for which treatment or prevention claims are made are illegal under US law.

Drugs

Stimulants

In 2015, systematic medical reviews and meta-analyses of clinical research in humans established consensus that certain stimulants, only when used at low (therapeutic) concentrations, unambiguously enhance cognition in the general population; in particular, the classes of stimulants that demonstrate cognition-enhancing effects in humans act as direct agonists or indirect agonists of dopamine receptor D_1, adrenoceptor A_2, or both receptors in the prefrontal cortex. Relatively high doses of stimulants cause cognitive deficits.

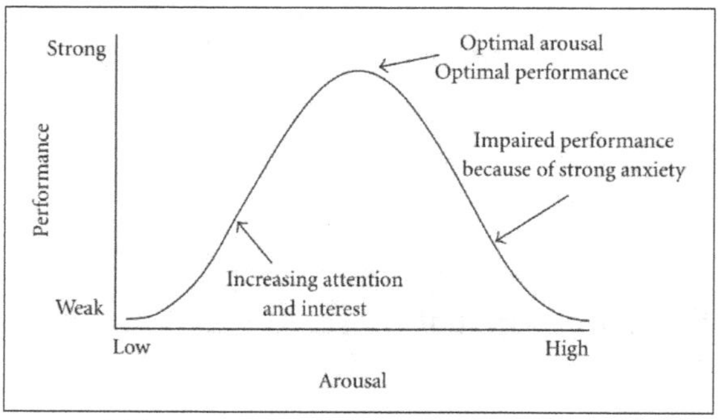

Hebbian version of the Yerkes–Dodson law.

- Amphetamine pharmaceuticals (e.g., Adderall, dextroamphetamine, and lisdexamfetamine [an inactive prodrug]) – systematic reviews and meta-analyses report that amphetamine benefits a range of cognitive functions (e.g., inhibitory control, episodic memory, working memory, and aspects of attention) in the general population, and these effects are especially notable in individuals with ADHD. A systematic review from 2014 noted that low doses of amphetamine also improve memory consolidation, in turn leading to improved recall of information in non-ADHD youth. It also improves task saliency (motivation to perform a task) and performance on tedious tasks that require a high degree of effort.
- Methylphenidate – a substituted phenethylamine that improves a range of cognitive functions (e.g., working memory, episodic memory, and inhibitory control, aspects of attention, and planning latency) in the general population. It also improves task saliency and performance on tedious tasks that require a high degree of effort. At above optimal doses, methylphenidate has off target effects that can decrease learning by activating neurons not involved in the task at hand.
- Eugeroics (armodafinil and modafinil) – wakefulness promoting agents; modafinil increases alertness, particularly in sleep deprived individuals, and was noted to facilitate reasoning and problem solving in a systematic review. They are clinically prescribed for narcolepsy, shift work sleep disorder, and daytime sleepiness remaining after sleep apnea treatments.
- Xanthines (most notably, caffeine) – shown to increase alertness, performance, and, in some studies, memory. Children and adults who consume low doses of caffeine showed increased alertness, yet a higher dose was needed to improve performance.
- Nicotine – A meta-analysis of 41 double-blind, placebo-controlled studies concluded that nicotine or smoking had significant positive effects on aspects of fine motor abilities, alerting and orienting attention, and episodic and working

memory. A 2015 review noted that stimulation of the α4β2 nicotinic receptor is responsible for certain improvements in attentional performance; among the nicotinic receptor subtypes, nicotine has the highest binding affinity at the α4β2 receptor (k_i=1 nM), which is also the biological target that mediates nicotine's addictive properties.

Racetams

Racetams, such as piracetam, oxiracetam, and aniracetam, are structurally similar compounds, which are often marketed as cognitive enhancers and sold over-the-counter. Racetams are often referred to as nootropics, but this property of the drug class is not well established. The racetams have poorly understood mechanisms of action; however, piracetam and aniracetam are known to act as positive allosteric modulators of AMPA receptors and appear to modulate cholinergic systems.

According to the US Food and Drug Administration, "Piracetam is not a vitamin, mineral, amino acid, herb or other botanical, or dietary substance for use by man to supplement the diet by increasing the total dietary intake. Further, piracetam is not a concentrate, metabolite, constituent, extract or combination of any such dietary ingredient. [...] Accordingly, these products are drugs, under section 201(g)(1)(C) of the Act, 21 U.S.C. 321(g)(1)(C), because they are not foods and they are intended to affect the structure or any function of the body. Moreover, these products are new drugs as defined by section 201(p) of the Act, 21 U.S.C. 321(p), because they are not generally recognized as safe and effective for use under the conditions prescribed, recommended, or suggested in their labeling."

Miscellaneous

- L-Theanine – A 2014 systematic review and meta-analysis found that concurrent caffeine and L-theanine use has synergistic psychoactive effects that promote alertness, attention, and task switching; these effects are most pronounced during the first hour post-dose.
- Tolcapone – a systematic review noted that it improves verbal episodic memory and episodic memory encoding.
- Levodopa – a systematic review noted that it improves verbal episodic memory and episodic memory encoding.
- Atomoxetine – can improve working memory and aspects of attention when used at an optimal dose.

Dietary Supplements

- *Bacopa monnieri* – A herb sold as a dietary supplement. There is some preliminary evidence for memory-enhancing effects.

- *Panax ginseng* – A review by the Cochrane Collaboration concluded that "there is a lack of convincing evidence to show a cognitive enhancing effect of Panax ginseng in healthy participants and no high quality evidence about its efficacy in patients with dementia." According to the National Center for Complementary and Integrative Health "Although Asian ginseng has been widely studied for a variety of uses, research results to date do not conclusively support health claims associated with the herb." According to a review published in the journal "Advances in Nutrition", multiple RCTs in healthy volunteers have indicated increases in accuracy of memory, speed in performing attention tasks and improvement in performing difficult mental arithmetic tasks, as well as reduction in fatigue and improvement in mood.
- *Ginkgo biloba* – An extract of *Ginkgo biloba* leaf (GBE) is marketed in dietary supplement form with claims it can enhance cognitive function in people without known cognitive problems. Studies have failed to find such effects on memory or attention in healthy people.

Null Findings in Systematic Reviews

- Omega-3 fatty acids: DHA and EPA – two Cochrane Collaboration reviews on the use of supplemental omega-3 fatty acids for ADHD and learning disorders conclude that there is limited evidence of treatment benefits for either disorder. Two other systematic reviews noted no cognition-enhancing effects in the general population or middle-aged and older adults.
- Folate – no cognition-enhancing effects in middle-aged and older adults.
- Vitamin B6 – no cognition-enhancing effects in middle-aged and older adults.
- Vitamin B12 – no cognition-enhancing effects in middle-aged and older adults.
- Vitamin E – no cognition-enhancing effects in middle-aged and older adults.
- Pramipexole – no significant cognition-enhancing effects in healthy individuals.
- Guanfacine – no significant cognition-enhancing effects in healthy individuals.
- Clonidine – no significant cognition-enhancing effects in healthy individuals.
- Ampakines – no significant cognition-enhancing effects in healthy individuals.
- Fexofenadine – no significant cognition-enhancing effects in healthy individuals.
- *Salvia officinalis* – Although some evidence is suggestive of cognition benefits, the study quality is so poor that no conclusions can be drawn from it.

Raw Foodism

Raw foodism (or following a raw food diet) is the dietary practice of eating only, or mostly, uncooked, unprocessed foods. Depending on the philosophy, or type of lifestyle and results desired, raw food diets may include a selection of fruits, vegetables, nuts, seeds, eggs, fish, meat, and dairy products.

It may also include simply processed foods such as various types of sprouted seeds, cheese, and fermented foods such as yogurts, kefir, kombucha or sauerkraut, but generally not foods that have been pasteurized, homogenized, or produced with the use of synthetic pesticides, chemical fertilizers, industrial solvents or chemical food additives.

Varieties

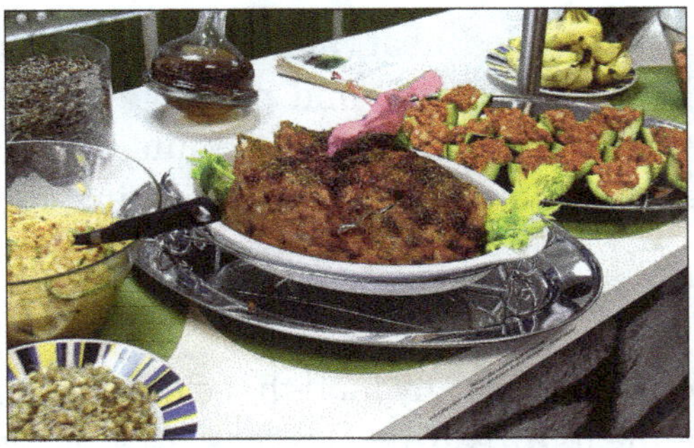

Raw Vegan "Thanksgiving Turkey".

Raw food diets are diets composed entirely or mostly of food that is uncooked or which is cooked at low temperatures.

Raw Veganism

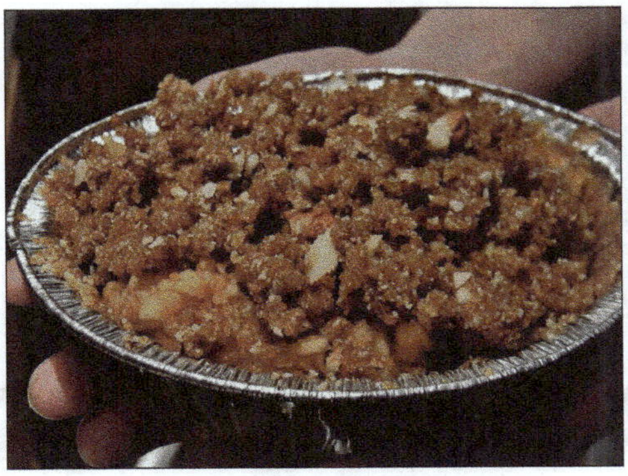

Raw vegan "apple pie".

A raw vegan diet consists of unprocessed, raw plant foods, that have not been heated above 40–49 °C (104–120 °F). Raw vegans such as Brian Clement, Gabriel Cousens, Thierry Browers a.k.a. "Superlight", and Douglas Graham believe that foods cooked above this temperature have lost much of their nutritional value and are less healthy or even harmful to the body. Advocates argue that raw or living foods have natural enzymes, which are critical in building proteins and rebuilding the body, and that heating these foods destroys the natural enzymes and can leave toxic materials behind. However, enzymes, as with other proteins consumed in the diet, are denatured and eventually lysed by the digestive process, rendering them non-functional. Typical foods included in raw food diets are fruits, vegetables, nuts, seeds, and sprouted grains and legumes.

Among raw vegans there are some subgroups such as fruitarians, juicearians, or sproutarians. Fruitarians eat primarily or exclusively fruits, berries, seeds, and nuts. Juicearians process their raw plant foods into juice. Sproutarians adhere to a diet consisting mainly of sprouted seeds.

Raw Vegetarianism

Vegetarianism is a diet that excludes meat (including byproducts like gelatin), fish (including shellfish and other sea animals), and poultry, but allows dairy and/or eggs. Common foods include fruit, vegetables, sprouts, nuts, seeds, grains, legumes, dairy, eggs, and honey. There are several variants of this diet, including raw versions.

Raw Animal Food Diets

Included in raw animal food diets are any food that can be eaten raw, such as uncooked, unprocessed raw muscle-meats/organ-meats/eggs, raw dairy, and aged, raw animal foods such as century eggs, fermented meat/fish/shellfish/kefir, as well as vegetables/fruits/nuts/sprouts/honey, but in general *not* raw grains, raw beans, and raw soy. Raw foods included on such diets have not been heated above 40 °C (104 °F). Raw animal foodists believe that foods cooked above this temperature have lost a lot of their nutritional value and are less bioavailable.

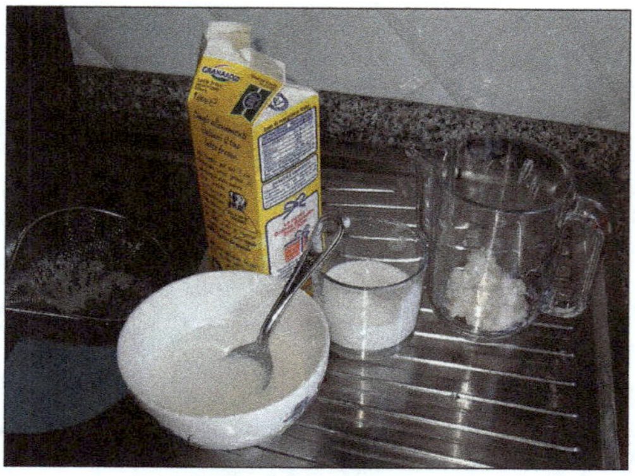

Kefir preparation.

Examples of raw animal food diets include the Primal Diet, anopsology (otherwise known as "Instinctive Eating" or "Instincto"), and the Raw Paleolithic diet (otherwise known as the "Raw Meat Diet").

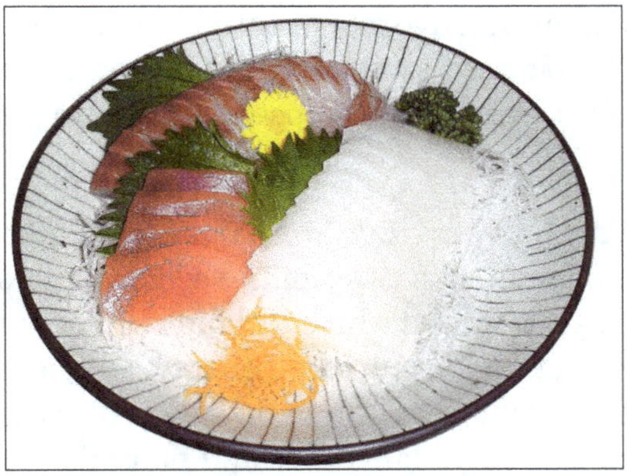

A sashimi dinner set.

The Primal Diet consists of fatty meats, organ meats, dairy, honey, minimal fruit and vegetable juices, and coconut products, all raw.

The "Raw Meat Diet", otherwise known as the "Raw, Paleolithic Diet", is a raw version of the (cooked) Paleolithic Diet, incorporating large amounts of raw animal foods such as meats/organ-meats, seafood, eggs, and some raw plant-foods, but usually avoiding non-Paleo foods such as raw dairy, grains, and legumes.

A number of traditional aboriginal diets consisted of large quantities of raw meats, organ meats, and berries, including the traditional diet of the Nenets tribe of Siberia and the Inuit people.

History

Contemporary raw food diets were first developed in Switzerland by Maximilian Bircher-Benner (1867 – 1939), who was influenced as a young man by the German *Lebensreform* movement, which saw civilization as corrupt and sought to go "back to nature"; it embraced holistic medicine, nudism, free love, exercise and other outdoors activity, and foods that it judged were more "natural". Bircher-Benner eventually adopted a vegetarian diet, but took that further and decided that raw food was what humans were really meant to eat; he was influenced by Charles Darwin's ideas that humans were just another kind of animal and Bircher-Benner noted that other animals do not cook their food. In 1904 he opened a sanatorium in the mountains outside of Zurich called "Lebendinge Kraft" or "Vital Force," a technical term in the Lebensreform movement that referred especially to sunlight; he and others believed that this energy was more "concentrated" in plants than in meat, and was diminished by cooking. Patients in the clinic were fed raw foods, including muesli, which was created there. These ideas were dismissed by scientists and the medical profession of his day as quackery.

Other proponents from the early part of the twentieth century include Ann Wigmore, Norman W. Walker (inventor of the Norwalk Juicing Press), and Herbert Shelton. Shelton was arrested, jailed, and fined numerous times for practicing medicine without a license during his career as an advocate of rawism and other alternative health and diet philosophies. Shelton's legacy, as popularized by books like *Fit for Life* by Harvey and Marilyn Diamond, has been deemed "pseudonutrition" by the National Council Against Health Fraud.

Leslie Kenton's book *Raw Energy - Eat Your Way to Radiant Health*, published in 1984, added popularity to foods such as sprouts, seeds, and fresh vegetable juices. The book advocates a diet of 75% raw food which it claims will prevent degenerative diseases, slow the effects of aging, provide enhanced energy, and boost emotional balance; it cites examples such as the sprouted-seed-enriched diets of the long-lived Hunza people and Gerson therapy, an unhealthy, dangerous and potentially very harmful raw juice-based diet and detoxification regime claimed to treat cancer.

Claims

Claims held by raw food proponents include:

- That heating food above 104–118 °F (40–48 °C) starts to degrade and destroy the enzymes in raw food that aid digestion. A few raw food proponents such as Douglas Graham dispute the importance of enzymes in foods, however, and it is commonly believed that enzymes in food play no significant role in the digestive process, prior to being digested themselves.
- That raw foods have higher nutrient and antioxidants values than foods that have been cooked. In reality, whether cooking degrades nutrients or increases their availability, or both, depends on the food and how it is cooked.
- That cooked foods, and especially meat, contain harmful toxins, which can cause chronic disease and other problems, including trans fatty acids produced by heating oil, acrylamide produced by frying, advanced glycation end products (AGEs), and polycyclic aromatic hydrocarbons. While it is true that a healthy diet minimizes fried food and red meat, not all cooked food contains harmful chemicals (a serving of french fries has 200 times the AGEs of a bowl of cooked oatmeal), and a diet containing a normal mix of cooked and raw food does not shorten life. High rates of some of these compounds formed by cooking meat can cause cancer in other animals; whether such an exposure causes cancer in humans remains unclear. According to the American Cancer Society it is not clear, as of 2013, whether acrylamide consumption affects people's risk of getting cancer.

Health Effects

A meta-analysis clinical trials and epidemiological studies published in 2004, and covering a broad range of cancers, found that it appears that there is an inverse relationship between the risk of developing certain types of cancer and eating both raw and cooked vegetables. Consumption of raw vegetables tended to be associated with decreased cancer risks somewhat more often than consumption of cooked vegetables. On the other hand, a raw food diet is likely to impair the development of children and infants.

Care is required in planning a raw vegan diet, especially for children. Dr. Joel Fuhrman, author of *Disease-Proof Your Child*, says there may not be enough vitamin B_{12}, enough vitamin D, and enough calories for a growing child on a totally raw vegan diet. Fuhrman fed his own four children raw and cooked vegetables, fruits, nuts, grains, beans, and occasionally eggs.

Food poisoning is a health risk for all people eating raw foods, and increased demand for raw foods is associated with greater incidence of foodborne illness, especially for raw meat, fish, and shellfish. Outbreaks of gastroenteritis among consumers of raw and undercooked animal products (including smoked, pickled or dried animal products) are well-documented, and include raw meat, raw organ meat, raw fish (whether ocean-going or freshwater), shellfish, raw milk and products made from raw milk, and raw eggs.

In his book *Health or Hoax*, nutritionist Arnold E. Bender has written that "Many raw foods are toxic and only become safe after they have been cooked. Some raw foods contain substances that destroy vitamins, interfere with digestive enzymes or damage the walls of the intestine. Raw meat can be contaminated with bacteria which would be destroyed by cooking; raw fish can contain substances that interfere with vitamin B1 (anti-thiaminases)".

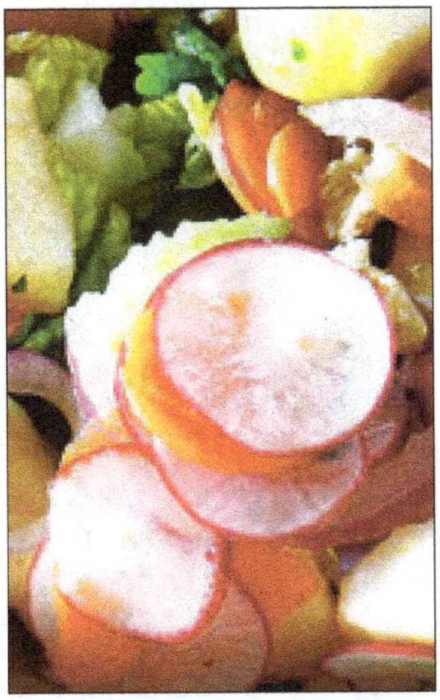

A close-up of a raw food dish.

Cooking and Global Warming

It has also been pointed out that cooking food, directly or indirectly, requires energy and may thus release gases associated with global warming. Raw diets mitigate the use of non-renewable resources, which results in raw diets being less environmentally deleterious than cooked food diets in this respect.

Role of Cooking in Human Evolution

Richard Wrangham, professor of biological anthropology at Harvard University, proposes that cooked food played a pivotal role in human evolution. Evidence of a cooked diet, according to Wrangham, can be seen as far back as 1.8 million years ago in the anatomical adaptations of *Homo erectus*. Reduction in the size of teeth and jaw in *H. erectus* indicate a softer diet, requiring less chewing time. This combined with a smaller gut and larger brain indicate to Wrangham that *H. erectus* was eating a higher quality diet than its predecessors. To explain a decreased gut providing the amount of energy required for an increased brain size, Wrangham links his research on the digestive effects of cooked versus raw foods with the lower reproductive abilities of female raw foodists, and BMI in both sexes, to support his hypothesis that cooked starches provided the energy necessary to fuel evolution from *H. erectus* to *H. sapiens*.

Theories opposed to Wrangham's include that of Leslie Aiello, professor of biological anthropology at University College London, and physiologist Peter Wheeler. Aiello and Wheeler believe it was soft animal foods, including bone marrow and brains, which contributed to humans developing the characteristics Wrangham attributes to cooked foods. Further, archaeological evidence suggests that cooking fires began in earnest only around 250 kya, when ancient hearths, earth ovens, burnt animal bones, and flint appear regularly across Europe and the Middle East. Two million years ago, the only sign of fire is burnt earth with human remains, which many anthropologists consider coincidence rather than evidence of intentional fire. Many anthropologists believe the increases in human brain-size occurred well before the advent of cooking, due to a shift away from the consumption of nuts and berries to the consumption of raw meat.

References

- Malenka RC, Nestler EJ, Hyman SE (2009). Sydor A, Brown RY, eds. Molecular Neuropharmacology: A Foundation for Clinical Neuroscience (2nd ed.). New York: McGraw-Hill Medical. p. 454. ISBN 9780071481274
- Kiefer, I. (2007). "Brain Food". Scientific American Mind. 18 (5): 58–63. doi:10.1038/scientificamericanmind1007-58. Retrieved November 1, 2009
- Food and Drug Administration (20 March 2014). "Q&A on Dietary Supplements". fda.gov. Archived from the original on 27 May 2014. Retrieved 26 June 2014
- Katz DL, Meller S (2014). "Can we say what diet is best for health?". Annu Rev Public Health. 35: 83–103. PMID 24641555. doi:10.1146/annurev-publhealth-032013-182351
- Palermo, M; Pellegrini, N; Fogliano, V (April 2014). "Review: The effect of cooking on the phytochemical content of vegetables.". Journal of the science of food and agriculture. 94 (6): 1057–70. PMID 24227349. doi:10.1002/jsfa.6478

- Fitzgerald M (2014). Diet Cults: The Surprising Fallacy at the Core of Nutrition Fads and a Guide to Healthy Eating for the Rest of US. Pegasus Books. ISBN 978-1-60598-560-2
- Griffith-Greene, Megan (November 13, 2015). "Marketplace: Some protein powders fail fitness test". CBC News. Retrieved December 11, 2015
- Macpherson, CN (2005). "Human behaviour and the epidemiology of parasitic zoonoses". International Journal for Parasitology. 35 (11–12): 1319–31. PMID 16102769. doi:10.1016/j.ijpara.2005.06.004
- Gazzaniga, Michael S. (2006). The Ethical Brain: The Science of Our Moral Dilemmas (P.S.). New York, N.Y: Harper Perennial. p. 184. ISBN 0-06-088473-8
- O'CONNOR, ANAHAD. "Herbal Supplements Are Often Not What They Seem". New York Times. Retrieved 12 November 2013

Permissions

All chapters in this book are published with permission under the Creative Commons Attribution Share Alike License or equivalent. Every chapter published in this book has been scrutinized by our experts. Their significance has been extensively debated. The topics covered herein carry significant information for a comprehensive understanding. They may even be implemented as practical applications or may be referred to as a beginning point for further studies.

We would like to thank the editorial team for lending their expertise to make the book truly unique. They have played a crucial role in the development of this book. Without their invaluable contributions this book wouldn't have been possible. They have made vital efforts to compile up to date information on the varied aspects of this subject to make this book a valuable addition to the collection of many professionals and students.

This book was conceptualized with the vision of imparting up-to-date and integrated information in this field. To ensure the same, a matchless editorial board was set up. Every individual on the board went through rigorous rounds of assessment to prove their worth. After which they invested a large part of their time researching and compiling the most relevant data for our readers.

The editorial board has been involved in producing this book since its inception. They have spent rigorous hours researching and exploring the diverse topics which have resulted in the successful publishing of this book. They have passed on their knowledge of decades through this book. To expedite this challenging task, the publisher supported the team at every step. A small team of assistant editors was also appointed to further simplify the editing procedure and attain best results for the readers.

Apart from the editorial board, the designing team has also invested a significant amount of their time in understanding the subject and creating the most relevant covers. They scrutinized every image to scout for the most suitable representation of the subject and create an appropriate cover for the book.

The publishing team has been an ardent support to the editorial, designing and production team. Their endless efforts to recruit the best for this project, has resulted in the accomplishment of this book. They are a veteran in the field of academics and their pool of knowledge is as vast as their experience in printing. Their expertise and guidance has proved useful at every step. Their uncompromising quality standards have made this book an exceptional effort. Their encouragement from time to time has been an inspiration for everyone.

The publisher and the editorial board hope that this book will prove to be a valuable piece of knowledge for students, practitioners and scholars across the globe.

Index

www.ingramcontent.com/pod-product-compliance
Lightning Source LLC
LaVergne TN
LVHW080628210926
848485LV00003B/230

* 9 7 8 1 6 3 9 8 7 4 0 6 4 *